2013 YEAR BOOK OF OTOLARYNGOLOGY–HEAD AND NECK SURGERY®

The 2013 Year Book Series

Year Book of Critical Care Medicine®: Drs Dries, Zanotti-Cavazzoni, Latenser, Martinez, Rincon, and Zwank

Year Book of Emergency Medicine®: Drs Hamilton, Bruno, Handly, Minczak, Quintana, and Ramoska

Year Book of Endocrinology®: Drs Schott, Apovian, Clarke, Eugster, Meikle, Oetgen, Ovalle, Schteingart, and Toth

Year Book of Hand and Upper Limb Surgery®: Drs Yao, Adams, Isaacs, Lee, and Rizzo

Year Book of Medicine®: Drs Barker, Garrick, Gersh, Khardori, LeRoith, Panush, Talley, and Thigpen

Year Book of Neonatal and Perinatal Medicine®: Drs Fanaroff, Benitz, Donn, Neu, Papile, and Van Marter

Year Book of Neurology and Neurosurgery®: Drs Klimo, Minagar, Gandhi, House, Kevill, Liu, Mazia, Panagariya, Ragel, Riesenburger, Robottom, Schwendimann, Shafazand, Uhm, and Yang

Year Book of Obstetrics, Gynecology, and Women's Health®: Drs Dungan and Shulman

Year Book of Oncology®: Drs Arceci, Bauer, Chiorean, Gordon, Lawton, Murphy, Thigpen, and Tsao

Year Book of Ophthalmology®: Drs Rapuano, Cohen, Flanders, Hammersmith, Milman, Myers, Nagra, Nelson, Penne, Pyfer, Sergott, Shields, Talekar, and Vander

Year Book of Orthopedics®: Drs Morrey, Huddleston, Rose, Swiontkowski, and Trigg

Year Book of Otolaryngology-Head and Neck Surgery®: Drs Sindwani, Balough, Franco, Gapany, and Mitchell

Year Book of Pathology and Laboratory Medicine®: Drs Raab and Bissell

Year Book of Pediatrics®: Dr Stockman

Year Book of Plastic and Aesthetic Surgery™: Drs Miller, Boehmler, Gosman, Gutowski, Ruberg, Salisbury, and Smith

Year Book of Psychiatry and Applied Mental Health®: Drs Talbott, Ballenger, Buckley, Frances, Krupnick, and Mack

Year Book of Pulmonary Disease®: Drs Barker, Jones, Maurer, Spradley, Tanoue, and Willsie

Year Book of Sports Medicine®: Drs Shephard, Cantu, Feldman, Galea, Jankowski, Janssen, Lebrun, and Nieman

Year Book of Surgery®: Drs Copeland, Behrns, Daly, Eberlein, Fahey, Huber, Klodell, Mozingo, and Pruett

Year Book of Urology®: Drs Andriole and Coplen

Year Book of Vascular Surgery®: Drs Moneta, Gillespie, Starnes, and Watkins

2013 The Year Book of OTOLARYNGOLOGY–HEAD AND NECK SURGERY®

Editor-in-Chief
Raj Sindwani, MD, FACS, FRCS(C)

Associate Editors
Ben J. Balough, CAPT, USN retired
Ramon A. Franco, Jr, MD
Markus Gapany, MD, FACS
Ron B. Mitchell, MD

ELSEVIER
MOSBY

ELSEVIER
MOSBY

Vice President, Continuity: Kimberly Murphy
Editor: Katie Saunders
Production Supervisor, Electronic Year Books: Donna M. Skelton
Electronic Article Manager: Mike Rainey
Illustrations and Permissions Coordinator: Dawn Vohsen

2013 EDITION

Printed and bound by CPI Group (UK) Ltd, Croydon, CR0 4YY

Transferred to digital print 2013

Editorial Office:
Elsevier
Suite 1800
1600 John F. Kennedy Blvd.
Philadelphia, PA 19103-2899

International Standard Serial Number: 1041-892X
International Standard Book Number: 978-1-4557-7284-1

Editorial Board

Editor-in-Chief

Associate Editors

Table of Contents

Journals Represented

Journals represented in this Year Book are listed below.

Acta Anaesthesiologica Scandinavica
Acta Oto-Laryngologica
American Journal of Emergency Medicine
American Journal of Otolaryngology
American Journal of Rhinology & Allergy
American Surgeon
Anaesthesia
Anesthesia & Analgesia
Annals of Otology Rhinology & Laryngology
Annals of Plastic Surgery
Annals of Surgical Oncology
Archives of Otolaryngology Head & Neck Surgery
Canadian Medical Association Journal
Cancer
Clinical Nuclear Medicine
Clinical Radiology
Gastrointestinal Endoscopy
Head & Neck
Intensive Care Medicine
International Forum of Allergy & Rhinology
International Journal of Cancer
International Journal of Oral and Maxillofacial Surgery
International Journal of Radiation Oncology *Biology* Physics
Journal of Allergy and Clinical Immunology
Journal of Clinical Endocrinology & Metabolism
Journal of Clinical Neuroscience
Journal of Drugs in Dermatology
Journal of Laryngology and Otology
Journal of Nuclear Medicine
Journal of Otolaryngology Head & Neck Surgery
Journal of Pediatric Surgery
Journal of Plastic, Reconstructive & Aesthetic Surgery
Journal of Surgical Research
Journal of Voice
Journal of the American College of Surgeons
Laryngoscope
Nature
Neurology
Neuroradiology
New England Journal of Medicine
Oral Oncology
Otolaryngology-Head and Neck Surgery
Otology & Neurotology
Plastic and Reconstructive Surgery
Rhinology
Surgery
Thyroid

World Journal of Surgery
World Neurosurgery

Standard Abbreviations

The following terms are abbreviated in this edition: acquired immunodeficiency syndrome (AIDS), cardiopulmonary resuscitation (CPR), central nervous system (CNS), cerebrospinal fluid (CSF), computed tomography (CT), deoxyribonucleic acid (DNA), electrocardiography (ECG), health maintenance organization (HMO), human immunodeficiency virus (HIV), intensive care unit (ICU), intramuscular (IM), intravenous (IV), magnetic resonance (MR) imaging (MRI), ribonucleic acid (RNA), and ultrasound (US).

Note

The Year Book of Otolaryngology–Head and Neck Surgery is a literature survey service providing abstracts of articles published in the professional literature. Every effort is made to assure the accuracy of the information presented in these pages. Neither the editors nor the publisher of the Year Book of Otolaryngology–Head and Neck Surgery can be responsible for errors in the original materials. The editors' comments are their own opinions. Mention of specific products within this publication does not constitute endorsement.

To facilitate the use of the Year Book of Otolaryngology–Head and Neck Surgery as a reference tool, all illustrations and tables included in this publication are now identified as they appear in the original article. This change is meant to help the reader recognize that any illustration or table appearing in the Year Book of Otolaryngology–Head and Neck Surgery may be only one of many in the original article. For this reason, figure and table numbers will often appear to be out of sequence within the Year Book of Otolaryngology–Head and Neck Surgery.

Preface

Each year the Associate Editors and I are charged with the task of examining the relevant articles within our sub-specialty areas and selecting those we wish to include in the YEAR BOOK. As you would imagine, combing through the world literature in a particular discipline is quite a daunting project. To help facilitate this search, each of us receives periodic updates of articles from a large array of international journals based on words which reflect topics in our given specialty areas. The Associate Editor then reviews the abstracts and/or articles identified. He is also free to select any other article that he may come across as well, independent of the list of journals mined by the YEAR BOOK's technology.

The articles ultimately included in this conglomeration are selected for a variety of reasons, including: they are seminal works in the field; they reflect a major shift in medical/surgical decision making or theory; they reflect meaningful progress in basic science research; they are thought-provoking, innovative, or controversial; and/or at the very least, they are considered to be entertaining for our readers.

The fruits of our annual labor are contained herein.

This issue of the YEAR BOOK of OTOLARYNGOLOGY – HEAD AND NECK SURGERY contains articles from 51 domestic and international journals representing authors from many institutions around the globe. I would like to congratulate the entire staff of the YEAR BOOK of OTOLARYNGOLOGY – HEAD AND NECK SURGERY for another remarkable job. We hope you enjoy the articles and commentaries in the current issue.

Raj Sindwani, MD, FACS, FRCS(C)

1 Allergy and Immunology

Outcomes

Efficacy of subcutaneous and sublingual immunotherapy with grass allergens for seasonal allergic rhinitis: A meta-analysis–based comparison

Di Bona D, Plaia A, Leto-Barone MS, et al (Università degli Studi di Palermo, Italy)

J Allergy Clin Immunol 130:1097-1107e2, 2012

Background.—Subcutaneous (SCIT) and sublingual (SLIT) immunotherapy are the 2 most prescribed routes for administering allergen-specific immunotherapy. They were shown to be effective in control of symptoms and in reducing rescue medication use in patients with allergic diseases, but their effectiveness has to be balanced against side effects. In recent years, SLIT has been increasingly prescribed, instead of SCIT, because of improved safety and easy administration.

Objective.—We assessed which route is the most effective in the treatment of patients with seasonal allergic rhinitis to grass pollen.

Methods.—An indirect meta-analysis–based comparison between SCIT and SLIT was performed. Treatment efficacy was determined as the standardized mean difference (SMD) in symptom and medication scores obtained with active treatment, SCIT or SLIT, compared with placebo. Studies were included if they were double-blind randomized controlled trials comparing SCIT or SLIT with placebo. Thirty-six randomized controlled trials (3014 patients; 2768 controls) were analyzed.

Results.—The overall effect size of SCIT for symptom score (SMD, −0.92; 95% CI, −1.26 to −0.58) was significantly higher than SLIT, both administered via drops (SMD, −0.25; 95% CI, −0.45 to −0.05) and tablets (SMD, −0.40; 95% CI, −0.54 to −0.27). Similar results were reported for medication score (SCIT: SMD, −0.58; 95% CI, −0.86 to −0.30. SLIT drops: SMD, −0.37; 95% CI, −0.74 to −0.00. SLIT tablets SMD, −0.30; 95% CI, −0.44 to −0.16).

Conclusions.—Our results provide indirect but solid evidence that SCIT is more effective than SLIT in controlling symptoms and in reducing the use of antiallergic medications in seasonal allergic rhinoconjunctivitis to grass pollen.

▶ Allergen-specific immunotherapy can be given through a variety of routes, including subcutaneous (SCIT) and sublingual (SLIT) immunotherapy, with considerable variability on preferences worldwide. In the United States, SCIT is the route approved by the Food and Drug Administration and is widely prescribed, although SLIT is gaining a great deal of interest. By contrast, in Europe SLIT is prescribed nearly as frequently as SCIT, primarily because of its safety profile and ease of administration. Several clinical trials have reported the efficacy of both SCIT and SLIT compared with placebo for seasonal allergic rhinitis to grass pollens. This study looked at published randomized controlled trials (RCTs) to assess which route is the most effective in the treatment of patients with seasonal allergic rhinitis (SAR) to grass pollen. An "indirect" meta-analysis–based comparison between SCIT and SLIT (each vs placebo) was performed. The study included 36 RCTs (3014 patients; 2768 controls) and determined that the overall effect size of SCIT for symptom score and medication score was significantly higher than SLIT (when administered via both drops and tablets). The authors argued that although this analysis was not a head-to-head comparison (ideally the next step required in settling this question), they provided "solid indirect evidence" that SCIT is more effective than SLIT in controlling symptoms and reducing medication usage SAR to grass allergens. Even if this were true, and further work is required to establish this, how much more effective is SCIT than SLIT? Depending on the answer to this, perhaps the favorable safety profile and ease of administration of SLIT still would make its use attractive. Further studies comparing the efficacy of these routes directly are needed.

R. Sindwani, MD

Nasal irrigation as an adjunctive treatment in allergic rhinitis: A systematic review and meta-analysis

Hermelingmeier KE, Weber RK, Hellmich M, et al (Univ of Cologne, Germany; Städtisches Klinikum Karlsruhe, Germany)

Am J Rhinol Allergy 26:e119-e125, 2012

Background.—Saline nasal irrigation (SNI) is often recommended as additional nonpharmacologic treatment, having proven its efficacy in acute and chronic rhinosinusitis and for therapy after sinonasal surgery. To date, however, no systematic review or meta-analysis exists showing the influence of SNI on allergic rhinitis (AR). This study aimed to establish the impact of SNI on symptoms of AR in different patient groups.

Methods.—We conducted a systematic search of Medline, Embase, Cochrane Central Register of Controlled Trials, and ISI Web of Science databases for literature published from 1994 to 2010 on SNI in AR. Prospective, randomized, controlled trials that assessed the effects of SNI on four different outcome parameters were included. The evaluation focused on primary (symptom score) and secondary parameters (medicine consumption, mucociliary clearance, and quality of life).

Results.—Three independent reviewers chose 10 originals that satisfied the inclusion criteria (>400 participants total) from 50 relevant trials. SNI performed regularly over a limited period of up to 7 weeks was observed to have a positive effect on all investigated outcome parameters in adults and children with AR. SNI produced a 27.66% improvement in nasal symptoms, a 62.1% reduction in medicine consumption, a 31.19% acceleration of mucociliary clearance time, and a 27.88% improvement in quality of life.

Conclusion.—SNI using isotonic solution can be recommended as complementary therapy in AR. It is well tolerated, inexpensive, easy to use, and there is no evidence showing that regular, daily SNI adversely affects the patient's health or causes unexpected side effects.

▶ Allergic rhinitis (AR) is a global health problem. Further, the prevalence of AR is felt to be increasing. Medical spending to treat AR almost doubled from $6.1 billion in 2000 to $11.2 billion in 2005, and the mean annual out-of-pocket expenses related to AR were $520 per person in 2005.[1] It is well established that AR affects social life, sleep, school, and work, making treatment imperative. Traditionally, the management of AR encompassed environmental controls, medical therapy, and immunotherapy. More recently, it has become popular for patients to use saline irrigations for a variety of conditions, including AR. Although nasal irrigation is cheap, readily available, and well tolerated, to date, no systematic review or meta-analysis exists showing the influence of saline nasal irrigation (SNI) on AR. This study aimed to establish the impact of SNI on symptoms of AR in different patient groups in prospective, randomized, controlled trials. The evaluation focused on primary (symptom score) and secondary parameters (medicine consumption, mucociliary clearance, and quality of life). The study comprised 10 articles (> 400 participants). SNI performed regularly was observed to have a positive effect on all investigated outcome parameters in adults and children with AR. SNI use was associated with a 28% improvement in nasal symptoms, a 62% reduction in medicine use, a 31% acceleration of mucociliary clearance time, and a 28% improvement in quality of life. No significant adverse events associated with SNI were identified. This study nicely establishes that using isotonic saline solution can be recommended as complementary therapy in AR.

R. Sindwani, MD

Reference

1. Blaiss MS. Allergic rhinitis: direct and indirect costs. *Allergy Asthma Proc.* 2010; 31:375-380.

Allergic rhinitis and its impact on work productivity in primary care practice and a comparison with other common diseases: The Cross-sectional study to evAluate work Productivity in allergic Rhinitis compared with other common dIseases (CAPRI) study

de la Hoz Caballer B, Rodríguez M, Fraj J, et al (Hospital Universitario Ramón y Cajal, Madrid, Spain; Hospital Universitario Príncipe de Asturias, Alcalá de Henares, Madrid, Spain; Hospital Clínico-Instituto de Investigación Sanitaria Aragón, Zaragoza, Spain; et al)

Am J Rhinol Allergy 26:390-394, 2012

Background.—Allergic rhinitis (AR) is a highly prevalent allergic disease and also counts among the 10 most frequent reasons for medical consultation. Its impact on quality of life (QoL) and work productivity has been established but comparisons with other diseases are rare in the literature. The aim of this study was to evaluate the impact of AR in health-related QoL (HRQoL) and work productivity in primary care patients, compared with other prevalent diseases such as hypertension, diabetes mellitus (DM) type II, and symptomatic depression.

Methods.—Six hundred sixteen patients were included in a multicenter cross-sectional observational study. A generic HRQoL questionnaire, 36-item Short Form, and a specific questionnaire, "Work Productivity and Activity Impairment" were handed out to measure QoL and work productivity impact of the diseases. To assess clinical severity with a comparable scale between diseases Clinical Global Impression (CGI) had been used.

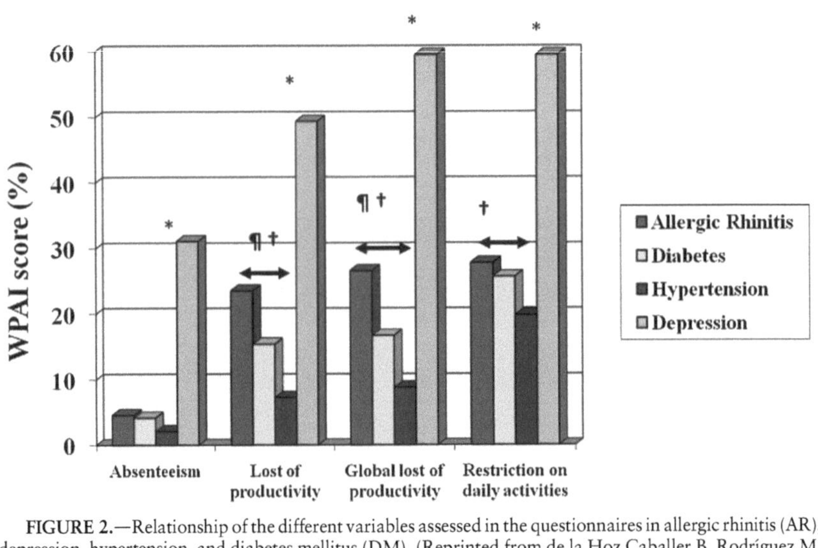

FIGURE 2.—Relationship of the different variables assessed in the questionnaires in allergic rhinitis (AR), depression, hypertension, and diabetes mellitus (DM). (Reprinted from de la Hoz Caballer B, Rodríguez M, Fraj J, et al. Allergic rhinitis and its impact on work productivity in primary care practice and a comparison with other common diseases: the Cross-sectional study to evAluate work Productivity in allergic Rhinitis compared with other common dIseases (CAPRI) study. *Am J Rhinol Allergy.* 2012;26:390-394, with permission from OceanSide Publications, Inc.)

Results.—Symptomatic depression was found to produce the greatest impairment on work productivity with a decrease of 59.5%, with significant differences compared with AR, hypertension, and DM type II ($p < 0.05$). Symptomatic depression was found to produce the highest negative impact on daily activities with a statistically significant reduction of 59.4% ($p < 0.05$) compared with AR (26.6% decrease), hypertension (8.8% decrease), and DM (16.7% decrease) patients. Differences between AR and DM or hypertension were also significant ($p < 0.05$). Restriction on daily activities for AR was 27.8%, which is significantly higher ($p < 0.05$) than hypertension (19.8% decrease) but not DM (25.7% decrease). Depression had the highest impairment on daily activities (59.4%), compared with the remaining three groups ($p < 0.05$).

Conclusion.—AR impairs work productivity in a greater magnitude than hypertension and DM type II (Fig 2).

► Allergic rhinitis (AR) is a very common disorder and one of the most common problems seen in a doctor's office. The aim of the CAPRI study was to evaluate the impact of AR in health-related quality of life and work productivity among primary care patients, compared with other diseases, such as hypertension, diabetes mellitus (DM) type II, and symptomatic depression. This multicenter, cross-sectional, observational study used a variety of surveys to evaluate 616 patients with AR. Of the disorders analyzed, symptomatic depression was found to produce the greatest impairment on work productivity and impact on daily activities. Surprisingly, however, AR was shown to impair work productivity more than DM or hypertension (Fig 2). This is an eye-opening finding, especially in light of how common a diagnosis AR is (approximately 1/10 people suffer with AR). Another interesting issue discussed in the article is the impact of sedative antihistamines that have been related to industrial accidents, yielding an estimated loss of productivity of 13%. Patients included in this study predominantly had moderate AR and most of them (80%) were taking medications for symptomatic relief. Approximately 19% of them admitted to suffering from somnolence, but no correlation with productivity loss was found. Overall, a very thought-provoking article.

R. Sindwani, MD

The risk and management of anaphylaxis in the setting of immunotherapy

Lieberman P (Allergy and Asthma Care, Germantown, TN)

Am J Rhinol Allergy 26:469-474, 2012

Background.—Anaphylactic events due to immunotherapy are probably not completely preventable. There is always an inherent risk surrounding the administration of an allergen to an individual who is sensitized to the substance administered.

Methods.—There are, however, effective measures to reduce the risk of these events, and to optimize the assurance of a good outcome in the face of such an event.

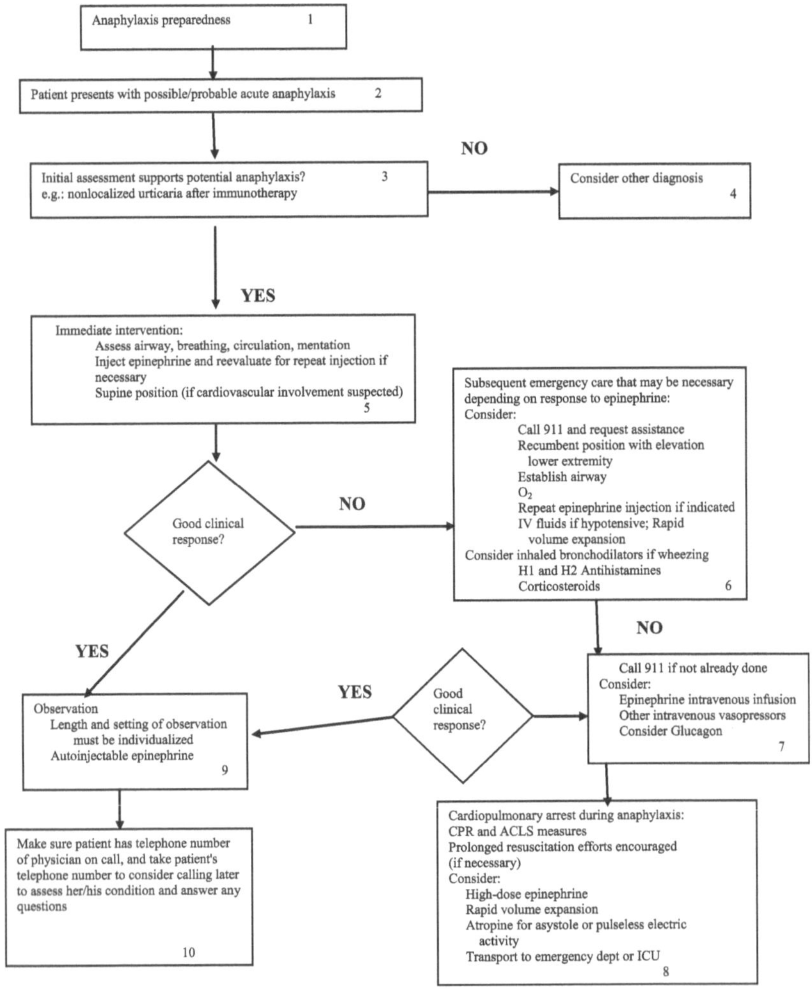

FIGURE 1.—Algorithm of the treatment of an anaphylactic event in the outpatient setting (i.v.). (Adopted from Ref. 2.) (Reprinted from Lieberman P. The risk and management of anaphylaxis in the setting of immunotherapy. *Am J Rhinol Allergy*. 2012;26:469-474, with permission from OceanSide Publications, Inc.)

Results.—Of prime importance in preventing these episodes is the regular assessment of the patient's health status, especially in regard to asthma, and the careful attention to the prevention of dosing errors.

Conclusion.—Of equal importance, in regard to assuring a good outcome should such an event occur, are the rapid recognition of symptoms and the immediate injection of epinephrine, the drug of choice for the treatment of any episode of anaphylaxis (Fig 1).

▶ By its very nature, immunotherapy is inherently dangerous because one is purposely introducing allergen into an allergic individual. To some extent, therefore, hypersensitivity reactions are unavoidable during the process of immunotherapy. There are, of course, specific measures to minimize the risk and effective therapy to treat any such reactions. The most dangerous form of reaction, anaphylaxis, must be avoided at all costs. This is a very well-written review article on the risk and management of anaphylaxis in the outpatient setting.

It draws heavily on the literature and consensus statements[1-3] to examine methods of minimizing risks of severe reactions and also presents protocols designed to treat such reactions if they do occur. The incidence of anaphylaxis suggested is approximately 5.4 per 1 million injections, but it carries with it a significant fatality risk. An excellent pathway for the management of severe reactions/anaphylaxis is presented in Fig 1. The author underscores that the best way of preventing fatal reactions during immunotherapy is the regular assessment of the patient's health status, especially with regard to asthma, and the careful attention to the prevention of dosing errors. These 2 issues are central to avoiding major issues in the outpatient setting. The management pathway and discussion of anaphylaxis in the report highlight the importance of rapid recognition of symptoms and the immediate injection of epinephrine, the drug of choice, for the treatment of any episode of anaphylaxis. A list of items to assure preparedness for such an event is also examined, so that if an event does occur, a favorable outcome is more likely. This is an excellent review on the topic of anaphylaxis and worth a read for those practicing allergy.

R. Sindwani, MD

References

1. Cox L, Nelson H, Lockey R, et al. Allergen immunotherapy: a practice parameter third update. *J Allergy Clin Immunol.* 2011;127:S1-S55.
2. Lieberman P, Nicklas R, Oppenheimer J, et al. The diagnosis and management of anaphylaxis practice parameter: 2010 Update. *J Allergy Clin Immunol.* 2010;126: 477-480.
3. Cox L, Larenas-Linnemann D, Lockey R. Speaking the same language: the World Allergy Organization subcutaneous immunotherapy systemic reaction grading system. *J Allergy Clin Immunol.* 2010;125:569-574.

Effects of montelukast on quality of life in patients with persistent allergic rhinitis

Cingi C, Ozlugedik S (Univ of Osmangazi, Eskisehir, Turkey; Numune Training and Res Hosp, Ankara, Turkey)

Otolaryngol Head Neck Surg 142:654-658, 2010

Objective.—To determine the effects of montelukast monotherapy on health-related quality of life (HRQL) in patients with persistent allergic rhinitis.

Study Design.—The study was placebo-controlled, randomized, and double blinded.

Setting.—Tertiary university hospital.

Subjects and Methods.—There were 46 patients in the study group and 24 patients in the control group, all of whom had a diagnosis of persistent

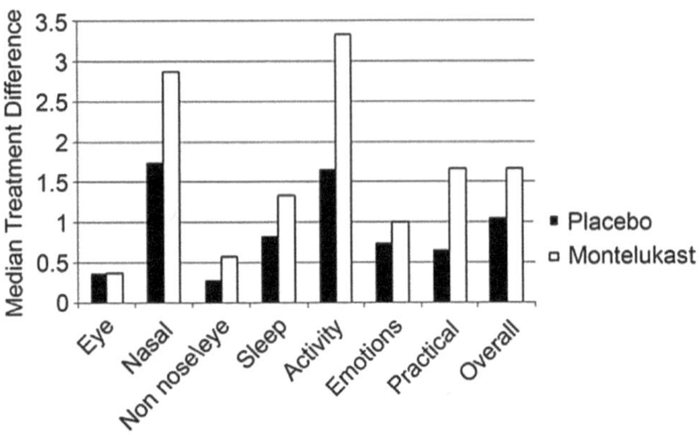

FIGURE 2.—Treatment difference was statically significant in favor of the study group compared with placebo for sleep, practical problems, nasal problems, activities that have been limited by nose or eye symptoms, non-nose/eye domains, and for overall score ($P < 0.001$, $P < 0.001$, $P = 0.003$, $P < 0.001$, $P = 0.012$, and $P < 0.001$, respectively). (Reprinted from Otolaryngology - Head and Neck Surgery. Cingi C, Ozlugedik S. Effects of montelukast on quality of life in patients with persistent allergic rhinitis. *Otolaryngol Head Neck Surg*. 2010;142:654-658, with permission from the American Academy of Otolaryngology-Head and Neck Surgery Foundation.)

allergic rhinitis of at least two years. The patients were evaluated at two control visits after the diagnosis. The study group was given 10-mg montelukast oral tablets, while the control group was given a placebo, and these were taken daily for one month. For evaluation of HRQL in both groups, the Rhinoconjunctivitis Quality of Life Questionnaire (RQLQ) was used.

Results.—There was a larger decrease in the overall RQLQ score for the group using montelukast compared with the placebo group ($P < 0.001$). The difference between scores at baseline versus the end of the first month for all domains was statically significant in both the placebo group and study group ($P < 0.001$). The difference in change from baseline to the end of the first month (treatment difference) between the placebo group and the study group was statically significant, in favor of the study group, for sleep, practical problems, nasal problems, and activities that have been limited by nose or eye symptoms, and for overall score ($P < 0.001$, $P < 0.001$, $P = 0.003$, $P < 0.001$, and $P < 0.001$, respectively).

Conclusion.—Montelukast is a drug that improves the disease-specific quality of life in patients being treated for persistent allergic rhinitis better than placebo (Fig 2).

▶ Pharmacotherapy for allergic rhinitis (AR) aims to reduce the effects of the inflammatory cells and mediators, which play a role in the early- and late-phase responses. Histamine and leukotrienes are important mediators that act in both phases. Whereas histamine is responsible for rhinorrhea, sneezing, and nasal itching, leukotrienes mainly cause nasal congestion. Montelukast is a leukotriene receptor antagonist commonly used in the treatment of asthma and/or AR as an effective adjunctive agent.[1] This randomized, double-blinded placebo-controlled trial sought to determine the effects of montelukast monotherapy on health-related quality of life in persistent AR. There were 46 patients in the study group who received 10 mg of montelukast daily for a month and 24 controls. The study found a significantly larger decrease in the overall Rhinoconjunctivitis Quality of Life Questionnaire score (for all domains) for the montelukast group compared with placebo. An important advantage of montelukast over other first-line AR medications that the authors highlight is that its side effects are the same as those seen with placebo. Specifically, montelukast does not have the side effect of sedation associated with most antihistamines,[2] and it tastes better, which may improve compliance in the pediatric population.[3] The authors conclude that montelukast is significantly better than placebo at improving the disease-specific symptoms of persistent AR and offers a more favorable side-effect profile than other agents.

R. Sindwani, MD

References

1. Meltzer EO, Malmstrom K, Lu S, et al. Concomitant montelukast and loratadine as treatment for seasonal allergic rhinitis: a randomized, placebo-controlled clinical trial. *J Allergy Clin Immunol.* 2000;105:917-922.
2. Lagos JA, Marshall GD. Montelukast in the management of allergic rhinitis. *Ther Clin Risk Manag.* 2007;3:327-332.
3. Chen ST, Lu KH, Sun HL, Chang WT, Lue KH, Chou MC. Randomized placebo-controlled trial comparing montelukast and cetirizine for treating perennial allergic rhinitis in children aged 2–6 yr. *Pediatr Allergy Immunol.* 2006;17:49-54.

2 Head and Neck Surgery and Tumors

Basic and Clinical Research

^{18}F-FDG Metabolic Tumor Volume and Total Glycolytic Activity of Oral Cavity and Oropharyngeal Squamous Cell Cancer: Adding Value to Clinical Staging

Dibble EH, Alvarez ACL, Truong M-T, et al (Boston Univ School of Medicine, MA; Harvard School of Public Health and Brigham and Women's Hosp, Boston)
J Nucl Med 53:709-715, 2012

^{18}F-FDG metabolic tumor volume (MTV) and total glycolytic activity (TGA) have been proposed as potential prognostic imaging markers for patient outcome in human solid tumors. The purpose of this study was to establish whether MTV and TGA add prognostic information to clinical staging in patients with oral and oropharyngeal squamous cell carcinomas (SCCs).

Methods.—The Institutional Review Board approved this Health Insurance Portability and Accountability Act–compliant single-institution retrospective study. Forty-five patients with histologically proven oral or oropharyngeal SCC underwent PET/CT for initial cancer staging and were included in the study. MTV was measured using a gradient-based method (PET Edge) and fixed-threshold methods at 38%, 50%, and 60% of maximum standardized uptake value (SUV). The TGA is defined as MTV × mean SUV. Bland–Altman analysis was used to establish the reliability of the methods of segmentation. Outcome endpoints were overall survival (OS) and progression-free survival. Cox proportional hazards univariate and multivariate regression analyses were performed.

Results.—In Cox regression models, MTV and TGA were the only factors significantly associated with survival outcome after adjusting for all other covariates including American Joint Committee on Cancer (AJCC) stage, with hazards ratio of 1.06 (95% confidence interval, 1.01–1.10; $P = 0.006$) and 1.00 (95% confidence interval, 1.00–1.01; $P = 0.02$). The model fit was significantly better when MTV was added to AJCC stage in model I (χ^2 value change, 1.16–6.71; $P = 0.01$) and when TGA was added to AJCC stage in model II (χ^2 value change, 1.16–4.37; $P = 0.04$).

The median cutoff point of 7.7 mL for primary tumor MTV was predictive of time to OS (log rank $P = 0.04$). The median cutoff point of 55 g for PET Edge primary tumor TGA was predictive of time to OS (log rank $P = 0.08$), though the result was not statistically significant.

Conclusion.—Gradient-based segmentations of primary tumor MTV and TGA are potential ^{18}F-FDG markers for time to survival in patients with oral and oropharyngeal SCC and may provide prognostic information in addition to AJCC stage. These exploratory imaging markers need validation in larger cohort studies.

▶ This selected study addresses an interesting question of whether metabolic tumor volume (MTV) and total glycolytic activity (TGA), as determined by fluorodeoxyglucose (FDG)-positron emission tomography (PET), could serve as a predictor of tumor biology and serve as prognostic markers in oropharyngeal cancer. This is a retrospective pilot study, and therefore the results are preliminary and need validation in a large, well-designed study. Nevertheless, the results are interesting in that, according to this study, both PET parameters can serve as independent prognostic markers and can prove to be of clinical value when used in conjunction with American Joint Committee on Cancer staging.

FDG-PET, especially when used in co-registration with computed tomography (CT), has already proven itself as the most accurate early diagnostic tool for determining response and recurrence of head and neck cancer treated with radiochemotherapy. The current protocol calls for the first posttherapy CT/PET at 12 weeks after completion of treatment, followed by 2 subsequent studies at 6 and 9 months. Radiation oncologists are also claiming that CT/PET is helpful in planning therapy. The question then arises how many PET scans will we obtain in the course of diagnosis and therapy of a single head and neck cancer patient? Is it cost-effective? Does it really improve patient survival or positively affect local and regional control of the cancer? All those questions have to be answered before we subject our patients to half a dozen PET scans and expect insurance to cover them.

M. Gapany, MD

Sentinel Lymph Node Biopsy Is Accurate and Prognostic in Head and Neck Melanoma

Erman AB, Collar RM, Griffith KA, et al (Univ of Michigan Health System, Ann Arbor; Univ of Michigan Comprehensive Cancer Ctr, Ann Arbor)

Cancer 118:1040-1047, 2012

Background.—Sentinel lymph node biopsy (SLNB) has emerged as a widely used staging procedure for cutaneous melanoma. However, debate remains around the accuracy and prognostic implications of SLNB for cutaneous melanoma arising in the head and neck, as previous reports have demonstrated inferior results to those in nonhead and neck regions. Through the largest single-institution series of head and neck melanoma patients, the authors set out to demonstrate that SLNB accuracy and prognostic value in the head and neck region are comparable to other sites.

Methods.—A prospectively collected database was queried for cutaneous head and neck melanoma patients who underwent SLNB at the University of Michigan between 1997 and 2007. Primary endpoints included SLNB result, time to recurrence, site of recurrence, and date and cause of death. Multivariate models were constructed for analyses.

Results.—Three hundred fifty-three patients were identified. A sentinel lymph node was identified in 352 of 353 patients (99.7%). Sixty-nine of the 353 (19.6%) patients had a positive SLNB. Seventeen of 68 patients (25%) undergoing completion lymphadenectomy after a positive SLNB result had at least 1 additional positive nonsentinel lymph node. Patients with local control and a negative SLNB failed regionally in 4.2% of cases. Multivariate analysis revealed positive SLNB status to be the most prognostic clinicopathologic predictor of poor outcome; hazard ratio was 4.23 for SLNB status and recurrence-free survival ($P < .0001$) and 3.33 for overall survival ($P < .0001$).

Conclusions.—SLNB is accurate and its results are of prognostic importance for head and neck melanoma patients.

▶ This is an excellent and important study establishing sentinel lymph node (SLN) biopsy for melanoma of the head and neck region as equally accurate and prognostic as SLN biopsies from the trunk and the extremities. In the past, the yield, the accuracy, and the predictive value of SLN biopsy from the head and neck region were considered inferior to that from other anatomic areas. It is very likely that the limited experience of individual surgeons, complex anatomy of the head and neck region, and the relatively small study groups were at fault for such conclusions. This large and well-conducted study convincingly dispels previously existing doubts about the validity of SLN biopsy for melanoma of the head and neck region. I agree with the authors that the most likely reason for the excellent accuracy of this series is the result of expert surgeons very familiar with the head and neck anatomy as well as close cooperation with an equally expert nuclear medicine and histopathology team. This is an important message for teams who lack the necessary expertise.

M. Gapany, MD

General

A Head and Neck Surgeon's Perspective on Best Practices for the Use of PET/CT Scans for the Diagnosis and Treatment of Head and Neck Cancers

Funk GF (Univ of Iowa Carver College of Medicine)

Arch Otolaryngol Head Neck Surg 138:748-752, 2012

Background.—The most useful applications for positron emission tomographic and computed tomographic (PET/CT) scans in pretreatment assessments of patients with head and neck squamous cell carcinoma (HNSCC) and in assessing patients with HNSCC and a clinically N0 (cN0) neck has been evaluated in several studies. In addition, the timing for PET/CT scanning in post-treatment surveillance programs for patients with HNSCC has been questioned. The current best practices for PET/CT in HNSCC were noted.

Methods.—Articles identified through a Medline search using PubMed. These were limited to adult human studies in the English language that involved clinical trials, meta-analyses, practice guidelines, and randomized controlled trials. Fifty-four articles were chosen, along with 12 documents from the Cochrane Database. Only the most relevant articles were cited.

Findings.—PET/CT has demonstrated superiority over either PET imaging or CT imaging alone in identifying and characterizing primary tumors, nodal disease, and distant metastasis. The use of contrast enhancement has further increased the abilities of PET/CT. Therapy has been altered based on PET/CT scans, especially when applied to imaging cystic lymph node metastasis from human papilloma virus-n-related oropharyngeal cancers.

Metabolic imaging with PET/CT in pretreatment regimens for advance-stage (III/IV) HNSCC offers the primary benefits of enhanced accuracy in staging and the ability to identify distant disease. These do not apply in patients with early-stage NHSCC or those with a low probability of distant disease. The negative predictive value (NPV) for low-volume disease is poor, and the positive predictive value (PPV) is consistently suboptimal for metabolic imaging in general. Taking time to investigate false-positive findings in patients with early-stage disease can be costly and delay treatment.

The results of PET/CT imaging in the diagnostic assessment of a cN0 neck are influenced by many factors. The central deficiency relates to the high frequency of occult metastasis smaller than 10 mm. Treatment decisions should not be based solely on PET/CT imaging. The definitive staging intervention for the cN0 neck should still be guided by pathologic evaluation.

Timing.—The optimal time to perform the first post-treatment PET/CT scan is not known, but many centers scan 12 or more weeks after treatment to reduce the number of false-positive scans and avoid detrimental survival effects if salvage surgery is needed. Insufficient data have been collected to determine the usefulness of additional scanning after a negative post-treatment PET/CT scan done at least 12 weeks after the last cancer-directed treatment.

Conclusions.—The use of PET/CT imaging for pretreatment analysis of patients with advanced-stage and recurrent HNSCC provides useful additional information that can guide management planning. Its usefulness in early-stage disease is limited, and it is not helpful for patients with cN0 necks. ^{18}F-fluorodeoxyglucose (^{18}F-FDG) has significant clinical usefulness when used in post-treatment analyses of patients with advanced-stage disease. The optimal time for such scans is at least 12 weeks after completing treatment.

▶ Fluoro-2-deoxy-D-glucose positron emission tomography/computed tomography (FDG-PET/CT) has emerged as the most sensitive imaging modality for detection of head and neck cancer. It has been used for initial staging of tumors, for detection of cancers with unknown primary sites, for detection of synchronous tumors, and for detection of metastatic disease at the time of the initial cancer workup. In addition, radiation oncologists have been using FDG-PET/CT for treatment planning, whereas oncologists have been relying on FDG-PET/CT for determining response to radiochemotherapy. To make things even more complicated, FDG-PET/CT appears to be an excellent study for posttherapy tumor surveillance monitoring in patients treated with chemoradiotherapy. Needless to say, FDG-PET/CT is an expensive imaging modality. The question that remains is whether the potential benefits of this imaging modality justify its significant cost. At the end of the day, how many FDG-PET/CT studies will we end up doing on every patient? Are all of these studies justified? Which studies are more important than others? This selected review article summarizes the available literature on this subject and makes recommendations on best practices for the use of FDG-PET/CT for the diagnosis and treatment of head and neck cancer. It is well worth reviewing!

M. Gapany, MD

Vitamin or mineral supplement intake and the risk of head and neck cancer: pooled analysis in the INHANCE consortium

Li Q, Chuang S-C, Eluf-Neto J, et al (Chinese Academy of Med Sciences, Beijing, China; International Agency for Res on Cancer, Lyon, France; Universidade de Sao Paulo, Brazil; et al)

Int J Cancer 131:1686-1699, 2012

To investigate the potential role of vitamin or mineral supplementation on the risk of head and neck cancer (HNC), we analyzed individual-level pooled data from 12 case–control studies (7,002 HNC cases and 8,383 controls) participating in the International Head and Neck Cancer Epidemiology consortium. There were a total of 2,028 oral cavity cancer, 2,465 pharyngeal cancer, 874 unspecified oral/pharynx cancer, 1,329 laryngeal cancer and 306 overlapping HNC cases. Odds ratios (OR) and 95% confidence intervals (CIs) for self reported ever use of any vitamins, multivitamins, vitamin A, vitamin C, vitamin E, and calcium, beta-carotene, iron, selenium and zinc supplements were assessed. We further examined frequency, duration and cumulative exposure of each vitamin or mineral when possible and stratified by smoking and drinking status. All ORs were adjusted for age, sex, race/ethnicity, study center, education level, pack-years of smoking, frequency of alcohol drinking and fruit/vegetable intake. A decreased risk of HNC was observed with ever use of vitamin C (OR = 0.76, 95% CI = 0.59–0.96) and with ever use of calcium supplement (OR = 0.64, 95% CI = 0.42–0.97). The inverse association with HNC risk was also observed for 10 or more years of vitamin C use (OR = 0.72, 95% CI = 0.54–0.97) and more than 365 tablets of cumulative calcium intake (OR = 0.36, 95% CI = 0.16–0.83), but linear trends were not observed for the frequency or duration of any supplement intake.

We did not observe any strong associations between vitamin or mineral supplement intake and the risk of HNC.

▶ Several recently published epidemiologic studies for the first time provided factual evidence in support of promoting a diet rich in fresh fruit, juices, vegetables, and vitamins for head and neck cancer patients and populations at risk for oral cavity premalignancy. This simple dietary modification may be the least expensive and most effective method of decreasing the risk of head and neck cancer (even in smokers). There are even data supporting the efficacy of green leafy vegetables in protection against the acquisition of gene promoter methylation in the upper aerodigestive tract epithelial cells, reducing the risk of lung cancer in smokers.

This selected study is based on the analysis of pooled data from the International Head and Neck Cancer Epidemiology Consortium and includes studies from Europe, Latin America, and the United States. In this study, reduction in head and neck cancer risk was observed for vitamin C and calcium supplementation but not for other vitamins and minerals.

After reviewing this new body of literature, I started to routinely recommend to my head and neck cancer patients to alter their dietary habits and include in their diet large amounts of vitamin C–rich fruits, juices, leafy green vegetables, and, based on the results of the current study, calcium supplements.

M. Gapany, MD

Head and Neck Carcinoma in the United States: First Comprehensive Report of the Longitudinal Oncology Registry of Head and Neck Carcinoma (LORHAN)

Ang KK, Chen A, Curran WJ Jr, et al (The Univ of Texas MD Anderson Cancer Ctr, Houston; American Cancer Society, Atlanta, GA; Emory Univ, Atlanta, GA; et al)

Cancer 118:5783-5792, 2012

Background.—Detailed information about how patients with head and neck carcinoma (HNC) are treated across practice settings does not exist. The authors conducted a prospective, observational study to examine the patterns of care for a series of patients with newly diagnosed HNC in the United States and to test 2 hypotheses: 1) There is no difference in the pattern of care between community and academic settings; and 2) the results of major randomized clinical trials will change the pattern of care in both practice settings within 1 year of publication in peer-reviewed journals.

Methods.—Patients aged ≥18 years were enrolled in the Longitudinal Oncology Registry of Head and Neck Carcinoma (LORHAN) after providing written informed consent if they had a confirmed diagnosis of new HNC and were scheduled to receive treatment other than surgery alone.

Results.—Between 2005 and 2010, 100 centers enrolled 4243 patients, including 2612 patients (62%) from academic investigators and 1631 patients (38%) from community centers. Initial treatments were radiation with concurrent chemotherapy (30%) or cetuximab (9%), adjuvant radiotherapy (21%), induction chemotherapy (16%), and other (24%). Intensity modulated radiation therapy was the dominant radiation technique (84%). Single-agent cisplatin was prescribed in nearly half of patients and more often in academic centers (53% vs 43% of patients; $P < .0001$). Single-agent cetuximab was the next most common drug used (19%) and was prescribed more frequently in community settings (24% vs 17%; $P = .0001$). The data rejected the 2 prospective hypotheses.

Conclusions.—LORHAN documented differences in patient characteristics and treatments between community and academic settings for a large series of patients in the United States.

▶ This is the second large epidemiologic study on head and neck carcinoma in the United States included in this Year Book. This one is based on the Longitudinal Oncology Registry of Head and Neck Carcinoma (LORHAN) database. This database was established in 2005 with the objective of collecting information on patterns of care for head and neck cancer. Unlike the National Cancer Institute's Surveillance, Epidemiology, and End Results registry, LORHAN collects data on all therapeutic modalities, toxicities, supportive care, and outcomes. In that respect, LORHAN is a more complete database. Furthermore, it has been designed to compare therapeutic patterns in the academic health care centers versus treatment methods used in the community. Another major task of LORHAN is to assess implementation of the newest trial results in the community and academic setting within a year of their publication in peer-reviewed journals. In general, this study contains very interesting and important epidemiologic data and is worth reviewing.

M. Gapany, MD

Venous thromboembolism in patients with head and neck cancer after surgery

Thai L, McCarn K, Stott W, et al (Oregon Health and Science Univ, Portland)
Head Neck 35:4-9, 2013

Background.—The purpose of this study was to report the incidence of venous thromboembolism (VTE) in patients with head and neck cancer after surgery.

Methods.—This was a single-institution, retrospective cohort: 134 patients underwent resection and simultaneous microvascular reconstruction. The primary endpoint was identification of confirmed or suspicious VTE within 30 days of surgery.

Results.—Two subjects (1.4%) with confirmed VTE (1 pulmonary embolism, 1 deep venous thrombosis) and 6 subjects (4.4%) with suspicious VTE (1 acute respiratory failure, 1 sudden cardiac arrest, and 4 cases of leg edema without imaging) were identified. The strongest predictors of possible VTE were prior VTE ($p = .004$; odds ratio [OR], 25.11; 95% confidence interval [CI], 1.13–556.40), red cell transfusion ($p = .009$; OR, 1.80; 95% CI,

1.16–2.80), high body mass index ($p = .015$, OR, 1.29, 95% CI, 1.05–1.58), and older age ($p = .046$; OR, 1.10; 95% CI, 1.00–1.19).

Conclusion.—The incidence of VTE in patients with head and neck cancer after resection and microvascular reconstruction ranged from 1.4% to 5.8%.

▶ This selected article underscores the importance of a frequently overlooked topic in otolaryngology-head and neck surgery: the importance of venous thromboembolism (VTE) prophylaxis. Although clinical research on this subject is sparse in otolaryngology, available data point to a relatively low incidence of VTE in otolaryngology as compared with other surgical specialties. Even in head and neck oncologic surgery, the incidence of reported VTE appears to be less than 0.5%. Because the use of pharmacologic thromboprophylaxis in head and neck tumor surgery, especially when flap reconstruction is involved, can be associated with increased risk of postoperative hemorrhage, many head and neck surgeons (including myself) opt for mechanical compression devices and early ambulation for VTE prophylaxis. It is entirely possible that true incidence of VTE in head and neck oncologic surgery could be underestimated. This article suggests exactly that: The reported incidence of VTE in patients with microvascular reconstruction ranged from 1.4 (confirmed VTE) to 5.8% (confirmed and suspicious VTE), which is in line with the incidence of VTE in other oncologic surgery subspecialties.

M. Gapany, MD

A Population-Based Study of Therapy and Survival for Patients With Head and Neck Cancer Treated in the Community

Ullmann CD, Harlan LC, Shavers VL, et al (Natl Cancer Inst, Bethesda, MD; et al)
Cancer 118:4452-4461, 2012

Background.—The objective of this study was to examine patterns of care and survival in a population-based sample of patients with head and neck cancer (HNC) who were treated in the community or in hospitals that had residency training programs.

Methods.—Data from the National Cancer Institute's Surveillance, Epidemiology, and End Results Program were used to sample 1317 patients aged ≥ 20 years with invasive squamous HNC who were diagnosed during 2004 and who had vital status available through 2008.

Results.—Treatment and survival were influenced by tumor site and disease stage. Patients who had stage I/II cancer of the oral cavity generally underwent surgery; patients with stage III oral cavity disease underwent surgery and received radiation; and patients with stage IV oral cavity disease underwent surgery and received chemoradiation. Patients with early stage cancer of the oropharynx either underwent surgery or received radiation and chemotherapy, and patients with late/unstaged oropharyngeal disease primarily received radiation and chemotherapy. Patients with early stage cancer of the larynx mainly received radiation alone, and patients with late stage laryngeal disease generally received chemoradiation. Cisplatin-based regimens were used most frequently. Overall, taxanes were used in 32% of regimens, and cetuximab was used in <3% of regimens. Patients aged ≥ 50 years, those with a Charlson comorbidity score ≥ 1, those with stage IV disease, and those with cancer located in the oral cavity or larynx had poorer survival. Although facilities with residency training programs treated more black patients and more patients with late stage disease, when adjusted for other factors, survival rates were similar to those reported in facilities with no such programs.

Conclusions.—Therapy generally followed accepted standards for 2004. Findings in particular tumor sites and stages may reflect the variability that still exists for the treatment of HNC. The use of taxanes and cetuximab is expected to increase based on new evidence of benefit. Reducing treatment-related toxicities and long-term functional deficits will be critical and especially important with the increase in human papillomavirus-related cancers. In addition, further attempts to improve survival for older patients are needed.

▶ This large epidemiologic study is based on the National Cancer Institute's Surveillance, Epidemiology, and End Results registry data. A total of 1317 patients diagnosed with head and neck cancer in 2004 were included and were followed through 2008. The study indicates the established use of chemoradiotherapy for head and neck cancer, primarily the combination of cisplatin and 5-FU. It provides very useful epidemiologic information on the therapy delivered and survival data according to the site and stage of the disease. The presented data do not as of yet completely reflect the introduction of taxanes and cetuximab into the most contemporary chemoradiotherapy protocols and are lagging behind the newest methodological advances in transoral robotic surgery. They are also not likely to reflect the unexpected epidemiologic change in the etiology of oropharyngeal cancer (ie, a shift toward human papillomavirus-related tumors as opposed to tobacco- and alcohol-associated oropharyngeal cancer), which so dramatically occurred in the last 6 or 7 years. Nevertheless, the study contains very interesting and important epidemiologic data and is worth reviewing.

M. Gapany, MD

Adenoid Cystic Carcinoma of the Head and Neck: Incidence and Survival Trends Based on 1973-2007 Surveillance, Epidemiology, and End Results Data

Ellington CL, Goodman M, Kono SA, et al (Emory Univ, Atlanta, GA)
Cancer 118:4444-4451, 2012

Background.—Adenoid cystic carcinoma (ACC) of the head and neck (ACCHN) is a rare tumor of minor salivary, parotid, and submandibular glands. The biologic behavior of the disease is poorly understood, and nonsurgical treatment strategies have yet to be standardized. The long-term prognosis continues to be guarded, with an estimated 10-year survival of <60%. Population-based studies examining ACC are scarce. The authors aimed to analyze incidence rates and survival outcomes for patients diagnosed with ACCHN using national population-based data.

Methods.—Data were obtained from the US National Cancer Institute's Surveillance, Epidemiology, and End Results (SEER) program. Newly diagnosed ACCHN cases reported to SEER from 1973 through 2007 were categorized according to their sex, race, age, year of diagnosis, marital status, treatment interventions, primary tumor site, and disease stage. Incidence of ACCHN and postdiagnosis survival were examined over time and compared across different demographic and disease-related categories.

Results.—The authors identified 3026 patients with ACCHN. The mean age at diagnosis among those cases was 57.4 years (range, 11-99 years). Analyses of incidence data demonstrated a decline in ACCHN rates between 1973 and 2007, noted across all sexes and races with no detectable inflexion points. The overall 5-year, 10-year, and 15-year survival outcomes for ACCHN patients were 90.3%, 79.9%, and 69.2%, respectively. Females, patients with localized disease, and younger patients were found to have significantly better survival across all time periods (all comparison-specific log-rank P values < 0.001). Multivariate analyses revealed better prognosis among women compared with men (hazard ratio [HR], 0.73; 95% confidence interval [CI], 0.65-0.82), among married compared with unmarried individuals (HR, 0.81; 95% CI, 0.71-0.91), with certain sites of origin and stage of disease (HR, 2.788; 95% CI, 2.36-3.29), and in those who had surgery of the primary tumor site (HR, 0.45; 95% CI, 0.37-0.54).

Conclusions.—The overall incidence of ACC is declining. The noted differences in survival based on sex, marital status, site of origin, and treatment intervention require further investigation.

▶ This selected article is a very large population-based epidemiologic study using the US National Cancer Institute's Surveillance, Epidemiology, and End Results (SEER) database. It focuses on adenoid cystic carcinoma of the head and neck—a tumor with unique and poorly understood biology. Data on this tumor are sparse, and therapeutic strategies are not well defined. Such large epidemiologic studies, thus, are very welcome and are important for practicing otolaryngologists and head and neck surgeons to review.

Adenoid cystic carcinoma is generally considered to be a radiosensitive tumor, and radiotherapy is generally recommended as an adjuvant modality to surgical extirpation of the tumor. It was interesting and surprising to learn from this study that adjuvant radiotherapy, according to the SEER database, confers little survival advantage to this disease. Not surprisingly, however, surgery remains the only truly effective therapeutic modality offering a survival benefit in adenoid cystic carcinoma of the head and neck. Unfortunately, the SEER database does not include information on chemotherapy. Its role in treating this cancer, therefore, has not been addressed by this study.

M. Gapany, MD

Cetuximab Therapy for Head and Neck Squamous Cell Carcinoma: A Systematic Review of the Data

Reeves TD, Hill EG, Armeson KE, et al (Med Univ of South Carolina, Charleston)

Otolaryngol Head Neck Surg 144:676-684, 2011

Objective.—To review the current state of the data on the use of cetuximab in head and neck squamous cell carcinoma (HNSCC).

Data Sources.—The National Center for Biotechnology Information's PubMed and the Cochrane collection.

Review Methods.—Search terms included *cetuximab* and *head and neck cancer.* These results were reviewed, and a second search was performed using limits: meta-analysis, randomized controlled trial, and clinical trial.

Results.—The literature search yielded 412 articles. Fifteen were identified for analysis. For patients with recurrent/metastatic disease who received combination chemotherapy in phase I/II trials, the overall response (OR) was 18.7% (95% confidence interval [CI], 10.4%-27.0%). Phase III trial data for combination chemotherapy in recurrent/metastatic disease showed OR to be 17.0% (95% CI, 12.6%-21.4%) for platinum-based regimens and 34.2% (28.6%-39.7%) for platinum-based regimens with cetuximab. For this same group, the estimated aggregate hazard ratio comparing platinum-based therapy plus cetuximab to platinum therapy alone was 1.10 (95% CI, 0.78-1.54), indicating no significant improvement in overall survival in the aggregate analysis. Combination chemoradiation with cetuximab in both phase I/II trials and the single phase III trial shows enhanced responsiveness, but the data are difficult to interpret because it is not used with standard-of-care regimens for advanced-stage disease.

Conclusion.—Early evidence has shown cetuximab to be effective in the treatment of HNSCC, and it should be used to enhance, but not replace, current treatment paradigms until further phase III data are available.

▶ This is a very useful literature review on the emerging role of cetuximab in treating head and neck squamous cell carcinoma. Cetuximab, an epidermal growth factor (EGF) receptor antagonist, appears to be an effective agent for the treatment of head and neck squamous cell carcinoma. EGF receptor antagonists are particularly appealing in head and neck oncology because of their relatively low side-effect profile compared with the standard chemotherapy agents. Nevertheless, current data in the literature do not provide enough support for substituting currently existing chemotherapy protocols with cetuximab, especially in broad use against a variety of head and neck subsites. The data, however, support its use to enhance standard chemotherapy regimens. It can also be used as an alternative to standard regimens in individuals who do not meet the criteria for standard therapy because of their poor performance status or poor general health. Furthermore, its role in treating human papillomavirus–associated head and neck carcinoma has not been fully elucidated and needs further studies.

M. Gapany, MD

Diagnosis and treatment of recurrent laryngeal cancer following initial nonsurgical therapy

Agra IM, Ferlito A, Takes RP, et al (Hosp Aristides Maltez, Salvador, Brazil)
Head Neck 34:727-735, 2012

Surgery is the preferred modality for curative treatment of recurrent laryngeal cancer after failure of nonsurgical treatments. Patients with initial early-stage cancer experiencing recurrence following radiotherapy often have more advanced-stage tumors by the time the recurrence is recognized. About one third of such recurrent cancers are suitable for conservation surgery. Endoscopic resection with the CO(2) laser or open partial laryngectomy (partial vertical, supracricoid, or supraglottic laryngectomies) have been used. The outcomes of conservation surgery appear better than those after total laryngectomy, because of selection bias. Transoral laser surgery is currently used more frequently than open partial laryngectomy for treatment of early-stage recurrence, with outcomes equivalent to open surgery but with less associated morbidity. Laser surgery has also been employed for selective cases of advanced recurrent disease, but patient selection and expertise are required for application of this modality to rT3 tumors. In general, conservation laryngeal surgery is a safe and effective treatment for localized recurrences after radiotherapy for early-stage glottic cancer. Recurrent advanced-stage cancers should generally be treated by total laryngectomy.

▶ This selected article is a useful review of the available surgical options for recurrent laryngeal cancer after radiation (or radiochemotherapy) failure. In my experience, the incidence of advanced laryngeal cancer has been steadily declining, with a clear predominance of early-stage tumors. In the state where I practice otolaryngology (Minnesota), I attribute it to great strides made in improving primary care. The occasional total laryngectomy that I have to perform is almost exclusively for salvage after organ-preservation failure. On the other hand, occasional radiation failure for early laryngeal cancer almost invariably can be tackled through an endoscopic, laser-assisted approach. Open laryngeal surgery is seldom indicated, with the exception of maybe radiation-failed anterior commissure tumors, which are very conveniently approached using open, anterior commissure laryngectomy. In properly selected cases, endoscopic, laser-assisted partial laryngectomy can be attempted even in radiation-failed T3 tumors, although such surgery should be performed only by very experienced endoscopic surgeons. The results of endoscopic salvage laryngeal surgery, according to the results reported in the literature, are at least as good as with open techniques. Endoscopic surgery is associated with substantially less morbidity and, therefore, is the preferred technique.

M. Gapany, MD

"Pharyngocise": Randomized Controlled Trial of Preventative Exercises to Maintain Muscle Structure and Swallowing Function During Head-and-Neck Chemoradiotherapy

Carnaby-Mann G, Crary MA, Schmalfuss I, et al (Univ of Florida, Gainesville; North Florida/South Georgia Veterans Health System, Gainesville, FL)

Int J Radiat Oncol Biol Phys 83:210-219, 2012

Purpose.—Dysphagia after chemoradiotherapy is common. The present randomized clinical trial studied the effectiveness of preventative behavioral intervention for dysphagia compared with the "usual care."

Methods and Materials.—A total of 58 head-and-neck cancer patients treated with chemoradiotherapy were randomly assigned to usual care, sham swallowing intervention, or active swallowing exercises (pharyngocise). The intervention arms were treated daily during chemoradiotherapy. The primary outcome measure was muscle size and composition (determined by T_2-weighted magnetic resonance imaging). The secondary outcomes included functional swallowing ability, dietary intake, chemosensory function, salivation, nutritional status, and the occurrence of dysphagia-related complications.

Results.—The swallowing musculature (genioglossus, hyoglossuss, and mylohyoid) demonstrated less structural deterioration in the active treatment arm. The functional swallowing, mouth opening, chemosensory acuity, and salivation rate deteriorated less in the pharyngocise group.

Conclusion.—Patients completing a program of swallowing exercises during cancer treatment demonstrated superior muscle maintenance and functional swallowing ability.

▶ Chemoradiotherapy for head and neck cancer has severe short-term and long-term detrimental effects on swallowing function in patients undergoing this treatment. It has long been observed that encouraging swallowing and swallowing exercises during chemoradiotherapy and avoiding percutaneous endoscopic gastrostomy (PEG) might improve functional outcome. So much so, that some authors have recommended avoiding routine pretherapy PEGs, arguing that they discourage swallowing.

This selected study is a first randomized controlled trial that demonstrated the clear-cut benefits of an intense preventative swallowing exercise program delivered over the course of radiochemotherapy. The results presented in this study speak for themselves. The timing and the intensity of therapy apparently play an important role in the success of such a program. The delivery of swallowing exercises is simple and does not require any additional resources beyond those available to an interdisciplinary head and neck oncology program. It thus appears to be an effective and a cost-effective way to mitigate the incapacitating swallowing impairment associated with radiochemotherapy for head and neck cancer.

M. Gapany, MD

Outcomes

Primary Surgical Treatment of T3 Glottic Carcinoma: Long-Term Results and Decision-Making Aspects

Mantsopoulos K, Psychogios G, Bohr C, et al (Univ of Erlangen-Nuremberg, Germany)
Laryngoscope 122:2723-2727, 2012

Objectives/Hypothesis.—The aim of this study was to assess the efficacy of primary surgical treatment in the management of T3 glottic carcinomas.

Study Design.—Retrospective clinical study.

Methods.—A retrospective evaluation of the records for all patients treated with primary surgery for T3 glottic carcinomas at a tertiary referral center between 1980 and 2005 was carried out. Data for the 5-year disease-specific survival (DSS) were assessed, as well as local control rates in relation to vocal cord immobility, N classification, choice of surgical modality, and adjuvant therapy. Patients who underwent partial laryngectomy were also evaluated in relation to organ preservation and the rate of permanent tracheotomies.

Results.—The 5-year DSS in the 120 patients was 78.3%. Positive neck disease was shown to be a significant negative prognostic factor. Organ preservation was achieved in 90.1% of the patients who underwent partial laryngectomy and in 50% of the overall patient group. The occult metastasis rate was 14%.

Conclusions.—Primary surgical treatment is an effective modality against T3 glottic carcinomas. Partial laryngectomy is a reliable method in carefully selected cases. Low complication rates can be expected.

▶ The concept of larynx preservation using radiochemotherapy was conceived more than 2 decades ago with quality of life (QOL) and improved organ function in mind. It is only recently that several studies have been published that objectively evaluated the impact of radiochemotherapy for laryngeal preservation on long-term QOL. So far, all studies have shown that laryngeal preservation did not result in any significant improvement in the QOL compared with total laryngectomy. Radiochemotherapy, on the other hand, resulted in significant acute and long-term toxicity and side effects.

As a result of these QOL outcomes, the question of laryngeal preservation using the newest surgical methods, such as endoscopic, laser-assisted partial laryngeal, and robotic, has gained renewed momentum. This selected study, which examined 25 years of single-institutional experience with treating T3 glottic cancer with primary surgical therapy, is timely and very relevant. The results of the study support the concept of partial laryngeal surgery for T3 glottic cancer in a carefully selected group of patients, offering acceptable oncologic and functional outcomes.

M. Gapany, MD

Functional outcomes after radiotherapy or laser surgery in early glottic carcinoma: A systematic review

van Loon Y, Sjögren EV, Langeveld TPM, et al (Leiden Univ Med Ctr, The Netherlands; et al)

Head Neck 34:1179-1189, 2012

Background.—Early glottic carcinoma is treated with laser surgery or radiotherapy, but which treatment has better functional outcomes is unclear. This systematic review compared functional outcomes (voice, swallowing, quality of life [QOL]) in more extended T1a and limited T2 tumors (1) between treatments and (2) between greater and lesser laser resections.

Methods.—A systematic literature search covered relevant databases from 1990 to 2009, combining all patient/problem, intervention, comparison, outcome (PICO) keyword variations.

Results.—A total of 19 papers met the inclusion criteria, all of which were level IV evidence. Papers reported only voice and QOL. Heterogeneity of outcome measures prevented data pooling. Uncertainty about tumor comparability (depth, extent) between the 2 treatments, small subject numbers, and poor-quality reporting hindered interpretation.

Conclusions.—To allow comparison of laser surgery versus radiotherapy, a standardized method is needed that accurately measures tumor extent and depth. Agreement on functional outcome measures is necessary to allow comparison of treatments and resection types. Multicenter studies should be encouraged to guarantee adequate subject numbers.

▶ Sometimes the importance of a study is not in what it was able to show, discover, or prove, but is exactly the opposite—what it failed to show, discover, or prove. This selected study is such an example; namely, the question remains: Which therapeutic modality for treating early cancer of the glottic larynx—endoscopic laser resection or radiotherapy—produces better functional outcome? A thorough meta-analysis of published data in the literature on this topic failed to produce conclusive answers to the above questions. So, based on the results of this study, it is fair to say that to date we do not have conclusive evidence to claim that radiotherapy or laser surgery renders better functional outcomes when it comes to quality of voice, swallowing function, or quality of life in general. The main problems preventing a meaningful analysis of the data remain a lack of standardization in measuring the depth and extension of the tumor, and a lack of uniform measurement criteria for functional outcomes.

M. Gapany, MD

Prognostic Factors and Survival Unique to Surgically Treated p16+ Oropharyngeal Cancer

Haughey BH, Sinha P (Washington Univ School of Medicine, St Louis, MO)

Laryngoscope 122:S13-S33, 2012

Objectives/Hypothesis.—Current head and neck epidemiology demonstrates a steadily increasing incidence of p16+ human papillomavirus-related oropharynx squamous cell cancer (OPSCC). This distinct tumor subtype is associated with better survival outcomes. There is a growing recognition of the need to define management regimens that take into account the inherent patho-biological attributes of these cancers and provide optimum oncological control with minimum morbidity. This is facilitated by a clear understanding of the prognostic variables that predict disease outcome in patients with p16+ OPSCC. To provide prognostic estimates, pathological staging and histopathological parameters are usually superior to clinical staging. However, knowledge of pathological predictors is sparse, mainly because of commonly employed nonsurgical management policies utilizing chemoradiotherapy. Minimally invasive approaches to the oropharynx, particularly transoral laser microsurgery (TLM), are well-reported effective primary treatments for oropharynx cancers. From such series, it is feasible to conduct a detailed appraisal based on pathologic information from surgical specimens of both the primary and neck, to establish prognosticators unique to p16+ oropharynx cancer patients.

Study Design.—A prospectively assembled database of oropharynx cancer patients treated with primary TLM ± neck dissection ± adjuvant therapy from 1996 to 2010, analyzed retrospectively for survival and recurrence.

Methods.—The fundamental inclusion criteria were: 1) previously untreated biopsy-proven OPSCC treated with primary TLM ± neck dissection, 2) diffuse p16 positivity in the surgical specimen, 3) availability for adjuvant therapy, if indicated, and 4), minimum follow-up of 12 months or to death. Cox proportional hazard regression analyses were used to identify variables that were prognostic for disease-free survival (DFS), the primary end point of the study, as well as disease-specific survival (DSS) and overall survival. Kaplan-Meier survival estimates and patterns of disease recurrence were also assessed. We also explored concordance for T and N staging, when assessed by clinical (cT, cN) and pathological (cT, pT) measures.

Results.—Of 211 patients in the TLM database, 171 met all the eligibility criteria. The median follow-up was 47 months. The 3- and 5-year Kaplan-Meier estimates for DFS were 91% and 88%, respectively, whereas for DSS they were 95.5% and 94.4%, respectively. A total of 12 (7%) recurrences occurred: two local, four regional, and six distant. Of all T-stage categories, pT4 tumors were strongest predictors of poorer DFS. cT4 tonsil primaries, ever smoking status, three or more metastatic nodes, pN2b+ stage, and radiation-based adjuvant therapy were other prognosticators for DFS. Angioinvasion and T3-T4 tumors were prognostic for reduced

DSS, although smoking parameters were not. Extracapsular spread, N stage, and margins were nonprognosticators. Recursive partitioning analysis defined high- and low-risk groupings of prognosticators. Downstaging of clinical T stage was observed for 31% of tumors on application of pathological classification.

Conclusions.—We document a well-delineated set of prognostic variables that specifically and accurately identify individuals at risk of reduced outcomes in an otherwise good prognosis p16+ OPSCC cohort. Based on these prognosticators, appropriate patient counseling, adjuvant treatment recommendations, and stratification for trials can more accurately be made. We also observed an additional edge conferred by TLM toward more accurate clinical as well as pathological T staging.

► Evidence has been mounting that human papilloma virus (HPV) infection constitutes an independent etiologic factor for causing oropharyngeal cancer and that HPV-associated oropharyngeal cancer has different epidemiologic, biologic, and clinical characteristics from non-HPV cancers. Epidemiologic implications of these findings are of utmost importance because it is likely that we are witnessing a new form of sexually transmitted disease from changes in sexual behavior. Furthermore, there is ample evidence in the literature that links HPV tumor status with relatively favorable clinical course of oropharyngeal cancer. This is in part because of different tumor biology of HPV-positive tumors compared with HPV-negative, smoking-linked, and alcohol-linked cancers. Of particular interest are most recent observations that surgery with adjuvant radiotherapy is equally as effective as radiochemotherapy in controlling HPV-positive cancer, suggesting that HPV-positive cancer will have a better prognosis regardless of the method of therapy.

This selected study is a significant contribution to the existing body of knowledge on the outcomes of therapy for HPV-positive oropharyngeal cancer with primary transoral laser microsurgery, neck dissection, and adjuvant radiochemotherapy. In their study, the authors were able to identify some prognostic indicators unique to this cancer that are counter to the established predictors of outcomes in tobacco- and alcohol-related oropharyngeal carcinoma. This study was published as a Triological Society candidate thesis and is strongly recommended for review.

M. Gapany, MD

Radiotherapy

Concurrent chemoradiation therapy with docetaxel (DOC) for laryngeal preservation in T2N0M0 glottic squamous cell carcinomas

Furusaka T, Matsuda A, Saito T, et al (Nihon Univ School of Medicine, Tokyo, Japan; Tokyo Univ of Agriculture and Technology, Japan; et al)
Acta Otolaryngol 133:99-112, 2013

Conclusion.—Concurrent chemoradiation therapy with docetaxel (DOC) at a dose of 10 mg/m^2 twice a week contributed to laryngeal preservation.

Objective.—To determine laryngeal preservation following concurrent chemoradiation therapy with DOC.

Methods.—A total of 141 patients with untreated T2N0M0 squamous cell carcinoma of the glottic larynx were included in the study. The treatments were either radiation therapy alone or DOC intravenously administered at a dose of 10 mg/m^2 once or twice a week during radiotherapy with 4 MV linac X-ray (total of 66 Gy for 33 days).

Results.—The response and CR rates were 100% and 90.5% in the once-weekly combination group, and 100% and 97.6% in the twice-weekly combination group, respectively. The 5-year survival rates were 76.8% in the once-weekly combination group and 96.8% in the twice-weekly combination group. The 5-year laryngeal preservation rates were 83.8% in the once-weekly combination group and 97.6% in the twice-weekly combination group. The most common side effects were mucositis, dermatitis, and alopecia. The patients who received DOC twice a week showed more severe cancer tissue degeneration, and pathological examination of serial sections indicated that the safety margin for partial laryngectomy was considered to be 3 mm from the gross tumor with good glottal closure.

▶ It is always interesting to review studies by our Japanese colleagues because of frequent conceptual differences, at times radical from our own, while presenting equally successful (or at times more successful) outcomes. In this selected article, the authors present their experience with concurrent chemoradiotherapy using docetaxel for laryngeal preservation in T2N0M0 squamous cell carcinoma of the glottis larynx. In the United States, the concept of laryngeal preservation for glottis cancer is applied only in cases in which the extent of the primary tumor would require total laryngectomy. It would never cross my mind to treat a respectable cancer of the glottis with anything else but organ-preserving partial laryngeal surgery (whether endoscopic or open, depending on the location of the tumor and the involvement of the anterior commissure), reserving radiotherapy for patients who for one reason or another are not surgical candidates. Based on the results presented in this study, the next time I have to offer an alternative to surgery in a case of T2N0M0 cancer of the larynx, I will strongly consider radiochemotherapy using docetaxel.

M. Gapany, MD

Impact of Radiotherapy on Laryngeal Cancer Survival: A Population-Based Study of 13,808 US Patients

Zhang H, Travis LB, Chen R, et al (Univ of Rochester Med Ctr, NY)

Cancer 118:1276-1287, 2012

Background.—Radiotherapy with its advantage of organ preservation has been used to treat laryngeal cancer (LC) for several decades. However, the impact of radiation on overall survival (OS) in a large population-based study has not been evaluated to date.

Methods.—The authors analyzed all patients who had localized and/or regional glottic and supraglottic cancer in the Surveillance, Epidemiology, and End Results Program by comparing treatment trends and OS for the periods 1988 to 1993, 1994 to 1999, and 2000 to 2006. Kaplan-Meier and logistic regression analyses were conducted to evaluate OS and the influence of patient demographics on treatment received.

Results.—Among 13,808 patients with LC, radiotherapy use increased over the 3 periods for localized glottic cancer (LGC) (94%, 97%, and 98% during 1988-1993, 1994-1999, and 2000-2006, respectively; $P < .001$); for regional glottic cancer (RGC) (53%, 66%, and 75%, respectively; $P < .001$), for localized supraglottic cancer (LSGC) (61%, 83%, and 94%, respectively), and for regional supraglottic cancer (RSGC) (43%, 55%, and 78%, respectively; $P < .001$). No significant decrease in 5-year OS was observed during the 3 periods (LGC: 73%, 76%, and 78%, respectively; RGC: 57%, 51%, and 56%, respectively; LSGC: 33%, 35%, and 39%, respectively; and RSGC: 36%, 36%, and 43%, respectively). Blacks were significantly less likely to receive radiotherapy than whites (odds ratio: LGC, 0.42; RGC, 0.76; RSGC, 0.68; all $P < .05$). Those in the lowest tertile of median household income, compared with highest tertile, received radiotherapy less frequently (odds ratio: LGC, 0.42; RGC, 0.57; RSGC, 0.57; all $P < .001$).

Conclusions.—The current results indicated that the increased use of radiation with its advantage of speech preservation had no adverse impact on the survival of patients with LC. Black race and low income status had significant, inverse relations with the receipt of radiotherapy.

► Since the landmark Veterans Affairs (VA) laryngeal preservation study was published in 1991, organ-sparing radiochemotherapy has become the standard of care for advanced laryngeal cancer. Although the functional results of this approach have been somewhat disappointing, long-term follow-up data of both the VA and Radiation Therapy Oncology Group studies confirmed survival equality with total laryngectomy followed by radiotherapy, adding the benefit of larynx preservation in about 50%–60% of patients. With the changing pattern of care for advanced-stage laryngeal cancer, some authors have voiced concern that laryngeal preservation is potentially adversely impacting survival. In this respect, this is a very important study, based on a very large epidemiologic database (Surveillance, Epidemiology, and End Results Program) and comparing survival of radiation-treated patients versus total laryngectomy-treated patients over a 19-year period. The results of this study showed no survival disadvantage in patients treated with radiotherapy, which is very encouraging. Unfortunately, the database used in the study does not collect information on chemotherapy. Nevertheless, the data presented in this study are the most solid data available, dispelling earlier voiced concerns about patient survival.

M. Gapany, MD

Surgical Technique

A retrospective evaluation of submandibular gland involvement in oral cavity cancers: a case for gland preservation

Okoturo EM, Trivedi NP, Kekatpure V, et al (Lagos State Univ College of Medicine (LASUCOM), Nigeria; Mazumdar Shaw Cancer Ctr, Bangalore, India)

Int J Oral Maxillofac Surg 41:1383-1386, 2012

The key factor mitigating against prognosis in head and neck cancer is nodal metastasis and its management. Neck dissection has been known to play an integral part in this type of cancer management. Submandibular gland preservation during neck dissection and post radiotherapy, have been known to improve subjective symptoms of xerostomia. The authors retrospectively surveyed the involvement of submandibular gland involvement in oral cancer with a view to confirm oncologic safety of submandibular gland preservation, as a first step in a quest to manage radiation induced xerostomia by submandibular gland transfer. The medical and pathological records of oral cancer patients who underwent surgical treatment at the authors' centre were reviewed retrospectively. 194 patients were included in the study. 229 submandibular glands were excised from the same number of neck dissections. 3 (1.3%) submandibular glands were involved with malignancies microscopically. The mode of involvement was by direct infiltration. In conclusion, no metastasis to submandibular gland was observed. This may suggest the oncologic safety of submandibular gland preservation and transfer.

▶ I have included this article in my selections not because of the novelty of the conclusion drawn by the authors, but rather because the premise of the study, namely that the "submandibular salivary gland is regularly excised in selective level IB neck dissection" came as a surprise to me. Ever since I grasped the concept of selective neck dissection, it became clear to me that a cervical lymphadenectomy can be performed without the need to sacrifice any of the neck structures, including the submandibular gland. The gland is invested in a sheath of superficial layers of deep cervical fascia and contains no lymph nodes in its parenchyma. On occasion, when the oral cavity tumor is extensive and a danger of direct tumor extension into the gland is real, the gland needs to be excised "en bloc" with the primary tumor as part of the oncologic operation. The data in this article are convincing and worth reviewing for those who still advocate routine submandibular gland resection as part of a selective cervical lymphadenectomy.

M. Gapany, MD

Closure of laryngectomy defects in the age of chemoradiation therapy

Hanasono MM, Lin D, Wax MK, et al (The Univ of Texas MD Anderson Cancer Ctr, Houston; Massachusetts Eye and Ear Infirmary, Boston; Oregon Health and Sciences Univ, Portland; et al)

Head Neck 34:580-588, 2012

The use of chemoradiation therapy in laryngeal cancer has resulted in significant reconstructive challenges. Although reconstruction of salvage laryngectomy defects remains controversial, current literature supports aggressive management of these defects with vascularized tissue, even when there is sufficient pharyngeal tissue present for primary closure. Significant advancement in reconstructive techniques has permitted improved outcomes in patients with advanced disease who require total laryngopharyngectomy or total laryngoglossectomy. Use of enteric and fasciocutaneous flaps result in good patient outcomes. Finally, wound complication rates after salvage surgery approach 60% depending on comorbid conditions such as cardiac insufficiency, hypothyroidism, or extent of previous treatment. Neck dehiscence, great vessel exposure, fistula formation, or cervical skin necrosis results in complex wounds that can often be treated initially with negative pressure dressings followed by definitive reconstruction. The timing of repair and approach to the vessel-depleted neck also present challenges in this patient population. Currently, there is significant institutional bias in the management of the patient with postchemoradiation salvage laryngectomy. Future prospective multi-institutional studies are certainly needed to more clearly define optimal treatment of these difficult patients.

▶ Salvage surgery for failed radiochemotherapy has become an integral part of head and neck oncologic surgery practice. With it, we have observed an increased incidence of pharyngocutaneous fistulae and other wound-healing problems. Salvage laryngectomy is associated with particularly high rate of such complications. In institutions where surgeons are subject to tight scrutiny using National Surgical Quality Improvement Program criteria, reducing the complication rate for salvage surgery after failed radiochemotherapy has become a goal in itself. This selected review article provides some great ideas on how to address those emerging reconstructive challenges. It is possible that in the future it will be recommended to preventively use flap reconstruction (microvascular or pedicle) to reduce the incidence of salivary leaks and wound breakdown. Another modality that is worth considering when faced with those complications is hyperbaric oxygen. It can be used as a single therapeutic option or in conjunction with a flap reconstruction.

M. Gapany, MD

3 Laryngology

Basic and Clinical Research

Development of a microclip for laryngeal microsurgery: initial animal studies

Lau DP, Chng CB, Choo JQ, et al (Singapore General Hosp)

Laryngoscope 122:1809-1814, 2012

Objectives/Hypothesis.—Mucosal closure following laryngeal microsurgery can be challenging due to limited access, and incisions are often left to heal without formal closure. This study explores the hypothesis that a bioabsorbable microclip can be developed as an alternative method to close mucosal incisions in laryngeal microsurgery.

Study Design.—Animal study.

Methods.—In vitro studies were performed to determine if a suitable clip could be designed using bioabsorbable materials. A porcine model was used to study behavior of the clip in vivo.

Results.—We initially studied poly-ϵ-caprolactone but encountered difficulty creating a small clip with the necessary material strength. Using magnesium we were able to produce a clip sufficiently small to close vocal fold incisions. Magnesium is biocompatible, bioabsorbable, and malleable, and has been used to manufacture vascular stents and sutures. The magnesium microclip could be deployed rapidly using modified 2-mm microlaryngeal cup forceps, which enable the clip to close in a circular shape. In vitro and in vivo tests showed the clip held securely to the vocal fold mucosa. Macroscopic and histologic studies showed no significant injury to the contralateral vocal fold. There was no evidence of lower airway injury after implanting clips into the lower airway.

Conclusions.—The bioabsorbable clip could be used to close selected incisions in laryngeal microsurgery. Currently we are working to further reduce the size of the clip and modify its bioabsorption properties to enable precise control of degradation.

▶ Phonomicrosurgical techniques were developed to try to limit the damage to the vibrating edge of the true vocal fold when removing true vocal fold lesions. When possible, primary closure of wounds is the most desirable way to close the epithelial flaps. The biggest problem in achieving this is the act of suturing down the barrel of a laryngoscope. Most laryngologists find it tedious and cumbersome, an exercise in frustration. There are alternative techniques, including the use of tissue glues, laser welding, and photochemical tissue bonding that have their own limitations. Tissue glues may cause scarring of the superficial lamina propria. Laser welding is a thermal process in which proteins are denatured and melt together—a very bad way to close a phonomicrosurgical wound! Photochemical tissue bonding does not rely on heat to bond the epithelial edges; it uses a dye that is activated by a laser to create strong covalent bonds between collagen fibers. This technique, although safe for the vocal fold superficial lamina propria layer, does require the use of a laser to activate the dye. Mechanical closure with a microclip is possible, but the clip needs to be made of a material that is biocompatible and reabsorbable without causing fibrosis. As can be seen in Fig 2 of the original article, the clips that were gold-coated reacted with the vocal folds. Histological evaluation demonstrated an increase in fibrosis around the clips (Fig 3 in the original article) compared with sutures (Fig 5 in the original article). It is important to remember that any technique that increases fibrosis is not worth using on the vibrating edge of the vocal fold.

R. Franco, MD

A new technique for percutaneous dilatational tracheostomy (G-Trach): preliminary experience in pigs

Guerra R, De Monte A, Girardis M (Univ of Udine, Italy)
Anaesthesia 67:968-972, 2012

Tracheostomies are currently used for airway management in patients requiring long-term respiratory assistance. The dilatational percutaneous technique of forming tracheostomies is a valuable alternative to traditional surgical 'open' techniques. In this study, we tested a new dilatational percutaneous tracheostomy device using a balloon dilator with a particular innovative shape (G-Trach). At the Autonomous University of Barcelona Veterinary Institute, eight pigs (weighing 20–40 kg) were anaesthetised and underwent tracheostomy using the novel G-Trach technique. The mean (SD) procedure time was 2.63 (0.64) min from tracheal puncture to ventilation through the tracheostomy tube, and the mean (SD) time from positioning the dilator balloon to introducing the cannula was 0.71 (0.38) min. Vital functions and oxygen saturation remained constant throughout the procedures. Postmortem examinations did not reveal any tracheal injury. The G-Trach seems to be a safe and easy new dilatational percutaneous technique for forming tracheostomies. The minimal subcutaneous tissue dissection could potentially decrease complications when compared with standard dilatational percutaneous tracheostomy methods. To confirm this hypothesis a human trial is ongoing.

▶ The field of medicine requires innovations to continue improving on proven techniques. Tracheostomy was once a procedure that was exclusively performed by surgeons, but because of the delay in obtaining tracheostomies, pulmonary, critical care, and emergency room physicians started doing percutaneous tracheostomies using a dilational technique with progressively larger dilators until the tracheostomy tube could be inserted over a wire (modified Seldinger technique). This resulted in injury to the tracheal cartilages that could later create a secondary tracheal stenosis that required surgical intervention to correct. Of course, what really matters in a percutaneous technique is safety and speed.

The authors tested a new percutaneous tracheostomy device named the G-Trach using eight 20- to 40-kg pigs. They were able to introduce the G-Trach into the tracheas of all 8 pigs without evidence for posterior wall damage or damage to the surrounding tracheal rings. The G-Trach uses a balloon dilator to exert radial force instead of the posterior forces typically used to force the trach through the tract (Fig 2 in the original article). They were able to complete the procedure in a total of 2.63 minutes, with 0.71 minutes from balloon dilation to insertion of the cannula into the airway. The authors are currently performing a human trial to show the safety and validity of this new modification to the percutaneous tracheostomy technique.

R. Franco, MD

Augmentation of Vocal Fold Using a Fat Block Implant Following Cordotomy Through a Minithyrotomy Approach in a Rabbit Model

Lee SW, Kim JW, Lee JY, et al (Soonchunhyang Univ College of Medicine, Bucheon, Korea; et al)

J Voice 26:521-525, 2012

Objectives.—Minithyrotomy is a novel approach that provides direct access to the lamina propria and vocalis muscle without requiring incision of the vocal fold mucosa. The aim of this study was to demonstrate the efficacy of minithyrotomy vocal fold augmentation in a rabbit model by comparing the vocal fold total square amount and the density of scars between the cordotomy with minithyrotomy group and a cordotomy without minithyrotomy group.

Study Design.—Animal study.

Methods.—Twenty adult laboratory-conditioned female rabbits were used for this study. Minithyrotomy vocal fold augmentation was performed using a single fat block implant 3 months after cordotomy. To compare total square amount and density of vocal folds between the minithyrotomy and cordotomy group, hematoxylin and eosin, Masson's trichrome, and alcian blue staining was used.

Results.—Histological examinations showed that minithyrotomy vocal fold augmentation postoperatively restored vocal fold bulkiness and maintained volume for up to 6 months, compared with the cordotomy group ($P < 0.05$). In light of the surgical manipulation, the procedure also did not aggravate scarring of the cordectomized vocal fold.

Conclusions.—Minithyrotomy vocal fold augmentation using an autologous fat block may soon be feasible in humans undergoing rehabilitation for postcordotomy dysphonia without causing additional damage to the vocal folds.

▶ Vocal fold augmentation after cancer resection poses a very big challenge for the treating otolaryngologist because of the destruction of normal tissue planes from resection and the subsequent scarring. Tissue that is normally very pliable becomes dense with fibrosis and adheres to the thyroid cartilage. Keys to reconstruction are to find materials that are biocompatible, are long-lasting in situ, and have viscoelastic properties similar to the normal, undamaged tissue. Autologous fat meets some of these requirements, approximating the viscoelastic properties of the native vocal fold and being supremely biocompatible. Its biggest failing to date is the unpredictable resorption of the fat cells injected into the vocal fold. This makes it impossible to know how much to inject to get a decent long-term result. Instead of harvesting fat cells via a liposuction technique, these authors harvested fat blocks about the length of the vocal fold and placed them into the superficial lamina propria via a minithyrotomy. A minithyrotomy uses an anterior access point though the thyroid cartilage to tunnel into the superficial lamina propria layer. They injured the vocal folds of the rabbits by using a Bovie electrocautery 3 times in a 25-watt cutting mode applied for 1 to 2 seconds. The authors delivered the fat blocks into the vocal folds of 20 rabbits and sectioned their larynges at 1, 4, 6, and 9 months to see how well the fat survived. They found the fat-augmented vocal folds were larger and retained viable fat at 6 months (Fig 3 in the original article). There were similar amounts of collagen density between the fat-reconstructed and non–fat-reconstructed specimen. The retention of viable fat makes this technique an alternative in the reconstruction armamentarium.

R. Franco, MD

Cervical osteophytes causing vocal fold paralysis: case report and literature review

Virk JS, Majithia A, Lingam RK, et al (Northwick Park Hosp, Harrow, UK)
J Laryngol Otol 126:963-965, 2012

Objectives.—To increase awareness of cervical osteophytes as an extremely rare cause of recurrent laryngeal nerve palsy; to outline the clinical approach to patients with unilateral vocal fold paralysis and to provide an update on the current management of osteoarthritis and osteophytes.

Case Report.—An elderly man presented with right unilateral vocal fold immobility and a small phonatory gap. By a diagnosis of exclusion, a cervical osteophyte at the level of the sixth and seventh cervical vertebrae was shown to be the cause. The patient responded to speech therapy and no further intervention was required.

Method.—A literature review, using Medline, identified only one previously published case of vocal fold paralysis due to osteophytes secondary to osteoarthritis.

Conclusion.—The aetiology of unilateral paralysis of the hemilarynx must be fully investigated, as the innervating system has a protracted course, particularly on the left side. Degenerative cervical spine disease, although rare, should be considered as part of the differential diagnosis.

▶ The value of this case report lies not in the description of the unilateral vocal fold immobility that was ascribed to the cervical osteophytes, but rather how it highlights the numerous and varied causes of vocal fold immobility that need to be kept in the differential diagnosis. The etiology of unilateral vocal fold immobility ranges from neurological (such as viral neuronitis, secondary to stroke or from compression/destruction from a tumor) to traumatic (iatrogenic vs blunt vs penetrating trauma, related to intubation) to systemic (lupus, rheumatoid arthritis, Lyme disease) and idiopathic. The typical workup after a detailed history and head and neck examination consists of a computed tomography scan from the skull base to the mediastinum assessing for tumors along the course of the nerve or vascular anomalies that could compromise the nerve. In light of the financial situation in health care today, the yields from these exams need to be systematically reviewed to see if they offer a benefit or if lower-priced alternatives should be employed.

There are those practitioners who perform serological testing with each case of vocal fold immobility, sending blood to test for rheumatoid factor, Lyme titers, and antinuclear antibodies. Laryngeal electromyography can be performed to establish the integrity of the nerve. Laryngeal electromyography is much better at predicting lack of return of function as opposed to predicting return of function. A nerve may be physically intact and capable of transmitting signals without having restoration of purposeful movement. The most common causes of vocal fold immobility are malignancy, iatrogenic injury, and idiopathic (likely viral).

As the authors mention in this case report, their diagnosis was one of exclusion. At most they established an association between the degenerative cervical spine disease and the immobility of the vocal fold, but they certainly could not establish cause and effect.

R. Franco, MD

Customization of the voice prosthesis to prevent leakage from the enlarged tracheoesophageal puncture: results of a prospective trial

Lewin JS, Hutcheson KA, Barringer DA, et al (The Univ of Texas MD Anderson Cancer Ctr, Houston)

Laryngoscope 122:1767-1772, 2012

Objectives/Hypothesis.—Customization of the tracheoesophageal (TE) voice prosthesis (VP) is often preferred over surgical closure to prevent

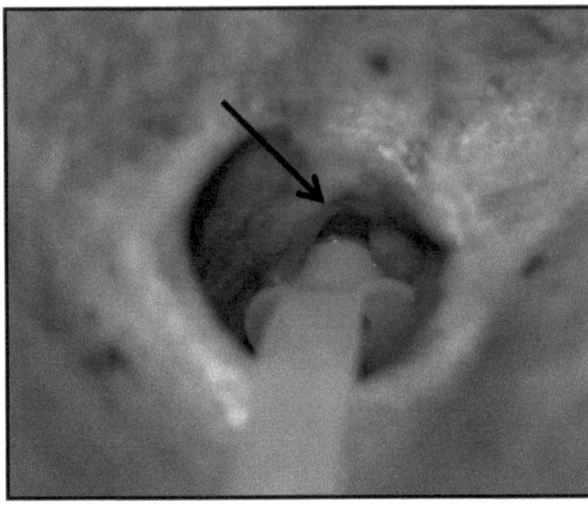

FIGURE 1.—Enlarged TE puncture. (Reprinted from Lewin JS, Hutcheson KA, Barringer DA, et al. Customization of the voice prosthesis to prevent leakage from the enlarged tracheoesophageal puncture: results of a prospective trial. *Laryngoscope*. 2012;122:1767-1772, with permission from Laryngoscope and John Wiley and Sons, www.interscience.wiley.com.)

aspiration around the VP in laryngectomized patients with an enlarged tracheoesophageal puncture (TEP), but it has not been thoroughly evaluated.

Study Design.—Single-institution prospective trial.

Methods.—A prospective trial was conducted to evaluate the effectiveness of a customized VP with the addition of an enlarged tracheal and/or esophageal collar in patients with leakage around an enlarged TEP. Absence of leakage around the VP after placement defined immediate effectiveness. Long-term success was defined by the prevention of adverse events related to leakage during the study period. Events that defined failure included: permanent gastrostomy dependence, aspiration pneumonia, and/or surgical TEP closure.

Results.—Twenty-one patients with enlarged TEP were enrolled (2003-2006). Insertion of a customized VP was unsuccessful in one patient; 145 customizations were performed in the remaining 20 patients (median, 3.5 customizations) during the trial period. Of the customizations, 77% (112/145) prevented leakage immediately after VP insertion. The most common adverse event was dislodgement of the prosthesis (11%) or the collar alone (7%) in 18% (26/145) of customized VP placements. Six patients who died of disease were not evaluable for long-term outcomes. Long-term success was achieved in 80% (12/15) of evaluable patients who avoided permanent gastrostomy, aspiration pneumonia, and surgical TEP closure.

Conclusions.—Prosthetic customization offers an effective method to prevent leakage around the VP in many patients with an enlarged TEP, thereby preserving TE voice while avoiding surgical closure in this high-risk population (Fig 1).

▶ The tracheoesophageal voice prosthesis has dramatically improved the quality of voice and life for the average total laryngectomy patient. It is much easier to produce consistent voice using the tracheoesophageal puncture (TEP) than using esophageal speech, and it produces much more natural voice than an electrolarynx. Because there is a fistulous tract between the trachea and esophagus, there is the ever-present risk of esophageal contents leaking anteriorly into the airway. Normally, this is dealt with by inserting a larger-sized TEP, but what happens when the leakage does not stop with the largest size in place?

The authors of this study customized commercially available TEPs by adding a silicone collar with medical-grade silicone glue, as seen in Fig 1. The collar was placed on the tracheal and esophageal sides in 60% (12 patients), just on the tracheal side in 35% (7 patients), and just the esophageal side in 5% (one patient). Most patients (80%, or 16 patients) required multiple customized prostheses during the study period, totaling 145 customizations. The modified devices prevented leaks for anywhere from 1 to 362 days, with a mean effectiveness of 56 days. Despite this, they were able to show that the modifications were able to immediately stop leaking in 77% of patients. Persistent leaking of esophageal contents into the airway can lead to pneumonia in a group in which the native risk of aspiration pneumonia after separation of the alimentary tract from the airway should be close to zero. These modifications were simple to institute and seemed to offer relief from the leaking in many cases. Their custom modifications allowed them to individualize the silicone collar to fit the defect in each patient's tracheoesophageal party wall. There were instances of failure in which the patient had to undergo surgical closure or have the placement of a feeding tube. There was aspiration pneumonia in 2 of these patients.

R. Franco, MD

A Method for Ultrasonographic Visualization and Injection of the Superior Laryngeal Nerve: Volunteer Study and Cadaver Simulation

Kaur B, Tang R, Sawka A, et al (Vancouver Coastal Health, British Columbia, Canada; et al)
Anesth Analg 115:1242-1245, 2012

Superior laryngeal nerve block is a valuable technique for provision of upper airway anesthesia. In bilateral scans of 20 volunteers, we developed a technique for ultrasonographic visualization of the superior laryngeal nerve and key anatomical structures using a hockey stick-shaped 8 to 15 MHz transducer (HST15 to 8/20 linear probe, Ultrasonix, Richmond, BC, Canada). Subsequently, we simulated superior laryngeal nerve scanning and injection in bilateral injections in 2 cadavers. Ultrasound-guided in-plane advancement of a needle toward the superior laryngeal nerve and injection of 1 mL of green dye was achieved in all 4 attempts and confirmed by a postprocedural dissection performed by an anatomist. We conclude that ultrasound-guided superior laryngeal nerve block in humans may be feasible (Figs 1 and 3).

▶ Outpatient awake procedures rely on the adequacy of anesthesia for success. Although endolaryngeal topical anesthesia with 4% lidocaine can provide the

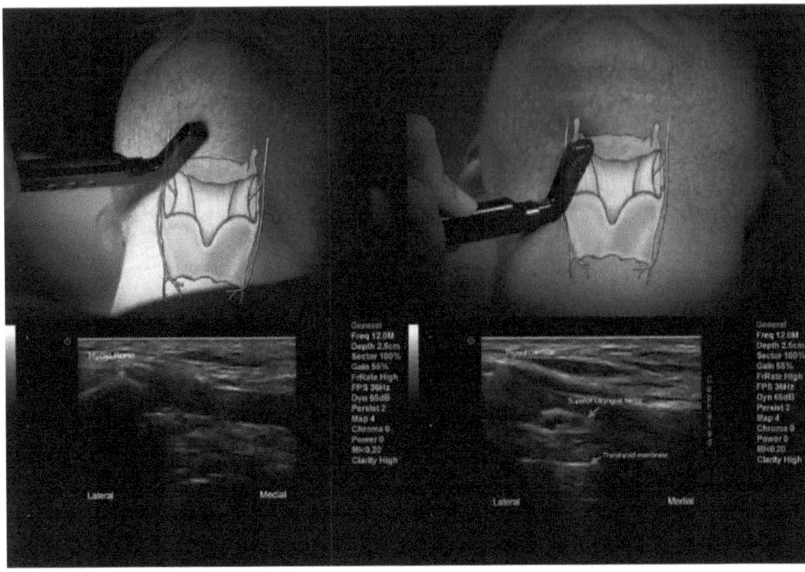

FIGURE 1.—Top left, probe orientation to view the hyoid bone with the corresponding ultrasound view in a volunteer. Top right, rotation of the probe obliquely to view the superior laryngeal nerve and landmarks with the corresponding ultrasound view below. (Reprinted from Kaur B, Tang R, Sawka A, et al. A method for ultrasonographic visualization and injection of the superior laryngeal nerve: volunteer study and cadaver simulation. *Anesth Analg*. 2012;115:1242-1245, with permission from International Anesthesia Research Society.)

proper amount of anesthesia, there are situations in which infiltration of the superior laryngeal nerves is desired to effect a profound and lasting anesthesia. Although the thyrohyoid space is easily palpated, the exact location of the nerve is difficult to know, making injection of it a process of trial and error. Because of this, currently the technique is mainly performed "blind," placing the needle in the region of the mid-thyrohyoid space and infiltrating a good quantity of local anesthetic to make sure to "get" the nerve.

The authors describe an ultrasound-guided technique using a hockey-shaped 8- to 15-MHz transducer (Fig 1) that allows visualization of the recurrent laryngeal nerve during attempted infiltration of analgesics. Ultrasound is an imaging modality that uses the reflections of sound returning from the tissues of interest to "see" structures. It has a history of use in the head and neck region for thyroid gland evaluation without the need for x-rays (radiation). Ultrasound is also employed in the aspiration and biopsy of cervical cysts and nodes. The authors identified the nerve bilaterally in 20 volunteers. They used this technique to successfully guide a percutaneous injection of 1 cc of dye into the area around the superior laryngeal nerve in 2 human cadaveric larynges (Fig 3). The authors did not inject analgesics into any of the volunteers — only into the 2 cadavers. Through the use of a visualizing technique, the accuracy of the injection could be improved, reducing the amount of local needed.

R. Franco, MD

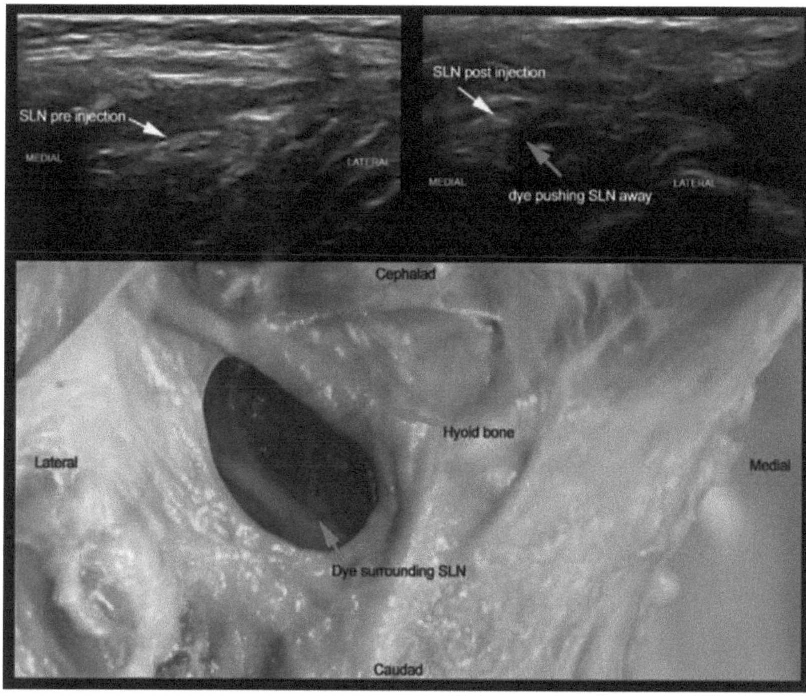

FIGURE 3.—(Cadaver) Ultrasound images: Top left/right, before superior laryngeal nerve dye injection/after injection dye surrounding superior laryngeal nerve (SLN). The photo corresponds to the dye surrounding the dissected superior laryngeal nerve in a cadaver. (Reprinted from Kaur B, Tang R, Sawka A, et al. A method for ultrasonographic visualization and injection of the superior laryngeal nerve: volunteer study and cadaver simulation. *Anesth Analg.* 2012;115:1242-1245, with permission from International Anesthesia Research Society.)

Microsuture after benign vocal fold lesion removal: a randomized trial

Yilmaz T, Sözen T (Hacettepe Univ Faculty of Medicine, Ankara, Turkey)
Am J Otolaryngol 33:702-707, 2012

Purpose.—Removal of benign vocal fold lesions results in small to moderate-sized mucosal defect on vocal fold, which heals by secondary intention. Microsuturing this defect leads to primary wound healing with fastened recovery and less scar. However, its value has not been determined.

Materials and Methods.—This is prospective, randomized, and controlled study performed in university hospital. Forty adults with vocal polyp, cyst, and Reinke's edema were included. Preoperatively, all patients completed VHI (Voice Handicap Index)—30, had acoustic analysis with continuous /a/ and videolaryngostroboscopy (VLS). The patients were randomly assigned to study group (with 1 or 2 6/0 vicryl suture) (n = 20) or control group (n = 20). Postoperative follow-up was done at the first,

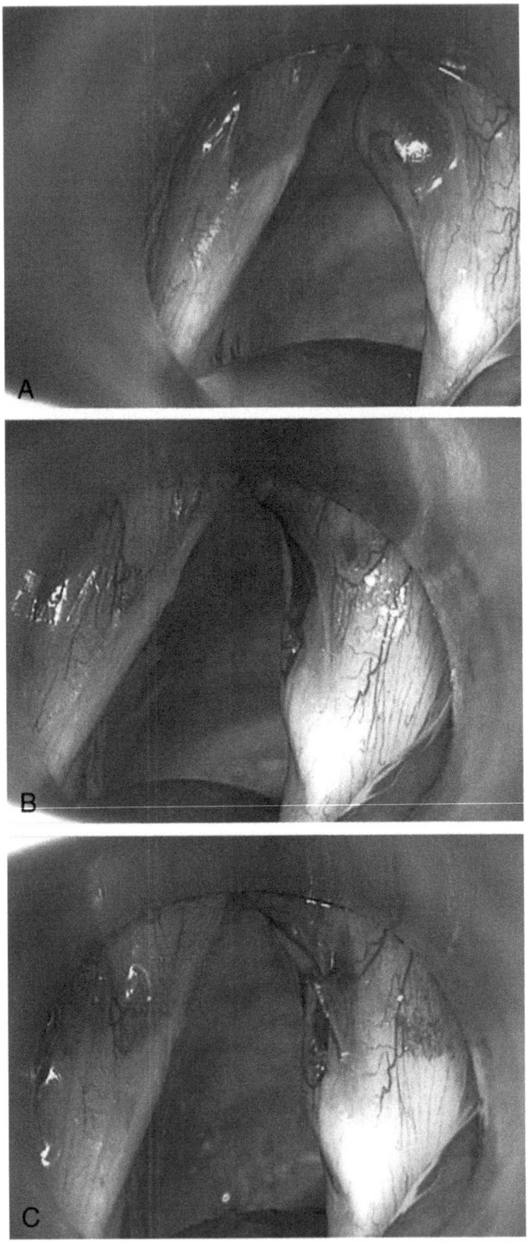

FIGURE 3.—A, Polyp of right vocal fold before removal. B, Polyp of right vocal fold, removed. C, Polyp of right vocal fold, mucosal defect sutured. (Reprinted from American Journal of Otolaryngology. Yilmaz T, Sözen T. Microsuture after benign vocal fold lesion removal: a randomized trial. *Am J Otolaryngol*. 2012;33:702-707, Copyright 2012, with permission from Elsevier.)

TABLE 2.—The Comparison of Preoperative and Postoperative Total VHI Scores and the Comparison of Total VHI Scores of Study and Control Groups

	Preoperative VHI	First Week		Student t Test for Paired Samples Second Week		Fourth Week	
No suture	55 ± 3.8	38 ± 4.1	$t = 2.54$, $P = .01$*	21 ± 2.8	$t = 2.86$, $P = .005$*	8 ± 2.5	$t = 3.88$, $P = .0005$*
Suture	58 ± 3.2	25 ± 3.6	$t = 2.82$, $P = .006$*	18 ± 3.0	$t = 3.01$, $P = .004$*	6 ± 2.7	$t = 3.92$, $P = .0004$*
Student t test for independent samples	$t = 0.52$, $P = .41$	$t = 2.02$, $P = .025$*		$t = 0.68$, $P = .25$		$t = 0.64$, $P = .32$	

Mean ± SD.
*Indicates statistical significance.

second, and fourth weeks. During follow-up examinations, VLS was repeated; the patients completed VHI-30 and had an acoustic analysis again.

Results.—All patients recovered with normal VLS and without complications; all were satisfied with the treatment result. The VHI results and acoustic analysis parameters of the study group were statistically significantly better than those of the control group at the first postoperative week ($P < .05$) but not at the second and fourth weeks ($P > .05$). Normal VLS was obtained significantly more early in the study group compared with the control group ($P < .05$).

Conclusions.—Microlaryngoscopic removal of benign vocal fold lesions is a safe, satisfying procedure with excellent to good results if done according to its principles. Microsuturing of the mucosal defect helps to speed up recovery, although final result remains to be clinically unchanged. It may be beneficial for professional voice users by making early return of vocal fold function possible (Fig 3, Table 2).

▶ To suture or not to suture; that is the eternal question in laryngeal microsurgery. Healing by primary intention is always preferred over the formation of granulation tissue to fill in the defect. This seems especially true when it comes to the delicate and normally pliable vocal folds where scar in many cases becomes translated into persistent hoarseness. The exceedingly low numbers of surgeons who routinely suture the vocal fold defects closed speaks to the frustrating experience of throwing 1 or 2 sutures into the vocal folds. The biggest question is whether the suturing will actually make a difference. We seem to get pretty good results now without suturing, so why bother? These authors bothered and created a randomized, controlled prospective trial with 20 patients in the control group and 20 in the experimental group. They used 6-0 Vicryl sutures (1 or 2) to close the mucosal defects in the experimental group, as can be seen in Fig 3. They took care to not include the vocal ligament while suturing, so as to not create an adynamic segment. They compared the videolaryngoscopic exams, Voice Handicap Index (VHI)-30 scores, and the acoustic analyses between the 2 groups. They found that the microsuture group had statistically better VHI-30 and acoustic results at 1 week compared with the control group, but that this difference disappeared by the second week. As can be seen in Table 2, by the fourth week, the results were statistically no different.

And so we return to the original question: Is it worth the extra effort to place sutures in the vocal folds? Is it worth the added operative time, the potential damage to the flaps from tearing through the mucosa, or the added frustration that comes from suturing in the larynx if the benefit is so short-lived? Although the sutures were usually gone by the time the of the first examination, there were a few that lasted 2 weeks and even 4 weeks. All of the patients in this study were satisfied with their voices in the end. The authors feel the suturing should still be done, especially for professional voice users, and in the case of overwhelmingly large mucosal flaps, such as during cytoreduction for Reinke's edema.

R. Franco, MD

Analysis of Vocal Fold Function From Acoustic Data Simultaneously Recorded With High-Speed Endoscopy

Döllinger M, Kunduk M, Kaltenbacher M, et al (Univ Hosp Erlangen, Germany; Louisiana State Univ, Baton Rouge; Alps-Adriatic Univ Klagenfurt, Austria)

J Voice 26:726-733, 2012

Summary.—Acoustic and endoscopic voice assessments are routinely performed to determine the vocal fold vibratory function as part of the voice assessment protocol in clinics. More often than not these data are separately recorded, resulting in information being obtained from two different phonation segments and an increase of time for the voice evaluation process. This study explores the use of acoustic data, simultaneously recorded during high-speed endoscopy (HSE), for the evaluation of vocal fold function.

Patients and Methods.—HSE and acoustic data were recorded from the subjects simultaneously during sustained phonation. The data included voices of 73 healthy subjects, 148 paresis, 210 functional dysphonias, and 119 benign lesions of vocal folds. For this study, only acoustic data were analyzed using *Dr. Speech* software (Tiger electronics Inc., MA). Twelve parameters were computed; 82% of the acoustic voice recordings could be analyzed. Statistical analysis was performed with *SPSS* 17.0.

Results.—Acoustic data was easily recorded simultaneously allowing analyses of the same phonation segment to determine vocal fold function and therefore eliminating the need for another voice recording. The acoustic voice parameters differed between genders in the healthy voice group. Most of the parameters showed significant differences between healthy and pathological groups.

TABLE 2.—Mean and STD for the 12 Computed Acoustic Parameters for the *Controls* are Given

	Controls			
	Female		Male	
Acoustic Values	Mean	STD	Mean	STD
Jitter (%)	0.31**	0.13	0.24	0.25
Shimmer (%)	2.83*	1.30	2.22	2.31
HNR (dB)	24.32*	4.25	26.81	5.19
SNR (dB)	24.36*	4.22	26.85	5.09
NNE (dB)	−9.26*	4.54	−12.67	4.51
STD F0 (Hz)	2.26**	1.06	1.59	1.34
Mode F0 (Hz)	260.44**	47.55	142.23	34.34
STD period (ms)	0.04**	0.02	0.08	0.04
Mean amplitude (%)	86.92*	5.28	90.42	4.30
STD amplitude (%)	5.63	2.05	5.17	2.82
F0 tremor (Hz)	6.44*	2.86	4.85	2.21
Amplitude tremor (Hz)	7.30**	3.45	4.17	1.83

Notes: The mean values under the female column marked with (*) show a significant and (**) shows a statistical highly significant difference between both gender groups within the *Controls*. The bold value is the only one that has no significant difference.

Abbreviations: STD, standard deviation; Mean, mean values; HNR, harmonic-to-noise ratio; SNR, signal-to-noise ratio; NNE, normalized noise error.

Conclusion.—Simultaneously recorded endoscopic and acoustic data is valuable. Differentiation between healthy and pathological groups was possible using acoustic data only. We suggest that the synchronously recorded acoustic signal is of sufficient quality for objective analysis yielding reduced examination time (Table 2).

► Voice analysis has been performed for many years to document the changes in the voice during and after treatment. There has been much debate over which parameters are the most meaningful (eg, jitter, shimmer, harmonic-to-noise ratio, maximum phonation time) and which ones can be used to describe a normal voice. Because of the complexity of the voice, multiple parameters are necessary to model normal voice and differentiate the normal from the abnormal. Another complicating factor is the impact lesion position has on the eventual acoustic signature, making it very difficult to differentiate some nodules from some polyps if they lead to the same voice alteration. Despite all of these hurdles, researchers are still attempting to categorize voices through their acoustic signature, especially disordered voices. The dream would be to be able to take a several-seconds-long high-quality sample of a voice and properly determine what is causing the disordered voice (eg, nodules, polyps, vocal fold weakness, scarring) without the need for endoscopy. High-speed endoscopy (video) is a technique that allows (mainly) researchers to capture several seconds of phonation at (typically) 4000 frames per second to analyze vocal fold vibration as it truly happens. Unlike stroboscopy, high-speed video can be used to analyze the initiation of phonation and can be used with disordered voices that cannot be tracked with stroboscopy. Unfortunately, high-speed video is still very cumbersome and takes time to interpret, making it mainly a research tool until computer algorithms improve in speed and accuracy.

The authors of this study captured audio during high-speed endoscopy for analysis. They had 4 groups, including controls (80 men and women), organic dysphonia (338 subjects subdivided into recurrent nerve pathology and anatomical changes such as nodules and polyps), and 254 functional patients. They were able to clearly differentiate the normal group from the disordered voice group. There were obvious gender differences in the normal group, as seen in Table 2, with higher fundamental frequency, jitter, and shimmer. The problem was that it remains difficult to differentiate between the disordered voices, and it still requires endoscopy to do so. At this time, acoustic evaluation is no better than the human ear—most of us can easily differentiate between normal voices and disordered voices without the need for any analyses. Despite these current limitations, researchers should still continue to find ways to describe the voice with a number of parameters so we can develop more noninvasive ways to diagnose and track patients with voice disorders.

R. Franco, MD

Diagnosis and Management of New-Onset Hoarseness: A Survey of the American Broncho-Esophagological Association

Paul BC, Branski RC, Amin MR (New York Univ School of Medicine)
Ann Otol Rhinol Laryngol 121:629-634, 2012

Objectives.—The recently published Clinical Practice Guideline raised issues related to the value and timing of laryngoscopy in patients with hoarseness. We sought to determine the extent to which these guidelines concur with clinical practice among members of the American Broncho-Esophagological Association (ABEA).

Methods.—A web-based survey was distributed to ABEA members, composed of four sections: 1) background and demographics; 2) information regarding the appropriate length of time that new-onset dysphonia may be managed before laryngeal visualization, given particular comorbidities; 3) the frequency and risks of office-based flexible transnasal laryngoscopy; and 4) the overall value of laryngoscopy and stroboscopy.

Results.—Seventy-one ABEA members completed the survey; they had a combined 1,468 years of post-residency experience. Approximately 75% of respondents were involved in a fully academic practice. Across all respondents, an average of 11 patients with new voice complaints were seen per week. Overall, 98.6% of respondents believe that laryngoscopy is very valuable. Stridor in a neonate and potential foreign bodies were both conditions necessitating laryngoscopy on the day of presentation. In patients with no serious underlying condition(s), the mean duration until laryngoscopy was 12.96 days (range, 0 to 30 days).

TABLE 2.—Reported Duration in Days Between Onset of Hoarseness and Laryngoscopy as Function of Underlying Comorbidities

	All Respondents	Respondents With >50% Laryngology Practice	*p*
History of tobacco or alcohol use	9.70 ± 8.78	9.84 ± 12.50	0.915
Associated dysphagia, odynophagia, or otalgia	4.06 ± 7.29	3.62 ± 7.55	0.405
Hemoptysis	1.72 ± 5.66	2.62 ± 7.53	0.496
Accompanying neurologic symptoms	3.90 ± 9.11	4.65 ± 12.02	0.724
Unexplained weight loss	4.66 ± 9.47	5.81 ± 14.50	0.299
Immunocompromised	4.63 ± 7.30	5.78 ± 8.05	0.469
Possible foreign body aspiration	0.11 ± 0.32	0.08 ± 0.28	0.595
New-onset stridor in neonate	0.59 ± 2.16	0.46 ± 2.30	0.777
Recent surgery involving intubation	3.85 ± 5.26	4.03 ± 5.66	0.872
No identified serious underlying history or comorbidity	12.96 ± 9.66	13.57 ± 9.42	0.753

Data are mean ± SD, and are presented from entire cohort, as well as those respondents who dedicate greater than 50% of their clinical practice to laryngology.

TABLE 3.—Responses Related to Value and Role of Laryngoscopy as Component of Initiation of Rehabilitation

	All Respondents				Respondents With >50% Laryngology Practice			
	0%	1%-49%	50%-99%	100%	0%	1%-49%	50%-99%	100%
How frequently do you determine that it is NOT appropriate to visualize the larynx in a patient with a complaint of acute voice changes or hoarseness?	69.00	25.35	2.82	2.80	72.97	18.92	2.70	5.41
How frequently do you visualize the larynx before prescribing treatment?	1.40	1.40	22.54	74.60	0	5.41	10.81	83.78
How frequently do you visualize the larynx before prescribing voice therapy?	2.80	0	9.86	87.90	5.41	0	2.70	91.89
How often does initial laryngoscopy help determine the next step in treatment?	1.40	2.80	52.10	43.70	0	5.41	40.54	54.05
How often do risks of flexible laryngoscopy outweight the benefits of the diagnostic capacity of laryngoscopy, such that you defer the examination?	47.90	12.68	26.76	11.30	51.35	18.92	18.92	10.81

Data are percentages, and are presented from entire cohort, as well as those respondents who dedicate greater than 50% of their clinical practice to laryngology.

TABLE 4.—Reported Value of Laryngoscopy and Stroboscopy as Function of Practice Setting

	Practice Setting		
	Academic	Mixed	Private
How valuable is laryngoscopy in your practice?			
Very	98	100	100
Moderately	2		
Not very			
Not at all			
How valuable is stroboscoopy in your practice?			
Very	55	33	13
Moderately	29	44	13
Not very	14	22	13
Not at all	2	0	63

Data are percentages.

Conclusions.—These data suggest that the current practice patterns among experts in the field are divergent from the recently published Guideline (Tables 2-4).

▶ The American Academy of Otolaryngology-Head and Neck Surgery Foundation produced a Clinical Practice Guideline (CPG) on the treatment of hoarseness in 2010 that was poorly received by the laryngology community. Much of the controversy centered around the assumption by the CPG authors that hoarseness could be treated as a clinical entity in itself, when in reality it is a symptom of true clinical entities. There is always a reason for hoarseness, be it infectious, traumatic, neoplastic, neurologic, or congenital. Two very distinct clinical lesions (a benign fibrovascular polyp and a T1 squamous cell carcinoma of the membranous vocal fold) may produce the same level of hoarseness but may lead to very different outcomes if left untreated. The only way to definitively and directly begin the process of understanding the cause of the hoarseness is to visually evaluate the larynx. Laryngoscopy, in all its forms (mirror, direct, microscope assisted, flexible fiberoptic, flexible distal-chip, and rigid transoral), along with the history, are the foundation of decision making and establishing a voice-related diagnosis. Without the use of this examination technique, a proper accounting for the hoarseness is impossible.

There are differences among the various methods and situations when one may be superior to the others. Although mirror examination has been touted as easy and cheap, it affords only a real-time view of the larynx without the possibility of careful review. It is also not well suited to documentation and review at a later date for comparison, relying on the memory or artistic/descriptive abilities of the physician for documentation. Children are also ill suited for this type of examination, as is anyone who has a profound gag reflex. Flexible laryngoscopy is the workhorse in establishing the cause for hoarseness. Flexible laryngoscopy can be coupled to a strobed light source and allow evaluation of the mucosal wave. It can be tolerated by many more people than the mirror examination and can be recorded for careful review and proper documentation of the patient's current situation. The power in the recording of examinations is that they can be reviewed at subsequent visits to establish direct comparisons and guide treatment.

The authors designed a survey to obtain the perceived value and timing of laryngoscopy within the membership of the American Broncho-Esophagological Society. Of the 358 members, only 71 (20%) responded to the survey. As could be predicted, most were in academic practices (72%), with 40% claiming fellowship training. Most also cared for adults only or mainly adults, and only 10% were exclusively pediatrics clinicians. As can be seen from Tables 2 and 3, there was astounding concordance among this cohort when it came to the timing and use of laryngoscopy in the different clinical scenarios. As is seen in Table 4, the disagreement was seen in the perceived value of stroboscopy. Fifty-five percent of those who identified as belonging to an academic practice reported stroboscopy to be very important, whereas 69% of the private practitioners reported stroboscopy had no value in their practices.

It is clear from these findings that laryngoscopy is viewed as an important part in the investigation of the hoarse patient. Stroboscopy does not give the same level of confidence in a subset of these 71 physicians. It would be interesting to know if these results hold true within the context of the greater membership of the Academy of Otolaryngology-Head and Neck Surgery.

R. Franco, MD

General

Direct health care costs of laryngeal diseases and disorders

Cohen SM, Kim J, Roy N, et al (Duke Univ Med Ctr, Durham, NC; Univ of Utah, Salt Lake City; et al)

Laryngoscope 122:1582-1588, 2012

Objectives/Hypothesis.—To estimate the annual direct costs associated with the diagnosis and management of laryngeal disorders.

Study Design.—Retrospective analysis of data from a large, nationally representative, administrative US claims database.

Methods.—Patients with a laryngeal disorder based on International Classification of Diseases, Ninth Revision-Clinical Modification codes from January 1, 2004 to December 31, 2008 and who were continuously enrolled for 12 months were included. Data regarding age, gender, geographic location, and type of physician providing the diagnosis were collected. Medical encounter, medication, and procedure costs were determined. Total and mean costs per person for 12 months were determined.

Results.—Of almost 55 million individuals in the database, 309,300 patients with 12 months follow-up, mean age of 47.3 years (standard deviation: 21.3), and 63.5% female were identified. Acute and chronic laryngitis, nonspecific causes of dysphonia, and benign vocal fold lesions were the most common etiologies. The total annual direct costs ranged between $178,524,552 to $294,827,671, with mean costs per person between $577.18 and $953.21. Pharmacy claims accounted for 20.1% to 33.3%, procedure claims 50.4% to 69.9%, and medical encounter claims 16.3%

to 8.6% of overall direct costs. Antireflux medication accounted for roughly 10% and antibiotics 6% of annual direct costs.

Conclusions.—This study establishes the economic impact of the assessment and management of patients with laryngeal disorders and permits cost comparisons with other diseases.

▶ A voice disorder can have a big public health effect because of the central role voice plays in the public and private lives of patients. Voice disorders can create depression, social isolation, and withdrawal in addition to decreasing work productivity and increasing absences from work. All of these together make for unhappier absentee employees who become a financial drain on the medical system and society at large. To get a handle on just how big this problem is, the authors used a large nationally representative administrative US claims database with 55 million entries to determine such features as the most common etiologies of voice disorders, the number of people who sought treatment for voice disorders, and the breakdown of the associated costs. Pharmaceutical spending and the top medications were also identified.

A total of 309 300 patients had a diagnosis associated with the symptom of dysphonia and had 12 months of follow-up. A total of 63.5% were women with a group mean age of 47.3 years. The total direct costs ranged from $178 million to $295 million over 12 months. Proton pump inhibitors accounted for 10% of the direct costs. When these figures are extrapolated to reflect the true population in the United States, and using prevalence rates of 6.6% to 7.5% of dysphonia among adults, we find that between 20 million and 23 million American adults may have a voice disorder. These figures translate into between 1.2 million and 5.2 million people actually seeking medical treatment in 12 months, resulting in direct costs from $702 million to $3 billion. The total potential direct costs (using the number of people who have voice disorders) would be between $12 billion and $13.5 billion a year, placing it between the annual direct costs for chronic obstructive pulmonary disease ($8–20 billion), asthma ($18 billion), diabetes ($14–100 billion), and allergic rhinitis ($1.6–5 billion). These figures should be a sobering reminder of the economic impact voice disorders have in the US.

R. Franco, MD

Characteristics of Vocal Fold Immobility Following Endotracheal Intubation

Xu W, Han D, Hu R, et al (Capital Med Univ, Beijing, China)

Ann Otol Rhinol Laryngol 121:689-694, 2012

Objectives.—We investigated the clinical and laryngeal electromyography (LEMG) characteristics and the outcome of closed reduction of arytenoid cartilage dislocation in patients with vocal fold immobility (VFI) following endotracheal intubation.

Methods.—Sixty patients with VFI following endotracheal intubation were included. Closed reduction was performed under local anesthesia in 54 cases. Another 6 patients did not undergo an intervention. Laryngeal behaviors and voice function were evaluated. Forty-five patients underwent LEMG testing.

Results.—All patients complained of persistent hoarseness immediately following surgery. The LEMG results for 29 of 45 patients showed normal patterns (15 cases) or mildly abnormal patterns (14 cases) on the affected side. Sixteen cases displayed apparent abnormal LEMG patterns on the affected side. The voices of all 54 patients improved after reduction. The movement of the affected vocal folds recovered to normal in 51 cases. One month after reduction, neuromuscular function had improved in 29 of 30 cases. Among the 6 patients who did not undergo intervention, 3 had normal or slightly hoarse voices, and 3 experienced moderate hoarseness.

Conclusions.—Vocal fold immobility following endotracheal intubation is typically caused by arytenoid dislocation. Some instances were accompanied by an abnormality of the recurrent laryngeal nerve. A timely closed arytenoid reduction should be performed to restore patients' normal voices and vocal fold mobility. Our reduction technique under local anesthesia can be performed easily and obtains satisfactory outcomes within 6 weeks after endotracheal intubation.

▶ Persistent hoarseness after orotracheal intubation can be broadly separated into mechanical disruptions of the arytenoid (dislocation), direct damage to the vocal folds, or a neurologic insult to the recurrent laryngeal nerve (RLN). Examination of the larynx allows the physician to assess the motion and location of the vocal fold and arytenoid cartilage and signs of direct damage to the vocal fold. Laryngeal electromyography (EMG) can be used to assess the neurologic status of the larynx to see if there is an RLN injury. If there is deemed to be normal or near-normal function of the nerve without movement, the authors recommend a closed reduction of the arytenoid cartilage. In their series of 60 patients, 54 underwent closed reduction of the dislocation and had improved voices after reduction. Despite the normal function, there were some abnormalities seen in the EMG signals with reduced amplitude and even 3 cases with no EMG signals or evoked potentials. They postulate that the reduction in signal might be accompanying hemorrhage into the thyroarytenoid muscle.

Although left-sided dislocations occurred more than right-sided ones, 5 of the 7 with long-term impaired mobility had right-sided dislocations. In their series, nearly 89% of patients achieved normal voice with the closed reduction. If the arytenoid seems very unstable at the time of reduction, they suggest performing a type I thyroplasty to maintain the arytenoid position. This seems curious, as one would not expect an unstable arytenoid to respond to a medialization of the membranous vocal fold. An adduction arytenopexy would seem like a good idea if any surgical procedure is to be used. Some would argue that surgical intervention in the form of an open laryngoplastic procedure is too aggressive when nerve function and, subsequently, muscle function may improve with a bit of time.

R. Franco, MD

Iatrogenic tracheal flap mimicking tracheal stenosis with resultant stridor

Tan KL, Chong AW, Amin MA, et al (Universiti Malaya Medical Centre, Kuala Lumpur, Malaysia)

J Laryngol Otol 126:751-755, 2012

Objective.—To illustrate a case of an iatrogenic mucosal tear in the trachea which caused a one-way valve effect, obstructing the airway and manifesting as post-extubation stridor.

Case Report.—We report a case of iatrogenic tracheal mucosal tear secondary to violent movement during intubation. The patient presented with post-extubation stridor that worsened over three days. Initial evidence suggested tracheal stenosis. Computed tomography scans revealed a mucosal tear at the level of the seventh cervical to second thoracic vertebrae. The tear was caused by forceful inflow of air as breathing became more and more difficult, resulting in a false tract. A tracheostomy changed the direction of airflow, bypassing the tear. The inflated tracheostomy tube cuff acted as a stent to keep the flap in place as healing occurred.

Conclusion.—Iatrogenic laryngotracheal injuries are common, especially when endotracheal intubation is performed under unfavourable emergency conditions. A tracheal mucosal tear is a rare entity which is almost always undiagnosed. However, a tracheal mucosal flap may be suspected when changes in patient position alter the nature and severity of the resultant stridor and/or respiratory distress. In such cases, an inflated tracheostomy tube cuff should be kept in place for an adequate period, to act as a stent and help keep the flap in place while healing occurs.

▶ Although normally seen as the benign start to a surgery, endotracheal intubation is a potentially traumatic procedure that carries risks such as direct laryngeal injuries to the arytenoid cartilages and compromising the integrity of the cricoarytenoid joints, blunt and penetrating injuries to the true and false vocal folds, abrasions and injuries to the subglottis, and mucosal injuries to the trachea. Typically, stenosis is the result of pressure necrosis from the cuff pressure exceeding the perfusion pressure of the tissue, rather than widespread denuding of tissue with healing by secondary intention. Granulation tissue forms and contracture of the nonviable or semiviable segment from collagen replacement of the soft tissue and cartilage causes the airway signs and symptoms of stridor and dyspnea. As with all pathologies, rapid recognition of the process can result in quicker institution of proper remedies.

The authors present the case of a 15-year-old girl who was traumatically intubated during an active seizure and was mechanically ventilated for 5 days. After going home, she presented with increasing stridor and labor of breathing that on lateral airway film (Fig 1 in the original article) was felt to be due to a long-segment tracheal stenosis. Flexible endoscopic evaluation of the airway was consistent with narrowing of the airway below the level of the vocal folds. Her condition eventually required tracheostomy placement in an emergent manner after initially refusing intervention. A computed tomography scan was performed revealing a double lumen, as seen in Fig 3 of the original article, indicating a posterior mucosal flap that dissected from the seventh cervical vertebra to the second thoracic vertebra (Fig 2 in the original article). This was likely a direct result from the traumatic intubation that was made worse with the increasing work of breathing, eventually resulting in this large flap that occluded the airway. The tracheostomy tube bypassed this area and allowed the mucosa to adhere to the posterior trachea.

A case such as this one reinforces the need for a thorough airway evaluation at the time of the initial contact. Instilling 4% lidocaine into the trachea and larynx would have made proper and thorough tracheal inspection possible, potentially immediately giving the otolaryngologists the proper diagnosis and defining the most appropriate clinical pathway.

R. Franco, MD

Age-dependent structural and radiological changes in the larynx

Türkmen S, Cansu A, Türedi S, et al (Karadeniz Technical Univ, Trabzon, Turkey; et al)

Clin Radiol 67:e22-e26, 2012

Aim.—To define radiological physiological changes in the larynx by establishing an age-related scale.

Materials and Methods.—The present retrospective study used radiological records of patients that had undergone lateral cervical imaging. Three hundred patients were included. Thyroid cartilage was divided into anatomical regions. The hyoid bone was evaluated as the body and greater horns. Cases were compared by grouping by age and gender.

Results.—Thyroid tissue and cricoid cartilage only became visible after the second decade. Ossification in the thyroid cartilage began in the posterior inferior horn and progressed to the superior horn and central lamina. It also began in the posterior part of the cricoid cartilage and moved forward with age. In the first decade, the body and greater horn parts of the hyoid bone could be seen more distinctly, and after the third decade the hyoid bone appeared as a single bone. The hyoid bone was the only structure ossified in the laryngeal region below the age of 20 and formed an image on direct imaging.

Conclusions.—Age-related changes to the laryngeal tissues are evident on radiographs. Clinicians should bear this in mind when evaluating neck radiographs (Fig 1).

▶ The laryngeal framework undergoes structural changes throughout life that need to be recognized to properly evaluate radiographic examinations. This is especially tricky when confronted with trauma in the setting of a young patient with nonossified cartilages or when deciding if there is cartilage invasion from a tumor in the paraglottic space because there is an area lacking ossification.

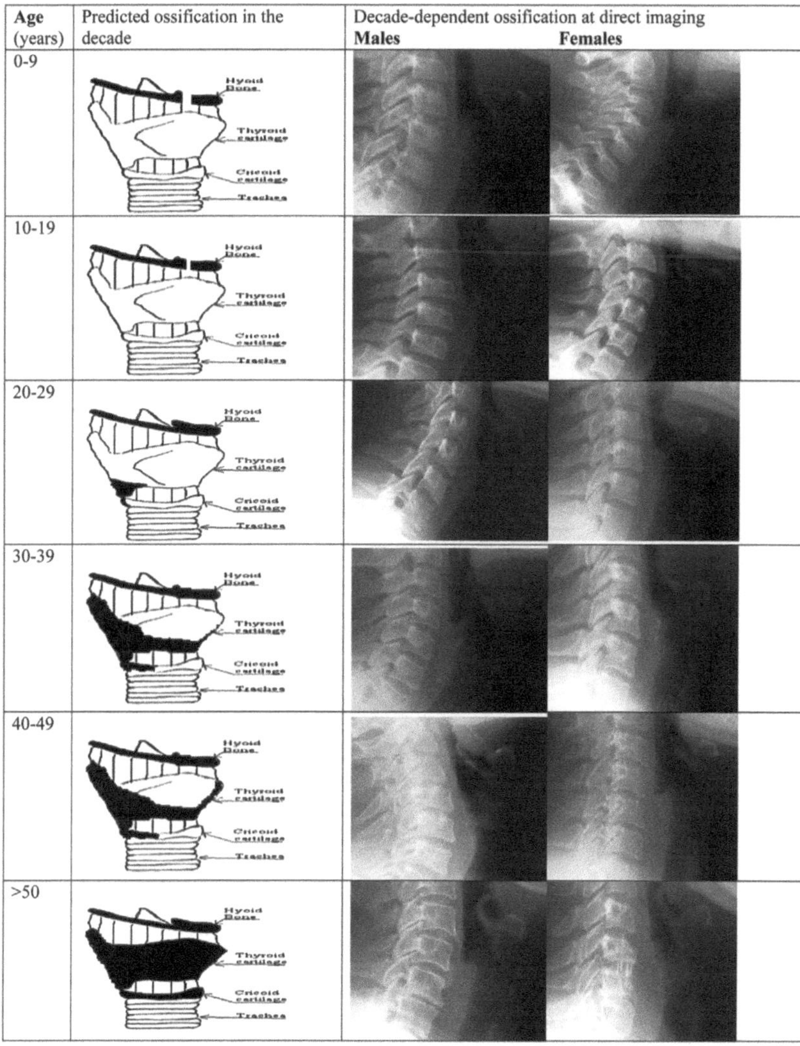

FIGURE 1.—Ossification level of the larynx by age in males and females. (Reprinted from Clinical Radiology. Türkmen S, Cansu A, Türedi S, et al. Age-dependent structural and radiological changes in the larynx. *Clin Radiol.* 2012;67:e22-e26, Copyright 2012, with permission from the Royal College of Radiologists.)

A proper accounting of the changes can be useful to forensic medicine in establishing an age based on the amount of thyroid cartilage ossification there is. The authors looked at 300 lateral cervical x-rays and found consistent, age-dependent changes to the hyoid bone, thyroid, and cricoid cartilages. As can be seen in Fig 1, the authors divided the findings into groups by decade.

The hyoid bone is the first structure to start ossifying during the first decade of life. It is located more cephalad in children compared with adults. The thyroid cartilage starts ossifying in the posteroinferior quadrant and progresses superiorly and anteriorly. Ossification in the cricoid also begins posteriorly but is more difficult to distinguish from the posterior and inferior thyroid cartilage. Ossification progresses anteriorly as the patient grows older.

R. Franco, MD

Laryngopyocoele: an unusual cause of a sore throat

Li SF, Siegel B, Hidalgo I, et al (Jacobi Med Ctr, Bronx, NY)

Am J Emerg Med 30:1655.e1-1655.e2, 2012

Laryngopyocoeles are rare entities that present as airway obstruction or as neck masses. We present a unique case of a laryngopyocoele in a young patient with a sore throat.

A 22-year-old man presented to the emergency department with a sore throat of 1-week duration. He had no other upper respiratory symptoms. His vitals were as follows: heart rate, 91; respiratory rate, 16; blood pressure, 119/60; and temperature, 36.8 (98.3°F). There were no signs of respiratory distress or airway involvement. The findings from his physical examination were normal except for tenderness on palpation of his larynx.

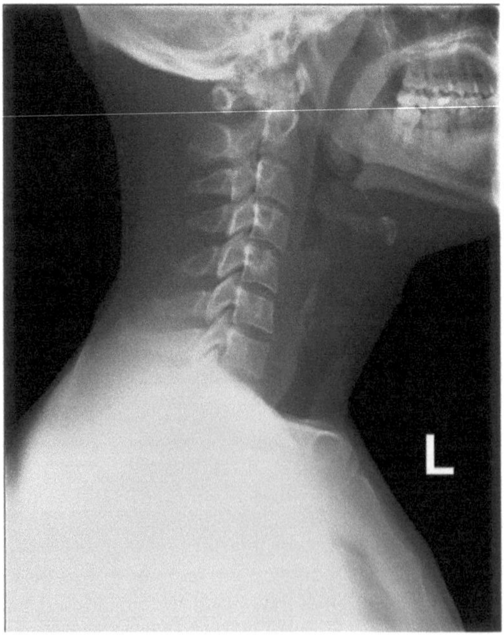

FIGURE 1.—Soft tissue neck x-ray suggestive of epiglottitis. (Reprinted from the American Journal of Emergency Medicine. Li SF, Siegel B, Hidalgo I, et al. Laryngopyocoele: an unusual cause of a sore throat. *Am J Emerg Med.* 2012;30:1655.e1-1655.e2, Copyright 2012, with permission from Elsevier.)

A soft tissue neck x-ray was suggestive of epiglottitis (Fig. 1). Fiberoptic laryngoscopy revealed a nonerythematous, edematous epiglottis and edema of the left arytenoid and aryepiglottic fold with slight bulging into the airway. A contrast neck computed tomography revealed a nonenhancing fluid collection at the level of the left arytenoid cartilage (Fig. 2). The diagnosis of a laryngopyocoele was made. The patient was admitted to the intensive care unit for airway monitoring and treated conservatively with intravenous antibiotics. The collection did not resolve by day 4, and the patient was taken to the operating room for incision and drainage of the laryngopyocoele. The patient made an uneventful recovery (Fig 1).

▶ Laryngoceles are air-filled sacs arising from the anterior ventricle, presumably from the saccule, which can extend under the false vocal fold and rise up and over the superior edge of the thyroid cartilage and through the thyrohyoid membrane into the neck. When they extend through the thyrohyoid membrane, they are called external or mixed laryngoceles (external and internal). Most laryngoceles are probably asymptomatic, but they come to medical attention either because of the compressive effects of the expanding sac (dysphonia, pain, or dysphagia) or because of an infection (laryngopyocele).

This case report highlights the importance of airway visualization over the use of a lateral neck x-ray. Fig 1 is the plain film where there was a thickening of the epiglottis (thumb sign): The true reason for the edema could not be ascertained. Flexible nasolaryngoscopy can be performed safely in the setting of acute infectious laryngitis, as long as the endoscopist does not irritate the larynx much. The inflamed left hemi-supraglottis was immediately identified as the source of the problem, with the epiglottic edema a secondary phenomenon. Antibiotics and steroids are the mainstay of treatment to help cool down the infection and inflammation. Surgery can be performed after several weeks to reduce the morbidity associated with the acute infection such as bleeding and improve the outcomes by avoiding overresecting inflamed but nonlaryngocele tissue.

R. Franco, MD

Gender differences in risk factors for airway symptoms following tracheal intubation

Jaensson M, Gupta A, Nilsson UG (Örebro Univ Hosp, Sweden)

Acta Anaesthesiol Scand 56:1306-1313, 2012

Background.—A common complaint after endotracheal intubation is sore throat and hoarseness. The aim of this study was to describe gender differences and independent risk factors in the development of postoperative sore throat and hoarseness after endotracheal intubation in adults.

Methods.—This prospective cross-sectional observational study was conducted at a university hospital in Sweden. A total of 495 patients were included (203 men and 292 women) and enrolled from a total of eight different surgical departments. Outcome variables were post-operative

TABLE 5.—Multivariate Analysis of Risk Factors for Post-Operative Sore Throat (POST) and Post-Operative Hoarseness (PH) in Men and Women

Explanatory Variables	Gender	Outcome	OR	95% CI	*P* Value
Less than 3 months' work experience	Men	POST	3.8	1.7–8.3	0.001
Cuff pressure < 20 cm H_2O	Men	PH	0.5	0.3–0.9	0.036
Two or more laryngoscopies	Women	POST	2.6	1.2–5.6	0.012
ETT size 7.0	Women	POST	2.2	0.97–4.9	0.059
Oesophageal temperature probe intraoperatively	Women	PH	4.8	1.4–16.9	0.014
ETT size 7.0	Women	PH	2.9	1.1–7.7	0.024
Cuff pressure < 20 cm H_2O	Women	PH	1.8	1.0–3.1	0.038

OR, odds ratio; CI, confidence interval; ETT, endotracheal tube.

sore throat and hoarseness evaluated post-operatively in the post-anaesthesia care unit. A total of 31 variables were recorded which described the intubation process, intraoperative factors as well as the extubation process. Bivariate and multivariate analyses were performed.

Results.—The overall incidence of post-operative sore throat was 35% and hoarseness 59%. The results show different predictors for men and women in the development of airway symptoms. The main risk factor for developing sore throat in men was intubation by personnel with <3 months' work experience. In women, it was endotracheal tube size 7.0 and multiple laryngoscopies during intubation. The main risk factors for hoarseness were cuff pressure for both men and women, and oesophageal temperature probe in women.

Conclusion.—Post-operative sore throat and hoarseness result from several factors, and the cause of these symptoms are multifactorial and differs by gender. Identification of these factors pre-operatively may increase awareness among anaesthesia personnel and possibly reduce the incidence of these minor but distressing symptoms (Table 5).

▶ One of the most common complications of general endotracheal anesthesia is postintubation hoarseness and soreness. Postoperative hoarseness has been reported as high as 50% with postoperative sore throat as high as 64%. Some of the hypothesized factors that lead to the soreness and hoarseness may be related to endotracheal tube size, the skill and training of the person placing the endotracheal tube, and the patient's particular anatomy. There are also established gender differences with respect to the chances of developing postoperative soreness and hoarseness.

The authors asked patients 2 hours postextubation to rate their soreness and hoarseness and found that 37% of women and 32% of men reported post-operative soreness. Overall, women were more susceptible to reporting more symptoms. As seen in Table 5, having greater than 2 laryngoscopies and an endotracheal tube larger than 7.0 resulted in postoperative soreness, whereas the presence of an esophageal temperature probe, an endotracheal tube larger than 7.0, and a low cuff pressure (less than 20 cm water) were associated with postoperative hoarseness in women. In men, a cuff pressure less than 20 cm water was associated with postoperative hoarseness, and inexperience on the part of the person performing the intubation caused postoperative sore throat.

Identifying these risk factors can help to mitigate the effects of the intubations and improve satisfaction with the surgical experience.

R. Franco, MD

Effect of a tracheostomy speaking valve on breathing–swallowing interaction

Prigent H, Lejaille M, Terzi N, et al (Hôpital Raymond Poincaré, Garches, France; INSERM, Caen, France)

Intensive Care Med 38:85-90, 2012

Purpose.—Expiratory flow towards the upper airway after swallowing serves to expel liquid or food particles misdirected towards the trachea during swallowing. However, expiration may not occur consistently after swallowing in tracheostomised patients with an open tracheostomy tube. We investigated the effect of a speaking valve (SV) on breathing–swallowing interactions and on the volume expelled through the upper airway after swallowing.

Methods.—Eight tracheostomised neuromuscular patients who were able to breathe spontaneously were studied with and without an SV. Breathing–swallowing interactions were investigated by chin electromyography, cervical piezoelectric sensor, and nasal and tracheal flow recording. Three water-bolus sizes (5, 10, and 15 mL) were tested in random order.

Results.—Swallowing characteristics and breathing–swallowing synchronisation were not influenced by SV use. However, expiratory flow towards the upper airway after swallowing was negligible without the SV and was restored by adding the SV.

TABLE 2.—Swallowing Variables per Bolus According to Bolus Size (5, 10, or 15 mL) and Test Condition: Without (SV−) and with (SV+) a Tracheostomy Valve

	5 mL		10 mL		15 mL		ANOVA (*p* Value)	
	SV−	SV+	SV−	SV+	SV−	SV+	SV Effect	Volume Effect
Duration of swallowing (s)	2.5 ± 2.4	2.9 ± 3.8	3.8 ± 2.7	4.4 ± 4.4	4.5 ± 3.2	4.6 ± 4.8	0.62	0.001
Number of swallows per bolus	1.6 ± 1.0	1.6 ± 1.1	2.2 ± 1.2	2.1 ± 1.4	2.6 ± 1.3	2.3 ± 1.7	0.37	0.001
Number of ventilatory cycles per bolus	1.0 ± 0.0	1.2 ± 0.4	1.3 ± 0.6	1.7 ± 1.0	1.3 ± 0.6	1.6 ± 1.1	0.44	0.006
% of swallows followed by expiration	65 ± 34	82 ± 24	72 ± 28	78 ± 21	62 ± 30	74 ± 28	0.37	0.51

Conclusion.—In tracheostomised patients, protective expiration towards the upper airway after swallowing is restored by the use of an SV (Table 2).

▶ Swallowing is thought to be highly dependent on the ability to create areas of high pressure and drive the bolus to the low-pressure environment of the esophagus. The lips and soft palate seal the potential leak of pressure to the outside world from the mouth or nose, whereas the tongue compresses against the hard palate and the posterior pharyngeal wall, driving the bolus down with a wave of high pressure. Tracheotomized patients are felt to be at a disadvantage when swallowing because of a limitation of laryngeal excursion from the tethering of the trachea to the skin, potentially decreased sensation, and the inability to provide proper subglottic pressure to prevent secretions from dripping into the subglottis. It is hypothesized that swallowing with a speaking valve on the tracheostomy tube should help to provide that missing subglottal pressure. The authors of this study evaluated tracheotomized patients swallowing with both the speaking valve on and off. To their surprise, they found no differences between the 2 groups with either the 5-cc, 10-cc, or 15-cc swallowing challenges. This is depicted in Table 2. There was a significant difference in the subglottal pressure that was generated at the end of the swallow in the patients wearing the speaking valve. The findings were somewhat surprising because it makes so much sense that swallowing during exhalation seems much safer—recreating that situation with the speaking valve and generating that subglottic pressure will prevent the passage of material through the glottis. The reality of this study was that despite these theoretical advantages for the speaking valve patients, there was no perceived benefit to the actual swallow.

R. Franco, MD

Cricopharyngeal Muscle Electromyography Findings in Patients with Gastroesophageal Reflux Disease

Alkan Z, Demir A, Yigit O, et al (Istanbul Training and Res Hosp, Turkey; et al)
Otolaryngol Head Neck Surg 147:295-301, 2012

Objective.—To analyze the grade of reflux and the behavior of the cricopharyngeal muscle (CPM) in patients with gastroesophageal reflux (GER) by means of electromyographic (EMG) analysis of CPM.

Study Design.—Prospective clinical study.

Setting.—Istanbul Training and Research Hospital.

Subject and Methods.—Motor unit potential (MUP) recordings and kinesiological recordings of CPM were performed using a concentric needle electrode during dry material swallowing and 3-, 5-, and 10-mL water swallowing. Twenty-four patients with GER were compared with 21 healthy volunteers.

Results.—GER was mild in 15 patients and moderate-to-severe in 9 patients. MUP recordings were normal in both groups during the preswallowing/postswallowing periods. Kinesiological investigations revealed that the number of patients who did not show a preswallow EMG burst had a positive correlation with the severity of reflux and the amount of liquid swallowed. Rebound bursts were observed in the patient and the control groups. Duration of preswallow and rebound bursts was similar in all groups. Duration of swallowing was shorter in mild GER patients compared with healthy volunteers and moderate-to-severe GER patients. Piecemeal deglutition during 10-mL liquid swallowing was higher in moderate-to-severe GER patients. We also found a positive correlation between the number of swallows and the severity of reflux.

Conclusion.—Needle EMG of the upper esophageal sphincter was normal in GER patients. Kinesiological evaluations showed increased piecemeal deglutition and number of swallows that correlated positively with the severity of GER.

▶ Laryngopharyngeal reflux is one of the terms used to describe a clinical entity that still does not have proper correlation to a defined and reproducible pathological process. The presumption is that the process is mediated by acid and enzymes from the stomach that make their way into the laryngopharynx and cause the changes that are seen (posterior edema, true vocal fold edema, excessive laryngeal mucus) and felt (chronic laryngeal irritation, need for throat clearing and cough) and are referable to the "throat." If one follows this line of reasoning, the upper esophageal sphincter becomes an important structure in the pathogenesis of laryngopharyngeal reflux symptoms. The cricopharyngeal muscle is tonically contracted and reflexively relaxes during swallowing and, therefore, it should normally act as a reflux barrier. There have been studies that reported an increase in manometric pressure in the region of the cricopharyngeal muscle (also known as the upper esophageal sphincter) when the upper esophagus was acidified intentionally or spontaneously. This activity would make sense because it should contract to ensure no gastric contents are refluxed up into the laryngopharynx. But there are conflicting studies that do not report this upper esophageal sphincter activity.

In this needle electromyography (EMG) study of 45 subjects (21 were normal [nonreflux] controls and 24 complained of gastroesophageal reflux symptoms), the authors were investigating the activity of the upper esophageal sphincter region during dry swallows and various defined volumes of water (3, 5 and 10 mL). They found no statistically significant differences between the controls and the reflux subjects by EMG. The differences that were identified were more piecemeal swallowing and a greater number of swallows necessary to clear the bolus correlated to the severity of the reflux by the reflux finding score and reflux severity index.

It is likely that the clinical entity we call laryngopharyngeal reflux (LPR) is a final common pathway that several pathological processes can take to the symptoms and signs we clinically associate with LPR. We still need to continue to resolve which patients have acid-related problems and separate those who have hypersensitivity and other problems so we can reliably treat these patients properly.

R. Franco, MD

Outcomes

Novel therapeutic approach to relieve pharyngoesophageal spasm after total laryngectomy

Kim HN, Lewin JS, Knott JK, et al (The Univ of Texas MD Anderson Cancer Ctr, Houston)

Gastrointest Endosc 76:193-196, 2012

Background.—Pharyngoesophageal spasm (PES) is the most common reason for tracheoesophageal (TE) speech failure in patients who have undergone total laryngectomy. PES increases peak intraesophageal pressure measurements during phonation and correlates with the levels of TE speech fluency. Chemical denervation of the PE segment using *Clostridium* botulinum toxin A (BTA) can prevent the release of acetylcholine at the neuromuscular junction and offers an effective way to facilitate TE speech and swallowing after total laryngectomy. BTA is usually injected percutaneously into the pharyngeal constrictor muscles along one side of the neopharynx just superior and lateral to the stoma. Electromyographic (EMG) guidance is used for the procedure. If percutaneous injection is not possible, the BTA injection may be delivered through the esophagogastroduodenoscope (EGD) for patients with PES. This method was used for several patients and the results reported.

Methods.—The four laryngectomized patients underwent eight sessions of BTA injections through the EGD. All the patients had TE speech problems, and three also had dysphagia. Videofluoroscopic examination was done before each injection to identify the site of the spasm. During endoscopy, nonstrictured smooth narrowing/spasticity above the TE prosthesis

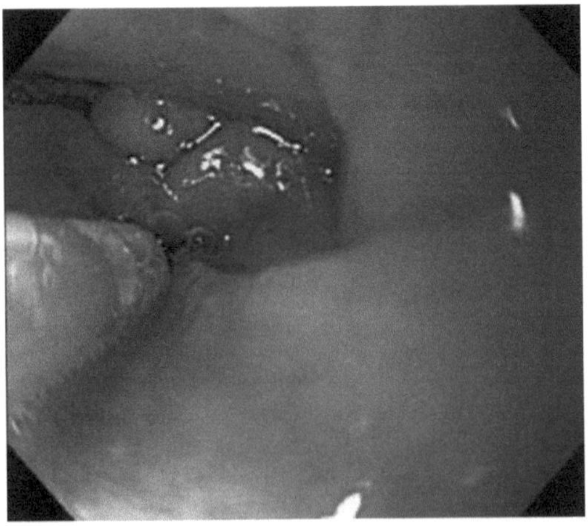

FIGURE 1.—Botulinum toxin A injection through a gastroscope. (Reprinted from Gastrointestinal Endoscopy. Kim HN, Lewin JS, Knott JK, et al. Novel therapeutic approach to relieve pharyngoesophageal spasm after total Laryngectomy. *Gastrointest Endosc.* 2012;76:193-196, Copyright 2012, with permission from the American Society for Gastrointestinal Endoscopy.)

was identified. BTA 100 IU was injected into four quadrants of the PES segment through the EGD, then gentle massage was performed using back-and-forth movement of an 18-mm controlled radial expansion (CRE) balloon dilator. TE speech fluency was rated before and after injection.

Results.—Local BTA injection improved speech and swallowing function in the four patients. The first patient did not improve with the initial procedure but responded to a second procedure. One patient at increased risk for pneumothorax related to percutaneous injection did well and had no complications after the BTA injection through the EGD.

Conclusions.—BTA injection through the EGD may minimize complications in at-risk patients. This procedure does not require general anesthesia, thereby avoiding the added cost and recovery time with such anesthesia. Patients whose speech difficulties and swallowing function fail to respond to percutaneous BTA injections and those for whom percutaneous injection is contraindicated or not tolerated should benefit especially from this novel approach (Fig 1).

▶ Post–total laryngectomy voice rehabilitation is dependent on the status of the newly reconstructed pharyngoesophageal segment. The tracheoesophageal puncture shunts air from the trachea into the esophagus and up into the pharyngoesophageal segment, causing it to vibrate and create the sound that the tongue, lips, and teeth modulate into voice. If the segment is too loose, it does not vibrate effectively, resulting in a weak voice. Too tight a segment and the air does not pass through to initiate vibration. This segment also has implications for swallowing function. When there is hypertonicity of the pharyngoesophageal segment, botulinum toxin can be injected to effect relation. These injections can be performed in the outpatient awake setting via a transcervical approach using an electromyographic setup to know when the needle tip is within muscle. The botulinum toxin can also be delivered through a long sclerotherapy needle passed through the working channel of a nasopharyngoscope and into the tight segment. The authors describe a technique using an upper gastrointestinal endoscopy scope used to deliver 100 units into 4 quadrants of the pharyngoesophageal segment under monitored anesthesia care in 4 patients (Fig 1). A Boston Scientific CRE 18-mm balloon was expanded to help massage the toxin through the tissues. They found that the botulinum toxin injection improved the tracheoesophageal speech anywhere from 10.5 months to 15 months. They also found that the swallowing difficulties from having a too-tight pharyngoesophageal segment preceded the eventual voice problems. This technique can be performed as needed by the gastroenterologist. Typically in the otolaryngology outpatient setting the procedure is performed with topical anesthesia, obviating the need for the monitored anesthesia care and sedatives, making it a safer, faster procedure.

R. Franco, MD

All-cause mortality after tracheostomy at a tertiary care hospital over a 10-month period

Kejner AE, Castellanos PF, Rosenthal EL, et al (Univ of Alabama-Birmingham)
Otolaryngol Head Neck Surg 146:918-922, 2012

Objective.—To evaluate perioperative mortality after tracheostomy in intensive care unit (ICU) patients undergoing routine tracheostomy over a 10-month period.

Study Design.—Case series with planned data collection.

Setting.—Tertiary care hospital.

Subjects.—Mechanically ventilated patients.

Methods.—Prospective analysis of ICU patients undergoing tracheostomy placement over 10 months was performed. Variables evaluated were demographics, pretracheostomy length of stay, time on ventilator, time to death, preoperative comorbidities, and cause of death.

Results.—There were 129 consultations resulting in 115 tracheostomies, of which 100 were included for study. The overall 30-day postoperative mortality rate was 25%, including palliative care deaths. Cause of death in all cases was due to a preexisting condition and not from tracheostomy. Patients who died within the 30-day postoperative period were found to have significant differences in age, pretracheostomy length of stay, location of tracheostomy, and preoperative comorbidity scores. No significant difference was found in time on ventilator, sex, or race/ethnicity. Mean time from consultation to tracheostomy was 2.5 days (range, 0-12 days).

Conclusion.—High rates of mortality after tracheostomy can possibly affect hospital quality ratings for surgical services. There were no deaths directly related to surgery. Despite this, the mortality rate in this population was quite high. This illustrates the significant disease burden in these patients and the need to stratify postoperative mortality as well as to consider comorbidity and age when evaluating patients for tracheostomy.

▶ Tracheotomy is a commonly performed procedure in the intensive care unit (ICU) setting with up to 24% of patients undergoing this procedure because of prolonged endotracheal intubation or the expected need for prolonged mechanical ventilation. The need for a tracheotomy is a bad prognostic indicator of health, and those who require them in the ICU setting have many intrinsic factors that make them very bad surgical candidates (eg, acid-base disorders, multiple organ failure, labile blood pressure, need for mechanical ventilation). These same factors also place these patients at risk for death.

Increasingly, payors are using defined metrics to determine reimbursement for procedures, with perioperative mortality a leading factor. The authors of this study evaluated some factors to try to understand some of the major ones that differentiated those who died within 30 days of the tracheotomy and those who lived. They found that intrinsic patient characteristics, such as greater age, length of hospitalization before tracheotomy, whether the tracheotomy was performed at the bedside, and the greater comorbidities, were associated with death within

30 days of the tracheotomy. They did not find time on the ventilator or the patient's sex to contribute to the mortality.

In this study, although 25% of the patients died within 30 days, there were no deaths caused by the tracheotomy itself. It seems important to have a way to recognize and control for the patient's comorbidities when assessing the 30-day postprocedure mortality. Of the 75 patients still alive after 30 days, another 33 subsequently died, leaving only 42 alive. Again, although none of these patients died because of the tracheotomy, it is incumbent on the ICU team members to evaluate and discuss the dire nature of the condition with the patient and his or her medical proxy. Of the original 100 patients, only 42% survived in this study.

R. Franco, MD

Analysis of pediatric direct laryngoscopy and bronchoscopy operative flow: opportunities for improved safety outcomes

Shah RK, Cohen J, Patel A, et al (Children's Natl Med Ctr, Washington, DC)

Arch Otolaryngol Head Neck Surg 138:624-627, 2012

Objective.—To study pediatric direct laryngoscopy and bronchoscopy operative flow.

Design.—Observational quality improvement initiative.

Setting.—Two freestanding tertiary care children's hospitals.

Patients.—Pediatric patients undergoing direct laryngoscopy and bronchoscopy.

Main Outcome Measures.—Trained medical students observed direct laryngoscopy and bronchoscopy operative flow. An audit tool containing 144 fields was completed during each encounter for the following domains: timing of the case, preoperative preparation, operative flow, and operating room personnel assessment.

Results.—Forty-one cases were observed. The mean time between the patient entering the operating room and the beginning of the case was 12 minutes. In all the patients, a complete history was obtained, and a physical examination was performed. The equipment was ready for 31 cases (76%) and was checked before 32 cases (78%). Anesthesia equipment was checked before 36 cases (88%). Issues with intravenous access were recorded for 19 cases (46%). The operating room orientation needed to be changed to accommodate the procedure in 11 cases (27%). Preoperative preparation of the patient proceeded smoothly in 16 cases (39%), and the operative flow proceeded without disruption in 19 cases (46%). The scrub nurse left the operating room in 2 cases (5%), the circulating nurse left in 15 cases (37%), and the anesthesiologist left in 9 cases (22%).

Conclusions.—Although a common pediatric otolaryngology procedure, direct laryngoscopy and bronchoscopy operative flow is ideal in less than half the cases. Areas for improvement include obtaining intravenous access, reducing operating room personnel turnover, verifying equipment, and educating staff on operating room setup. To our knowledge, this is the first observational quality improvement initiative in otolaryngology to study the operative flow of a specific procedure and provide insight into areas of patient risk and opportunities for improvement in efficiency.

▶ The continuing changes to the way the medical system is financed in the United States require optimization of the way the medical system utilizes its resources. There have already been several waves of change in the delivery of health care in otolaryngology, with some procedures that were once considered to be appropriate for the operating room, like treatment of laryngeal papillomatosis and keratosis, airway dilation of stenosis, and injection for glottal insufficiency, moving to the outpatient clinic setting. These changes have resulted in improved safety for the patients through the avoidance of general anesthesia, improved efficiency for the surgeons by allowing multiple procedures to be performed because of elimination of anesthesia preparation time (induction and emergence) and reduction in turnover time between patients, and a reduction in the cost per procedure for the system as a whole.

Not all procedures are candidates for the move from the operating room to the outpatient setting. In the operating room, time really does represent money, as there is a charge even if no active intervention is being performed. Because of this, it is vital to optimize the procedures to minimize the waste of valuable resources. An optimized system will also be a safer one, in which all of the proper instrumentation is available when it is needed, without having to wait for it. In this study, the authors evaluated the operative flow of one of the most common pediatric otolaryngologic procedures, direct laryngoscopy and bronchoscopy. The raters were asked to observe but not intervene during the course of the procedure using a 144-point audit tool to assess the communication between team members, the time of the case, and the overall flow of the case. They found the preoperative flow was uninterrupted in 39% of cases with proper flow during the operative case 46% of the time. There was significant disruption caused by operating team members leaving the room, with circulating nurses leaving the room in 37% of the cases and the anesthesiologists leaving in 22% of the cases. Although the average procedure was 22 minutes long, this represents less than half of the time (47%) in the operating room. Optimization of the preoperative environment means making sure the consents and intravenous placement are ready, and optimization in the operating room requires that the surgical sets contain all of the instruments the surgeon needs and requested. There is no doubt that any inquiry into the optimization of other procedures will reveal we have very far to go in nearly every surgery before being considered to be operating at peak efficiency.

R. Franco, MD

Early Postoperative Vocal Function Evaluation After Thyroidectomy Using Thyroidectomy Related Voice Questionnaire

Chun B-J, Bae J-S, Chae B-J, et al (The Catholic Univ of Korea, Seoul)

World J Surg 36:2503-2508, 2012

Background.—The objectives of this study were to evaluate a screening method for detecting postoperative vocal cord palsy and lower-pitched voice and to identify how a pre-thyroidectomy laryngeal disorder affects post-thyroidectomy voice change by using our subjective voice questionnaire.

Methods.—We examined 300 consecutive patients scheduled to undergo thyroidectomies between November 2010 and August 2011. Laryngoscopic examination, thyroidectomy-related voice questionnaire (TVQ) administration, and acoustic and perceptual analyses were performed preoperatively and 2 weeks after thyroidectomy.

Results.—Ninety-eight (32.6%) patients had a preoperative laryngeal disorder. Postoperatively, 31 (10.3%) patients had vocal cord palsy and 54 (18%) had a lower-pitched voice 2 weeks after thyroidectomy. Postoperative TVQs classified 25 (8.4%) patients as normal and 275 (91.6%) patients as abnormal, including 79 (26.3%) mild, 131 (43.6%) moderate, and 65 (21.6%) severe cases. Of the patients with vocal cord palsy, 80.6% belonged to the severe group, and 92.6% of patients with lower-pitched voices belonged to the moderate and severe groups. Fundamental frequency and speaking fundamental frequency were decreased significantly in women. The most efficient TVQ cutoff values for detecting post-thyroidectomy vocal cord palsy and postoperative lower-pitched voice were 35 (87.1% sensitivity, 79.9% specificity) and 25 (75.9% sensitivity, 56.5 % specificity), respectively. Total TVQ scores increased more in the nonlaryngeal than in the laryngeal disorder group.

Conclusions.—During the early postoperative period, 28.3% of patients had vocal cord palsy or lower-pitched voices, which could be evaluated using a simple questionnaire. Therefore, early postoperative voice evaluation is important. Patients with nonlaryngeal disorders may be more sensitive than those with laryngeal disorders to laryngeal symptoms.

▶ Many consider thyroidectomy to be a high-risk surgery for compromising vocal function. This surgery places the superior and recurrent laryngeal nerves, strap muscles and their innervation, and the vascular supply to the larynx in peril. This is also a surgery that is performed by many general surgeons and nonotolaryngologists around the world and in the United States. These other specialists may not have the proper training to perform detailed examinations of the larynx (such as nasolaryngoscopy) before and after thyroidectomy, making mild impairments to the larynx difficult to diagnose objectively. A surrogate, in the form of a questionnaire, would be much easier to administer and noninvasive and may alert the physician to the possibility of a change that deserves to be worked up. Why is this important? As many as 33% of postthyroidectomy patients have voice changes with most reporting a lowering of the pitch of the voice.

The authors evaluated 300 patients who underwent thyroidectomy with fiber-optic laryngoscopy, stroboscopy, perceptual voice analysis, computerized voice analysis, and the thyroidectomy-related voice questionnaire (TVQ) before and after surgery. They found laryngeal lesions in 98 of the 300 (32%) preoperatively. Postoperatively 31 (10%) were found to have vocal fold impairment, and 54 (18%) had a drop in pitch. Women seemed to be more afflicted by the pitch drop. Only about 8% of patients' scores remained in the normal range (< 5 on the TVQ), meaning there was a change in score in about 92%! TVQ scores greater than 35 predicted vocal fold movement impairment. The TVQ was previously used in a series of 500 thyroidectomies to determine the normal values. It might have a role as part of the pre- and postoperative thyroidectomy visits.

R. Franco, MD

Clinical and Histologic Predictors of Voice and Disease Outcome in Patients With Early Glottic Cancer

Chang J, Fang T-J, Yung K, et al (Univ of California, San Francisco; Chang Gung Univ, Taoyuan, Taiwan)

Laryngoscope 122:2240-2247, 2012

Objectives/Hypothesis.—To determine preliminarily if clinical or histological features of patients with laryngeal dysplasia/early carcinoma correlate with voice and disease outcomes.

Study Design.—Retrospective case series.

Methods.—All UCSF Voice Center patients treated with endoscopic surgery for severe dysplasia or early laryngeal cancer between 2004 and 2010 were identified. Preoperative stroboscopy, intraoperative appearance, and histologic characteristics (pattern of invasion, degree of inflammation, and degree of keratinization) of the neoplastic lesions were compared with cordectomy type and the outcomes of voice quality and disease-free interval.

Results.—Eighteen patients were evaluated. Increased stromal chronic inflammation correlated with longer disease-free interval ($r(2) = 0.38$). Cordectomy type correlated with both preoperative and postoperative voice parameters ($r(2) = 0.42–0.68$ and $0.33–0.39$).

Conclusion.—Increased stromal chronic inflammation correlates with improved disease outcome. Voice outcome correlates with the amount of tissue removed. The clinical appearance of the lesion did not correlate with disease or voice outcome.

► The larynx is a dynamic organ with incredible capacity to function despite absorbing various insults. Even in the face of cancer, the voice may not portray the seriousness of the problem it is harboring. As in other branches of medicine, we use the TNM classification to stage malignant tumors. The TNM is a somewhat incomplete staging system because it is an anatomical staging system that does not take into consideration other tumor-host characteristics. The authors of this study sought to discover those other characteristics, be they clinical or histological, to correlate with voice and disease outcomes. They reviewed the tumors of 18 patients who underwent transoral resection of the tumors. They reviewed the images taken at the start of the endoscopic resection for the size and location of the lesion, whether it was endophytic or exophytic, and whether there was associated inflammation. The histologic tissue was reviewed for the presence of keratinization, the pattern of invasion, the severity of dysplasia or cancer, and the degree of lymphocytic infiltration. The strobe exams were also reviewed for all of the relevant vibratory characteristics and voice quality based on a spoken sample of the rainbow passage (severity, roughness, breathiness, strain, pitch, and loudness). These characteristics were reviewed by 2 blinded pathologists, 2 blinded laryngologists, and 2 blinded speech pathologists. None of the characteristics was statistically correlated with the outcomes, but there was an association of greater lymphocytic infiltration in the sample with greater disease-free intervals. The greater the voice dysfunction preoperatively, the more chance there was that patients would need an extended surgery to resect the cancer. Although of the 18 patients, 4 had either Cis or severe dysplasia, there were 6 recurrences, including 2 in the "precancer" subset.

The authors found that the low inter-rater reliability for the clinical characteristics was very disappointing, making the case for the urgent need for new instruments that can objectively assess the vibratory characteristics.

R. Franco, MD

Laryngeal edema after radiotherapy in patients with squamous cell carcinomas of the larynx and hypopharynx

Bae JS, Roh J-L, Lee S-W, et al (Univ of Ulsan College of Medicine, Songpa-gu, Seoul, Republic of Korea)

Oral Oncol 48:853-858, 2012

Objectives.—Significant laryngeal edema (SLE) after radiotherapy for squamous cell carcinoma of the larynx and hypopharynx may be associated with upper airway obstruction or tumor recurrence. We assessed the risk factors predictive of SLE and those differentiating tumor recurrence from SLE.

Patients and Methods.—We evaluated 127 patients with laryngohypopharyngeal squamous cell carcinomas who were primarily treated with radiotherapy with/without chemotherapy, had no previous major head and neck surgery, and underwent laryngoscopic examinations after radiotherapy. SLE was defined as RTOG grades ≥ 2 and patient characteristics and imaging, treatment and survival results were compared in patients with and without SLE.

Results.—Of the 127 patients, 56 (44%) had SLE. Univariate analyses showed that tumor location, T and N classifications, overall stage, pathologic differentiation, and chemotherapy were significantly predictive of SLE ($P < 0.05$). Multivariate analysis revealed that T classification remained an independent predictor of SLE (T1 *vs.* T2–4; odds ratio = 5.070, 95% confidence interval = 1.999–12.857; $P = 0.001$). Twenty-seven (21%)

patients had tumor recurrences, diagnosed by PET/CT (sensitivity 88%; specificity 92%) and CT (sensitivity 68%; specificity 88%). Twenty-seven patients with severe SLE were treated but only 9 (33%) had improvement. Tumor recurrence rate was higher (39% *vs.* 7%, $P < 0.001$) and 3-year overall survival rate lower (54% *vs.* 87%, $P < 0.001$) in patients with than without SLE.

Conclusion.—Patients with T2–4 laryngohypopharyngeal cancers are at higher risk of SLE development and tumor recurrence after radiotherapy that can be properly detected by ^{18}F-FDG PET/CT.

▶ Any otolaryngologist who has ever cared for patients with laryngeal cancer treated by radiation therapy will have seen persistent edema and wondered how best to manage this vexing consequence of treatment. The biggest fear is that there is persistent cancer that is masked by the edema that will continue to grow and potentially become clinically evident at a late stage. The authors of this study evaluated 127 patients with severe laryngeal edema (SLE) who met their inclusion criteria from 2005 to 2010. Of all of the variables they evaluated, the T stage (TNM staging) was found to be an independent predictor of SLE through multivariate analysis. Patients with T2-T4 had the highest rates of persistence/recurrent cancer. They found treatment for SLE to be difficult with very limited responses. Of 27 patients with SLE grade 3 and 4, they found only 9 who responded positively to treatment (33%). Treatment consisted of antibiotics, steroids, and hyperbaric oxygen treatment. What is very important to remember is that SLE can be a sign that cancer is still present in the larynx, although it cannot easily be seen. Tumor recurrence rates were higher in the SLE group compared with the non-SLE patients (33% versus 7%, $P = .001$) with a statistically significant reduction in the 3-year survival rate of 54% vs 87% ($P < .001$).

These findings beg the question, "What can we do to detect the cancers in the setting of severe laryngeal edema?" Repeated blind biopsies of the larynx in the setting of full-course radiation therapy may induce a nonhealing area, with the potential for chondroradionecrosis. This may be read as a positive area for cancer on subsequent computed tomography (CT) scans or positron emission tomography (PET) scanning, resulting in further unnecessary surgical interventions that may compromise voice, breathing ability, and swallowing function without improving survival. The authors looked at CT vs positron emission tomography-computed tomography (PET/CT) scanning and found the PET/CT to have a sensitivity of 88% with a specificity of 92% vs the CT's sensitivity of 68% and specificity of 88%. Clearly PET/CT is superior and should be used in cases in which persistent tumor is suspected, before biopsy.

Persistent significant edema lasting more than 3 months should be viewed as troublesome and potentially signaling persistent tumor. The authors found persistent or recurrent tumor in 22 of 56 (39%) SLE subjects, with higher rates in those who did not improve after instituting treatment. They found the negative predictive value of PET/CT to be as high as 98%, meaning that if a PET/CT scan is negative, there is a very good chance it truly is negative for cancer. PET/CT positive scans should prompt biopsy to rule out recurrence/persistent tumors.

R. Franco, MD

A New Method of Reconstructing the Human Laryngeal Architecture Using Micro-MRI

Chen T, Chodara AM, Sprecher AJ, et al (Fudan Univ, Shanghai, China; Univ of Wisconsin School of Medicine and Public Health, Madison; et al)

J Voice 26:555-562, 2012

Objectives/Hypothesis.—A realistic three-dimentional (3D) model of the larynx could be of value for the understanding of normal laryngeal motion and for studying pathological changes as well as in modeling potential therapy outcomes. The objective of this research was to present a new method of creating a computer model of the human larynx using data obtained through micro-magnetic resonance imaging (MRI) scanning.

Study Design.—Prospective study.

Methods.—A 7-T micro-MRI scanner was used to scan an excised larynx obtained postmortem from a 68-year-old woman. MRI data was manually segmented and compiled into 3D images using *Mimics12.1* reconstruction software. Measurements of the reconstructed structures were also calculated using *Mimics12.1*.

Results.—The 3D laryngeal model contained the thyroid, cricoid, and arytenoid cartilages. Nearly all of the intrinsic muscles could be segmented. Although the cricoarytenoid joint could be visualized, the features of the

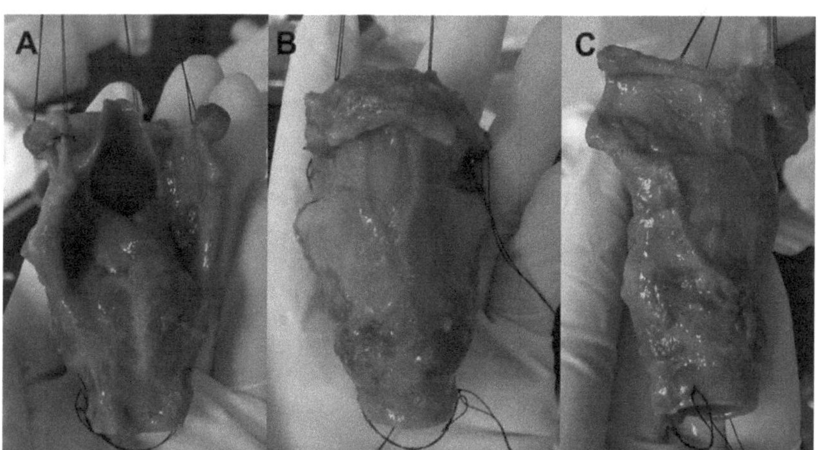

FIGURE 1.—Posterior (A), anterior (B), and lateral (C) views of the excised human larynx after dissection. All cartilages and intrinsic muscles were maintained intact. Reprinted from Journal of Voice. Chen T, Chodara AM, Sprecher AJ, et al. A new method of reconstructing the human laryngeal architecture using micro-MRI. *J Voice*. 2012;26:555-562, Copyright 2012, with permission from The Voice Foundation.)

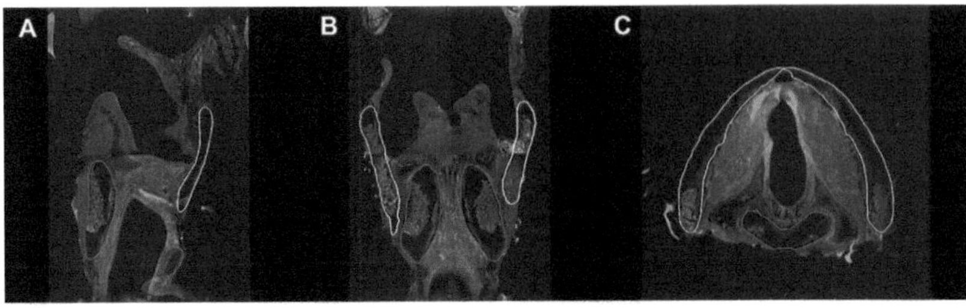

FIGURE 2.—MRI images from the sagittal (A), coronal (B), and transverse (C) planes, showing the tracing of cartilage boundaries for compilation and 3D reconstruction. Outlined in yellow is the thyroid cartilage, in blue the arytenoids, and in lavender the cricoid cartilage. (Reprinted from Journal of Voice. Chen T, Chodara AM, Sprecher AJ, et al. A new method of reconstructing the human laryngeal architecture using micro-MRI. *J Voice*. 2012;26:555-562, Copyright 2012, with permission from The Voice Foundation.)

TABLE 2.—Volumes of Intrinsic Laryngeal Muscles and LP as Calculated by *Mimics12.1*

Tissues	Left Volume (mm^3)	Right Volume (mm^3)
Thyroarytenoid muscle	862.75	851.56
Posterior CA muscle	605.10	599.02
Cricothyroid muscle	586.11	566.61
Lateral CA muscle	192.16	188.45
LP	95.65	92.34

cricothyroid joint were not clear. Muscle and cartilage volumes and surface areas were calculated from the 3D model.

Conclusions.—The combination of MRI and 3D reconstruction generates promising results in the hopes of creating a highly realistic and detailed model of the human larynx (Figs 1 and 2, Table 2).

▶ The larynx is a compact, complicated organ that is unbelievably dynamic. The striking surfaces of the vocal folds regularly experience forces upward of 6 Gs during phonation. Because of its importance to swallowing, breathing, and phonating, a detailed understanding of the anatomy is essential to refining our ideas about how the larynx works. Since invasive experimentation is very difficult, having a detailed and accurate model can allow us to postulate questions that can be answered through simulation. Accurate models can also be used to educate medical students, residents, and fully trained physicians, allowing them to appreciate subtleties that cannot be easily demonstrated in the intact larynx.

The authors used a high-resolution, 7-tesla micro-magnetic resonance imager to scan an excised human larynx. Using specialized software, the magnetic resonance imaging (MRI) data was converted into a 3-dimensional model that could be manipulated. They were able to clearly demonstrate all of the laryngeal cartilages (Fig 1), visualize the extent and fiber orientation of the intrinsic laryngeal musculature (Fig 2), and determine the volume of the muscles and the surface areas of the cartilages (Table 2). Even at 7 tesla, the MRI was unable to discriminate the different layers of the lamina propria. This is a tall task for a space that is less than 200 microns in depth and is composed of fibers of collagen and elastin in a bed of hyaluronic acid, water, and glycosaminoglycans. Because the water content is so high, regardless of the magnetic strength, we may never be able to properly resolve the lamina propria into its constituent histologic layers.

Models such as this one allow researchers to perform more complex and realistic simulation of the dynamic process of phonation.

R. Franco, MD

Surgical Technique

Acoustic and Perceptual Aspects of Vocal Function in Children With Adenotonsillar Hypertrophy—Effects of Surgery

Lundeborg I, Hultcrantz E, Ericsson E, et al (Linköping Univ, Sweden)
J Voice 26:480-487, 2012

Objective.—To evaluate outcome of two types of tonsil surgery (tonsillectomy [TE]+adenoidectomy or tonsillotomy [TT]+adenoidectomy) on vocal function perceptually and acoustically.

Study Design.—Sixty-seven children, aged 50–65 months, on waiting list for tonsil surgery were randomized to TE (n = 33) or TT (n = 34). Fifty-seven age- and gender-matched healthy preschool children were controls. Twenty-eight of them, aged 48–59 months, served as control group before surgery, and 29, aged 60–71 months, served as control group after surgery.

Methods.—Before surgery and 6 months postoperatively, the children were recorded producing three sustained vowels (/a/, /u/, and /i/) and 14 words. The control groups were recorded only once. Three trained speech and language pathologists performed the perceptual analysis using visual analog scale for eight voice quality parameters. Acoustic analysis from sustained vowels included average fundamental frequency, jitter percent, shimmer percent, noise-to-harmonic ratio, and the center frequencies of formants 1–3.

Results.—Before surgery, the children were rated to have more hyponasality and compressed/throaty voice ($P < 0.05$) and lower mean pitch ($P < 0.01$) in comparison to the control group. They also had higher perturbation measures and lower frequencies of the second and third formants. After surgery, there were no differences perceptually. Perturbation measures decreased but were still higher compared with those of control group ($P < 0.05$). Differences in formant frequencies for /i/ and /u/ remained. No differences were found between the two surgical methods.

Conclusion.—Voice quality is affected perceptually and acoustically by adenotonsillar hypertrophy. After surgery, the voice is perceptually normalized but acoustic differences remain. Outcome was equal for both surgical methods.

▶ It is commonly believed that surgery of the upper airway, especially the oropharynx and nasal cavities, can have profound effects on the sound of the voice. The pharynx is the resonating chamber that enhances some frequencies and filters out others to shape the raw sound that emanates from the larynx. Many singers will not undergo tonsillectomy or correct nasal deformities for fear of altering their voice detrimentally.

In this study, the authors compared tonsillectomy with tonsillotomy (complete removal of the tonsils vs removal of enough to relieve the obstruction) and the effects on the voice. Before surgery, the hypertrophic adenotonsillar children had higher jitter and shimmer and lower frequencies of the second and third formants. Reviewers described their voices as compressed/throaty and hyponasal. After surgery, the jitter and shimmer were reduced but still elevated compared with the control group. The tonsillectomy and tonsillotomy groups were statistically the same.

It is interesting to see that there was a normalization of the voice parameters after adenotonsillectomy (and tonsillotomy) but that they never reached the same level of pertubation measurements as the normal controls. The perceived voices were considered normal after surgery. This should be comforting to those parents who are contemplating surgery for their hyponasal-sounding, mouth-breathing children, that they have a good chance of sounding more like the normal controls.

R. Franco, MD

Analysis of Pitch Range After Arytenoid Adduction by Fenestration Approach Combined With Type I Thyroplasty for Unilateral Vocal Fold Paralysis

Tokashiki R, Hiramatsu H, Shinada E, et al (Tokyo Med Univ, Japan)
J Voice 26:792-796, 2012

Objective.—The purpose of this study was to determine the postoperative pitch range acquired in cases of unilateral vocal fold paralysis, as well as factors affecting outcomes.

Subjects and Methods.—We analyzed 39 cases of unilateral vocal fold paralysis for which surgery was performed between January 2006 and January 2009 and for which pitch ranges and the items listed below were measured preoperatively and 1 year postoperatively. Arytenoid adduction (AA) and type I thyroplasty were performed simultaneously in all cases regardless of preoperative severity. AA was performed by the fenestration approach as previously reported. In this procedure, the cricoarytenoid and cricothyroid joints are not released. Correlations between pitch range acquired postoperatively and the following items were examined: (1) pre- and postoperative maximum phonation time (MPT), (2) pre- and postoperative mean airflow rate (MFR), and (3) preoperative pitch range. Furthermore, patients were surveyed regarding their ability to sing after surgery, and the pitch range cutoff value dividing ability and inability to sing was calculated.

Results.—Pitch range increased significantly from 3 ± 4.47 halftones (mean ± standard deviation) preoperatively to 17.5 ± 5.80 halftones postoperatively. Preoperative MPT, MFR, and pitch range did not correlate with postoperative pitch range. Postoperatively, only MPT correlated with the width of postoperative pitch range. Twenty-three of 39 subjects (59%) responded that they were able to sing, and the pitch range cutoff value dividing the two groups was 22 halftones.

Conclusion.—AA and type I thyroplasty significantly expanded postoperative pitch range. There was no correlation between preoperative severity and width of pitch range acquired postoperatively.

▶ Optimization of voice requires the establishment of proper vocal fold height, appropriate tension, and closure to allow for the generation of subglottal pressure to achieve a loud voice. The quantitative measures maximum phonation time (MPT) and mean airflow rate (MFR) are reflections of the degree of closure, whereas pitch range tells something about the tension in the reconstructed vocal fold. The authors feel that arytenoid adduction can be helpful in nearly any type of unilateral vocal fold immobility case to improve the vocal outcomes. They looked at 39 patients in whom they performed arytenoid adduction and type I thyroplasty and recorded the patients both preoperatively and at 1 year postoperatively. They found statistically increased MPT (2.8–19.1 seconds), statistically decreased MFR (922.2–153 mL/s), and a significant increase in the pitch range from 3 semitones preoperatively to 17.5 semitones at the 1-year mark.

There is no doubt that controlling the position of the arytenoid aids in the closure of the larynx and in turn helps to achieve a louder and more substantial voice. With the vocal processes coming together in the midline and the tension somewhat matched, the patient is able to use the larynx in a more natural way with much higher dynamic range. Of all of the parameters, postoperative MPT correlated to improved pitch range. No preoperative data, no matter how good or bad, correlated this way.

In much the same way, surgically addressing the arytenoid is the proper thing to do to bring the cartilaginous vocal fold to the midline, and no cases were performed without the addition of a type I thyroplasty. The medialization aids substantially in the ability for the immobile membranous region to resist subglottic air pressure, ensuring a louder, more consistent voice. The idea that an arytenoid procedure should be done with each case of medialization is provocative and should warrant further investigation by other groups around the world.

R. Franco, MD

Application of Natural Orifice Transluminal Endoscopic Surgery (NOTES) Instrumentation to the Endolarynx

Tan M, Prufer N, Chinosornvatana N, et al (Mount Sinai School of Medicine, NY)
Ann Otol Rhinol Laryngol 121:435-441, 2012

Objectives.—RealHand instruments are high-dexterity instruments that have been designed for natural orifice transluminal endoscopie surgery applications. They provide dexterity by offering a full range of motion to endoscopie instruments. We hypothesize that RealHand instruments will resolve some of the limitations encountered in traditional endolaryngeal surgery. They have the potential to do so in the following ways: 1) they negate the limitation of mobility of traditional laryngoscopy instrumentation, which is rigid and fixed; 2) they maintain the ability of direct visualization through a telescope while precluding the need for an operating microscope; 3) they provide the dexterity to perform tasks that are otherwise not possible with traditional instrumentation; and 4) they provide flexibility that can be advantageous in difficult foreign body retrieval from distal airways.

Methods.—To test this hypothesis, we developed and optimized a cadaveric lamb larynx model for endolaryngeal microsurgery. To evaluate the feasibility of the RealHand instruments in their application to laryngeal surgery, we had 2 otolaryngology senior residents and 2 laryngology fellows-in-training perform 5 different endoscopic tasks: 1) foreign body removal; 2) arytenoidectomy; 3) microfiap elevation; 4) cricopharyngeal myotomy; and 5) endoknot suture tying.

Results.—Experience with RealHand instruments demonstrated that although they are limited in application to phonosurgery, they have the potential for more facile tissue manipulation in the supraglottic and hypopharyngeal structures. Endoscopic suturing ability is enhanced.

Conclusions.—RealHand high-dexterity instrumentation allows for full range-of-motion instrumentation and, with modification, has potential for wider application in endoscopie laryngeal surgery.

▶ As laryngeal surgeons, we have taken advantage of the natural entry into the larynx. Endoscopic laryngeal surgery is dependent on access to the endolarynx and the proper instrumentation to facilitate the intended procedure. The instruments currently in use are modified otologic instruments, elongated to accommodate the increased working distance to the larynx compared with the ear. Although they are specialized for working down the barrel of a laryngoscope, there are limitations to their use that transoral robotic surgery has highlighted. These include the incredible difficulty most people encounter when attempting suturing through the laryngoscope, the steep learning curve to properly using the instruments without tearing the mucosa from unwanted hand tremors, and the fulcruming that is used to stabilize the tips but results in the opposite movement distally (when the instrument handle is pushed down it results in tip elevation distally).

Natural orifice transluminal endoscopic surgery (NOTES) is a technique similar to laparoscopic that uses natural orifices to access the peritoneum via the stomach, the vagina, and the rectum. This approach minimizes incisions and decreases scarring and healing times. The authors of this study investigated the utility of using RealHand instruments designed for NOTES in the larynx. As can be seen in Fig 1 of the original article, RealHand instruments are full-range instruments that are capable of 360° of rotation and 70° of flexion. They devised a head-to-head competition that evaluated the time it took to remove a foreign body, elevate a microflap, perform an arytenoidectomy and, cricopharyngeal myotomy, and place a suture through the barrel of the endoscope. Although the tasks were completed with similar speed, and some were accomplished faster with the traditional instruments, the comments recorded revealed the longer the participants used the RealHand instruments, the more comfortable they felt using them. It seems the 15-minute tutorial was not enough to overcome the learning curve. The biggest limitation in the use of the RealHand instruments is the 5-mm size, making it necessary to use a rigid telescope to visualize the larynx because the line of sight is obscured by the 2 instruments. With the eventual modifications to decrease the profile of the instruments, the RealHand instruments may spawn new instruments that may help improve endolaryngeal surgery without the need for an expensive robot.

R. Franco, MD

Coblation of the Canine Vocal Fold: A Histologic Study

Divi V, Benninger M, Kiupel M, et al (Drexel Univ College of Medicine, Philadelphia, PA; Cleveland Clinic Foundation, OH; Michigan State Univ, East Lansing; et al)
J Voice 26:811.e9-811.e13, 2012

Controlled ablation (coblation) is a radiofrequency bipolar method of tissue ablation, which destroys tissue at very low temperatures. It has been used in a variety of clinical settings and is most frequently used by the otolaryngologist for tonsillectomy. In this study, we have examined the effect of coblation on the canine larynx by applying coblation to the vocal fold and harvesting the larynx on postoperative days (PODs) 0, 4, and 7. Histologic examination was performed with a variety of stains to examine the healing process. Coblation injury demonstrated complete epithelialization by POD 7. No injury to the underlying vocalis muscle was seen. The inflammatory response demonstrates less inflammation than previously reported with CO_2 laser injury. Coblation is a viable method for removal of tissue from the vocal fold resulting in minimal scar formation and a controlled depth of injury. Further studies should be performed to determine clinical utility in the removal of lesions such as respiratory papillomatosis (Figs 1 and 5).

► Coblation (controlled ablation) is a surgical cutting technique in which electric current is passed through irrigating saline, resulting in the polarization of the sodium ions. This occurs in a bipolar manner, causing destruction of tissue at the tip of the coblation wand. Coblation has been used in the removal of tonsils because of its superior thermal profile over electrocautery: 60° Celsius for coblation versus 400° Celsius for electrocautery. The belief is that less thermal injury results in less postoperative pain and an acceleration of the healing process. For tonsillectomy, the major factor limiting clinical improvement after surgery is the amount of pain because patients tend to become dehydrated when they do not drink because of the odynophagia. Keeping these patients pain-free goes a long way to giving them a rapid recovery. The hope is that this technology can be transferred to the vocal folds to allow resection of masses with less tissue damage.

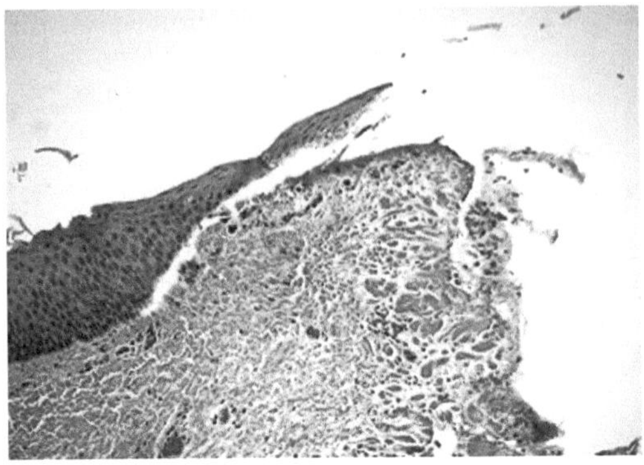

FIGURE 1.—Hematoxylin and eosin stain destruction of the superior surface of the epithelium on initial 7/3app injury. (Reprinted from Journal of Voice. Divi V, Benninger M, Kiupel M, et al. Coblation of the canine vocal fold: a histologic study. *J Voice.* 2012;26:811.e9-811.e13, Copyright 2012, with permission from The Voice Foundation.)

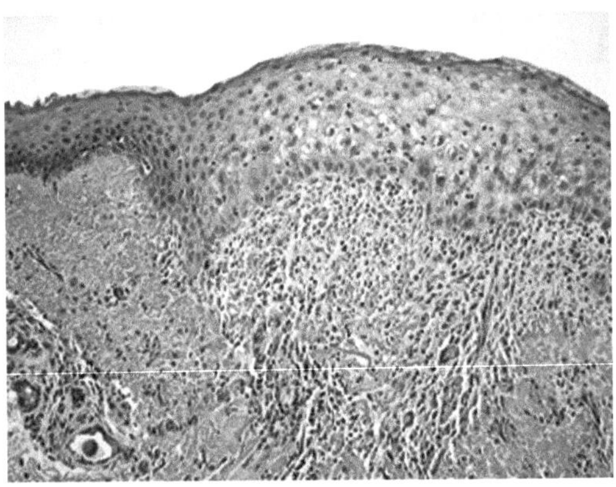

FIGURE 5.—Initial reepithelialization is complete by POD #7. (Reprinted from Journal of Voice. Divi V, Benninger M, Kiupel M, et al. Coblation of the canine vocal fold: a histologic study. *J Voice.* 2012;26:811.e9-811.e13, Copyright 2012, with permission from The Voice Foundation.)

The authors used the coblator at a setting of 7 to create injury to the vocal folds in a canine model. The dogs were sacrificed on Days 0, 4, and 7 after injury and the larynx analyzed histologically. Initially there were coagulative changes to the sample with inflammatory cells present on Day 4 and by Day 7 complete epithelialization in the sample. There was also less inflammation seen compared with using a carbon dioxide (CO_2) laser. Fig. 1 shows the initial injury with a hematoxylin and eosin stain, whereas Fig. 5 depicts postprocedure Day 7 with complete reepithelialization.

The major implications are for those patients who have recurrent diseases, notably bulky papilloma, who require multiple surgeries to debulk disease. For these patients, each surgical intervention potentially removes more superficial lamina propria, placing the voice at extreme risk. A technique that limits thermal damage is ideal. Cold instrument resection is the preferred method when possible, but the coblator could facilitate the removal of large amounts of disease in a reasonable amount of time without the risk profile (and thermal profile) of a CO_2 laser.

R. Franco, MD

A Transthyroidal Method for Arytenoid Adduction: A Basic Anatomical Study

Friedrich G, Gugatschka M, Kiesler K, et al (Med Univ Graz, Austria; et al)
J Voice 26:526-529, 2012

Introduction.—Arytenoid adduction is a very effective procedure for medializing the posterior part of the vocal fold in vocal fold paralysis. Major drawback of the method is the technically sometimes-difficult access to the arytenoid with increased postoperative morbidity. Aim of this study was to provide basic anatomical data regarding the accessibility of the arytenoid cartilage through a thyroplasty window. Furthermore, to investigate the feasibility of an arytenoid adduction by fixation of a surgical screw to the arytenoid cartilage by using this approach.

Materials and Methods.—10 cadaver larynges, six female and four male, were dissected and measured for our points of interest. A standard manufacture-made surgical screw attached to a suture was anchored to the fovea oblonga of the arytenoid cartilage.

Results.—Our anatomical measurements proved a mean distance from the posterior edge of the thyroid window to the arytenoid of about 8–9 mm in male larynges and 7–8 mm in female larynges. The distances did not differ significantly between the sexes. Pulling the anchored surgical screw medializes the posterior part of the vocal fold.

Discussion.—Our data showed that there is a very constant morphometric relation between the thyroplasty window and the arytenoid cartilage. It is known that gender-related differences result in a veritable laryngeal dimorphism in nearly all absolute laryngeal dimensions. These differences appear to a much lesser extend in the distances from the surface to the depth, as was confirmed in our series. Using these findings led us to identification of the fovea oblonga near the muscular process as the most favorable point for fixation of a surgical screw through a conventional thyroplasty window. Pulling the attached suture medializes the arytenoid cartilage.

▶ Reconstruction of paralytic dysphonia requires assessment of not only the degree of closure of the musculomembranous region, but also of any height discrepancies, differences in tension between the folds, and the position of the arytenoid cartilages. Arytenoid adduction is a method described by Isshiki to control the arytenoid cartilage to close the cartilaginous opening when, because of neurologic insult, the arytenoid moves lateral and inferior. As with many surgical techniques, numerous modifications have been made to the way the arytenoid is approached, including resection of a large posterior thyroid cartilage window and disarticulation of the cricothyroid joint. The authors in this article used the thyroplasty window to access the anterior face of the arytenoid without the need for a posterior approach. Although there are morphometric differences between male and female larynges, the distance from the posterior edge of the thyroplasty window to the fovea oblonga (Fig 3 in the original article) (midportion of the body of the arytenoid body) was between 7 and 9 mm (female-male), regardless of sex. Through this access window, a 2.4-mm × 7.5-mm metal suture anchor with 2 suture limbs was screwed into the fovea oblonga to allow the limbs to recreate the pull of the lateral cricoarytenoid (LCA) muscle. This causes the vocal process to move medially and the muscular process to swing laterally, effectively closing the posterior gap in many cases.

The theoretical disadvantage to the arytenoid adduction is the vector formed by recreating the action of the LCA muscle: It is an anterior and inferior pulling force that can take a denervated arytenoid away from its phonatory position to an inferior and anterior location. This anterior pull could also potentially make the musculomembranous region slack from a reduction in tension. The adduction arytenopexy, a procedure that sutures the arytenoid into place, has the effect of bringing the body of the arytenoid medial, pulled posteriorly and superiorly, effectively elongating the vocal fold and restoring tension. The reality is that either technique in the proper surgical hands has proven successful.

R. Franco, MD

Anatomical variations of the external branch of the superior laryngeal nerve in relation to the inferior constrictor muscle: cadaveric dissection study

Patnaik U, Nilakantan A, Shrivastava T (Base Hosp and Army College of Med Sciences, New Delhi, India)

J Laryngol Otol 126:907-912, 2012

Objectives.—To determine anatomical variations in the external branch of the superior laryngeal nerve in relation to the inferior constrictor muscle, and to propose a rational approach for the preservation of the nerve in thyroid surgery based on anatomical principles.

Method.—A cadaveric dissection study of the anatomy of the external branch of the superior laryngeal nerve in relation to the inferior constrictor muscle was conducted. Twenty-nine formalin-fixed cadavers of both sexes (age 50–70 years), with normal necks, were examined.

Results.—In relation to the Friedman classification, three anatomical variations of the external branch of the superior laryngeal nerve were found. Type 1 variation was found in 57.1 per cent of cases, type 2 in 26.8 per cent and type 3 in 16 per cent.

Conclusion.—The prevalence of type 3 variation of the external branch of the superior laryngeal nerve suggests that the nerve will not be encountered in a certain percentage of individuals as it lies under the cover of the

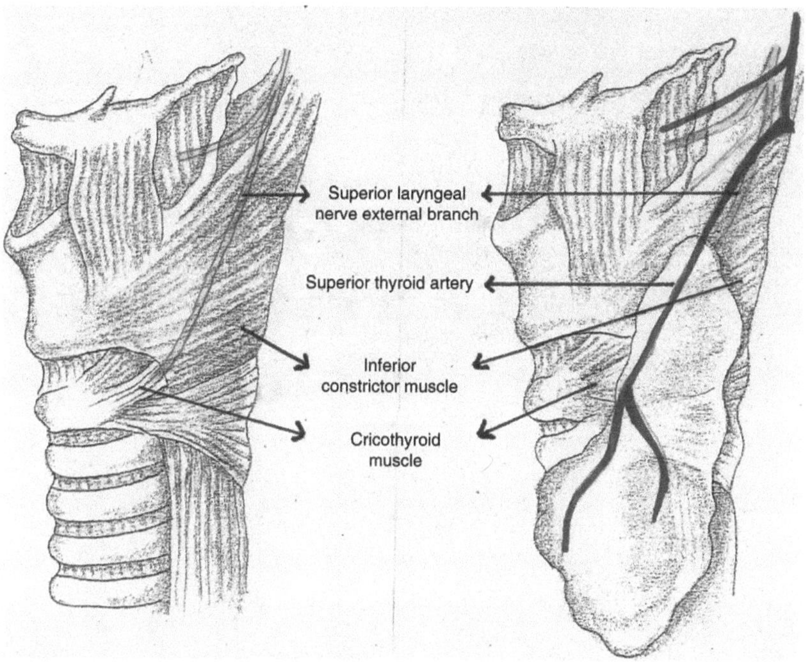

FIGURE 4.—Anatomical diagram showing type 1 Friedman variant: the external branch of the superior laryngeal nerve runs superficial to the inferior constrictor muscle. (Reprinted from Patnaik U, Nilakantan A, Shrivastava T. Anatomical variations of the external branch of the superior laryngeal nerve in relation to the inferior constrictor muscle: Cadaveric dissection study. *J Laryngol Otol.* 2012;126:907-912, with permission of Cambridge University Press.)

inferior constrictor. Therefore, there is no justification for attempting to identify the nerve in all cases (Figs 4-6).

▶ Thyroidectomy is a commonly performed procedure by otolaryngologists that potentially has big implications for the function of the voice postoperatively. Most of the time, it is the recurrent laryngeal nerve that grabs the headlines, considering it is the major nerve that controls the motor function to the larynx. It innervates all of the intrinsic muscles of the larynx, including the very important posterior cricoarytenoid muscle, the only abductor muscle in the larynx, making it a very important nerve to preserve. Almost all of the attention during surgery is given to the identification and preservation of the recurrent laryngeal nerve through nerve monitoring and stimulation, careful dissection when close to the expected course of the nerve, and pericapsular dissection of soft tissue when removing the gland. The problem is that during thyroidectomy, because of the focus on the recurrent laryngeal nerve, the superior laryngeal nerve is many times forgotten. The superior laryngeal nerve bifurcates into the internal and external branches. The internal branch pierces the thyrohyoid membrane and gives sensation to the endolarynx. The external branch has to make its way to the cricothyroid muscle, placing it at risk of injury when the superior thyroid

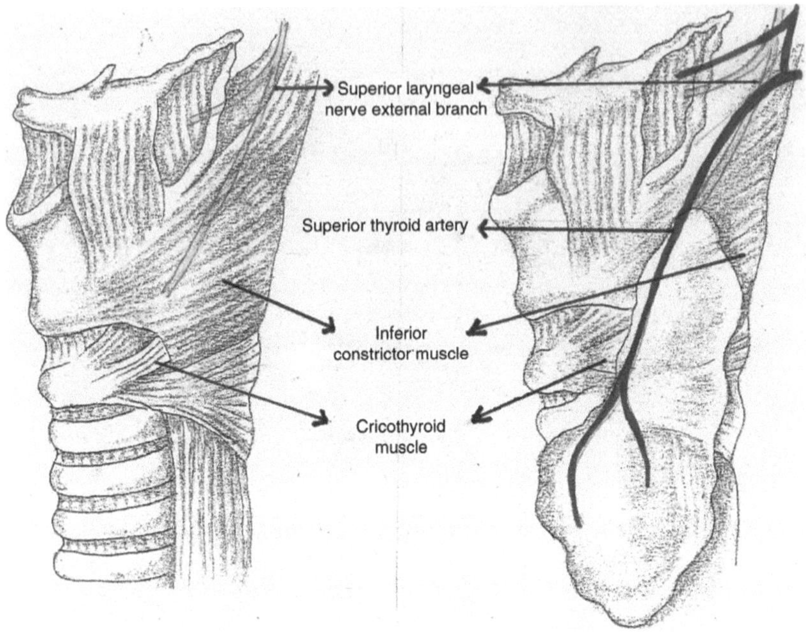

FIGURE 5.—Anatomical diagram showing type 2 Friedman variant: the external branch of the superior laryngeal nerve runs partly under the cover of the inferior constrictor muscle. (Reprinted from Patnaik U, Nilakantan A, Shrivastava T. Anatomical variations of the external branch of the superior laryngeal nerve in relation to the inferior constrictor muscle: Cadaveric dissection study. *J Laryngol Otol.* 2012;126:907-912, with permission of Cambridge University Press.)

vessels are ligated. Dysfunction of the superior laryngeal nerve also causes dysfunction and decreased quality of life, but in more subtle ways than a dysfunctional recurrent nerve. The external branch of the superior laryngeal nerve innervates the cricothyroid muscle that is responsible for the tension of the vocal fold and effecting register transitions. The voice issues after injury are not as dramatic and include subtle dysphonia, a deepening of the voice, loss of the ability to hit higher notes, and easy voice fatigue/inability to get loud. It also carries sensory information from the supraglottis to the level of the glottis, making injury to the internal branch of the superior laryngeal nerve a potentially disabling cause of aspiration.

The authors dissected cadavers to identify the course of the more vulnerable external branch of the superior laryngeal nerve as it relates to the inferior constrictor muscle and the superior thyroid pole. As can be seen in Figs 4-6, they found that in most cases (57%), the nerve runs external to the inferior pharyngeal constrictor (Fig 4), just under the superior thyroid vessels, making it easy to identify and preserve. In 27% of cases, it pierces the inferior constrictor muscle (Fig 5), making it more difficult to identify, whereas in 16% of cases, it is completely under the inferior constrictor throughout its journey to the cricothyroid muscle (Fig 6). These anatomic variations have been previously described and make it difficult to prescribe one way to proceed without potentially

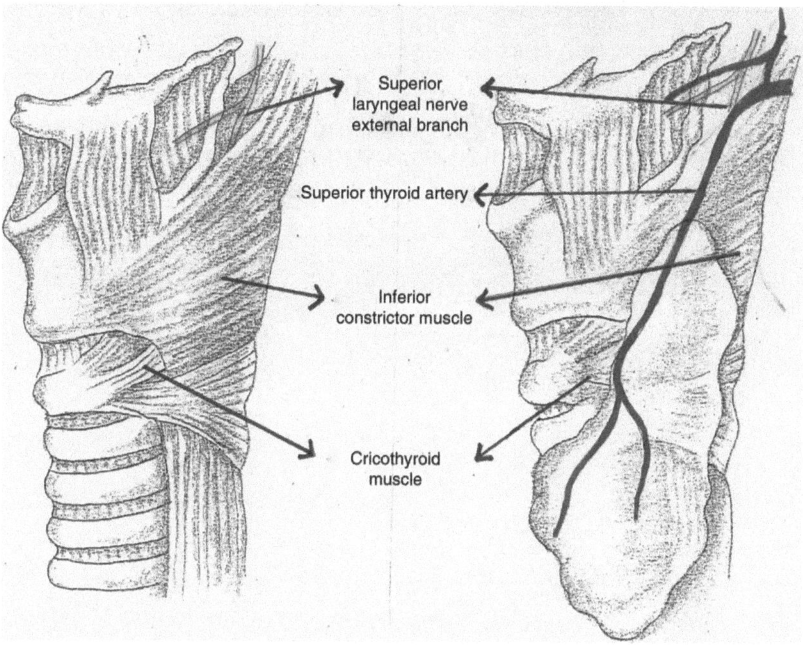

FIGURE 6.—Anatomical diagram showing type 3 Friedman variant: the external branch of the superior laryngeal nerve runs deep to the inferior constrictor muscle. (Reprinted from Patnaik U, Nilakantan A, Shrivastava T. Anatomical variations of the external branch of the superior laryngeal nerve in relation to the inferior constrictor muscle: Cadaveric dissection study. *J Laryngol Otol.* 2012;126:907-912, with permission of Cambridge University Press.)

injuring the nerve. The authors advocate that the external branch of the superior laryngeal nerve not be discretely identified (because of the anatomic variations). The best bet is still to take the superior thyroid vessels at the junction with the superior thyroid pole and dissect away any other soft tissue (ie, stay directly on the thyroid capsule).

R. Franco, MD

4 Otology

Basic and Clinical Research

Ototoxic Effect of Topical Oxiconazole and Terbinafine in Rats

Aydın E, Tastan E, Aydoğan F, et al (Ankara Training and Res Hosp, Turkey; et al)

J Otolaryngol Head Neck Surg 41:78-83, 2012

Objective.—To assess the ototoxic effects of topically applied oxiconazole and terbinafine by means of auditory brainstem responses in rats.

Design.—Nonrandomized, controlled trial.

Setting.—Tertiary referral centre.

Material and Methods.—The experiment was performed in 36 mature male Wistar albino rats. The study was conducted on four groups of rats: 10 rats received 1% oxiconazole cream, 10 rats received 1% terbinafine cream, 8 rats had gentamicin solution (40 mg/mL), and 8 rats had saline solution. A total perforation was created on the left tympanic membrane. The agents used in the study were administered to the left middle ears of the animals twice daily through a transcanal route, in doses of 0.1 cc, for 10 days.

Main Outcome Measures.—Auditory brainstem response thresholds were obtained before the treatment and 7 days after termination of the application.

Results.—The differences in pre- and posttreatment thresholds for all stimuli (click, 1000 Hz, 4000 Hz) in auditory brainstem responses were statistically significant in the oxiconazole, terbinafine, and gentamicin groups ($p < .0125$). When the saline and gentamicin groups were compared to the other groups, auditory brainstem response threshold findings for all stimuli after the treatment showed statistically significant differences ($p < .05$).

Conclusion.—Oxiconazole and terbinafine showed ototoxic effects reflected by elevated auditory brainstem response thresholds at the speech frequencies after being topically applied to the middle ear of rats. Further studies are needed to determine whether these auditory brainstem response threshold shifts are permanent.

▶ Treatment of otomycosis can be difficult, particularly if there is a coexistent perforation. As the authors state in their introduction, the wide use of broad-spectrum topical antibiotic preparations used for otorrhea from middle ear infections can, not infrequently, result in this situation. This is particularly true if the antibiotic used has a neutral pH, such as ofloxacin, which further promotes the growth of fungal organisms such as yeast. Further, it is the otolaryngologist who is faced with this situation after primary treatment. Although the ototoxic potential of antibacterials has been well studied, the toxicity of antifungals, particularly the newer ones, has not, hence, the importance of this article. Their methods are straightforward and standard for this type of work. Inner ear histology is not presented, which is a limitation of the study. The results demonstrate essentially equal toxicity for these antifungal agents as that of the control aminoglycoside. The authors acknowledge that the analysis is only short term—7 days posttreatment. A longer time point will be useful to determine if the effects are temporary or permanent. However, in the case of aminoglycosides, these have been used for decades in infected ears with little incidence of ototoxicity. This is thought to be from inflammation of the middle ear, which may provide a protective effect to the inner ear. Thus, this study may overestimate the ototoxic effect, as the middle ears of the animals used were not inflamed (in fact, Gelfoam was placed as a depot reservoir). This is the major limitation of the study. These factors are not mentioned by the authors and should temper the strength of their findings.

B. J. Balough, MD

Otologic Safety of Manuka Honey

Aron M, Victoria Akinpelu O, Dorion D, et al (Université de Sherbrooke, Quebec, Canada; Montreal Children's Hosp, Quebec, Canada)

J Otolaryngol Head Neck Surg 41:S21-S30, 2012

Objective.—To investigate the possible ototoxic effects of a 50% concentration of manuka honey in a chinchilla animal model.

Study Design.—A prospective, controlled animal study.

Setting.—The Research Institute of the Montreal Children's Hospital, McGill University Health Centre.

Subjects and Methods.—Eight animals had myringotomy incisions in both ears. One ear was randomly assigned to receive the 50% manuka honey solution. The contralateral ear received saline and served as the control ear.

Outcome Measures.—Auditory brainstem evoked responses (ABRs) were measured bilaterally for a wide range of frequencies (between 8 and 25 kHz) before and 2 weeks after transtympanic manuka honey and saline application. The animals were sacrificed, and all cochleae were dissected out and processed for light and scanning electron microscopy (SEM).

Results.—The measured ABR thresholds after the application of 50% concentration of manuka honey revealed severe ototoxicity in all honey-exposed ears. This was accompanied by gross physical changes and histologic evidence of hair cell toxicity on SEM and light microscopy. The control ears remained unchanged during the period of the experiment.

Conclusion.—Although 50% concentration of manuka honey is the proven concentration to have bactericidal properties against biofilms of

Pseudomonas aeruginosa and *Staphylococcus aureus*, this concentration appeared to have caused severe or intense inflammatory changes that produced facial paralysis, vestibulotoxicity, and hearing loss.

▶ "Without failure there can be no success," is an oft-reported adage in sport, politics, and science. Unfortunately, in medical literature, success is frequently reported while failure less so. In this article, the authors report their failure, but the abstract alone does little to emphasize the significance of what they are trying to achieve or where this failure may lead to success and why continuing to try is important. From the background, the following points are made: First, chronic suppurative ear disease shares many similarities with chronic sinonasal disease, not the least of which is that biofilm plays a significant role. Second, in many countries where this disease is most prevalent, access to antibiotics or long-term intravenous administration of antibiotics to eradicate biofilm is very limited, as is surgical care to remove disease. Thus, an effective, topically applied agent is very attractive, particularly if readily available. Manuka honey fits this profile and has been effective for treating chronic skin wounds. Regarding the study itself, a few criticisms of their methodology to establish ototoxicity can be made. First, the frequency range used is typical for most rodent species, but an advantage of the chinchilla model is that the hearing range is very similar to that of humans. This higher frequency range may lead to errors in the responses and overestimation of the losses. Second, insert earphones were used to deliver the stimulus and not bone conduction. The authors acknowledge this second limitation. However, these methodologic issues of auditory measurement are countered by the histologic evidence of toxicity as well as the universal presence of facial nerve paralysis and labyrinthine dysfunction. Despite this failure, it is in the discussion in which the foundation for further work and possible success can be found. A detailed examination of causal factors for the toxicity that was seen is explored with pH and osmolality being most likely. Further, a lower 4% solution in 2 pilot animals did not seem to produce the same toxic effects. What remains unknown is the lowest concentration that will provide beneficial antimicrobial action. If that lower concentration is proven to be safe, then a tremendous success will have been achieved starting from this initial spectacular failure.

B. J. Balough, MD

Transtympanic balloon dilatation of eustachian tube: a human cadaver pilot study

Kepchar J, Acevedo J, Schroeder J, et al (Walter Reed Natl Military Med Ctr, Bethesda, MD)

J Laryngol Otol 126:1102-1107, 2012

Objective.—To determine the feasibility and safety of transtympanic balloon dilatation of the eustachian tube.

Methods.—Transtympanic eustachian tube dilatation was performed on six cadaver heads using balloon catheters. Catheters were placed in each eustachian tube and the head scanned by computed tomography.

Randomised, blinded dilatation of one balloon in each head was performed, followed again by a second computed tomography scan. The scans were reviewed by a neurotologist and neuroradiologist who were blinded to previous treatment, and measurable dilatation and incidental damage noted.

Results.—There was adequate placement of the balloon catheter beyond the bony isthmus in 6 of 10 eustachian tubes. There was one insufficient catheter placement and three adverse placements (one into the petrous carotid canal and two into the vidian canal). Only one dilated tube showed a measurable increase in diameter.

Conclusion.—This experiment revealed serious safety issues with transtympanic eustachian tube dilatation. Therefore, this approach should not be considered feasible at this time.

▶ Improper functioning of the eustachian tube is thought to be the source for many ear-related symptoms. Though much of its course is relatively inaccessible, both the nasal and tympanic apertures provide a route for access. The authors provide a good review of the recent nasal approaches and treatments, many of which have shown promise. However, for the otologist, an approach via the tympanic opening that could be performed concurrently during reconstructive or other middle ear procedures is attractive; thus, this study explores using balloon dilation from this approach. Unfortunately, the results were poor both in terms of successful dilation and in terms of potential severe complications. The authors do admit the intubations of the carotid and vidian canals were in specimens with occult temporal bone fractures. However, in many cases, the bony lamina between the carotid and eustachian tube is very thin, making the likelihood of carotid injury from balloon inflation very real. Additionally, the bony portion of the tube is unlikely to be the cause of obstruction given that it is static, and as long as there is no complete obstruction, airflow should not be affected. Thus, addressing the dynamic nasal side is much more likely to provide benefit. Nonetheless, these negative results that highlight the potential problems are important to review to temper trial studies in patients.

B. J. Balough, MD

Dorsolateral Prefrontal Cortex Transcranial Magnetic Stimulation and Electrode Implant for Intractable Tinnitus

De Ridder D, Vanneste S, Plazier M, et al (Univ Hosp Antwerp, Belgium; Univ Hosp Louvain, Belgium)

World Neurosurg 77:778-784, 2012

Objective.—Tinnitus is a distressing symptom that affects up to 15% of the population; no satisfactory treatment exists. We present a novel surgical approach for the treatment of intractable tinnitus based on electrical extradural stimulation of the dorsolateral prefrontal cortex via an electrode implant. Tinnitus can be considered an auditory phantom phenomenon similar to deafferentation pain in the somatosensory system. It is characterized by gamma-band activity in the frontal cortex that can be visualized with the use of electroencephalography, magnetoencephalography, and functional magnetic resonance imaging (fMRI).

Case Description.—Transcranial magnetic stimulation (TMS) is a noninvasive technique capable of modulating the ongoing activity of the human brain. When linked with a neuronavigation system, fMRI-guided frontal cortex TMS can be performed in a placebo-controlled way. If it is successful in suppressing tinnitus, this focal and temporary effect can be maintained in perpetuity by implanting a cortical electrode. A neuronavigation-based auditory fMRI-guided frontal cortex TMS session was performed in a patient experiencing intractable tinnitus, yielding 50% tinnitus suppression. Two extradural electrodes were subsequently implanted, also based on auditory fMRI-guided navigation. Postoperatively the tinnitus has improved by 66.67% and progressively continues to improve for more than one year.

Conclusion.—Focal extradural electrical stimulation of the dorsolateral prefrontal cortex at the area of cortical plasticity is capable of suppressing contralateral tinnitus partially. TMS might be a possible method for noninvasive studies of surgical candidates for implantation of stimulating electrodes for tinnitus suppression.

► Despite being a common symptom affecting a large portion of the population, our understanding of tinnitus pathophysiology remains limited, as does the efficacy of our treatments. The concepts discussed in this article and the accompanying commentary move toward a more fundamental unified framework for the underlying mechanism of tinnitus. Benign tinnitus is a very crude definition for those suffering at the extremes of this disorder, and it doesn't help to categorize a malady that can range from a mild distraction to severe discomfort, with hearing ranging from normal to profound loss and unilateral or bilateral symptoms. Likewise, a simple model of loss of afferent input leading to cortical reorganization does not address the psychological symptoms accompanying tinnitus that seem to be independent of other characteristics such as loudness. In this case, the authors combine advanced neuroimaging, neuronavigation, and noninvasive temporary treatment to better tailor surgical intervention for tinnitus control. What emerges is a theory of tinnitus generation that relies not solely on the auditory cortex (a necessary, but not sufficient condition), but rather involves the active participation of other regions such as the prefrontal cortex as well as cortical regions. This emergent network as described not only better defines what causes tinnitus but also the variation seen in its manifestations. It also opens new areas for better diagnostic quantification, which in turn allows quantification of response to treatment. It is through multidisciplinary approaches to tinnitus such as this where real advances will be made; hence, it is worthy for the otolaryngologist to stay abreast of these findings.

B. J. Balough, MD

Restoration of auditory evoked responses by human ES-cell-derived otic progenitors

Chen W, Jongkamonwiwat N, Abbas L, et al (Univ of Sheffield, UK)
Nature 490:278-282, 2012

Deafness is a condition with a high prevalence worldwide, produced primarily by the loss of the sensory hair cells and their associated spiral ganglion neurons (SGNs). Of all the forms of deafness, auditory neuropathy is of particular concern. This condition, defined primarily by damage to the SGNs with relative preservation of the hair cells, is responsible for a substantial proportion of patients with hearing impairment. Although the loss of hair cells can be circumvented partially by a cochlear implant, no routine treatment is available for sensory neuron loss, as poor innervation limits the prospective performance of an implant. Using stem cells to recover the damaged sensory circuitry is a potential therapeutic strategy. Here we present a protocol to induce differentiation from human embryonic stem cells (hESCs) using signals involved in the initial specification of the otic placode. We obtained two types of otic progenitors able to differentiate *in vitro* into hair-cell-like cells and auditory neurons that display expected electrophysiological properties. Moreover, when transplanted into an auditory neuropathy model, otic neuroprogenitors engraft, differentiate and significantly improve auditory-evoked response thresholds. These results should stimulate further research into the development of a cell-based therapy for deafness (Fig 4).

▶ For those interested in keeping up with the latest developments in hearing regeneration but not interested in reviewing multiple scientific reports, this article provides an excellent update on the state of the technology. Communicated in the form of a letter, the scientific approach and rationale for a series of experiments are provided, with the ultimate goal being regeneration of functional auditory neurons. This provides an excellent overview to the current state of the science without the need to review multiple separate studies. The scientific approach is well discussed, providing the logic behind the clinical need for regeneration of spiral ganglion cells as well as the basic science challenges to achieve this goal. The methods are well detailed, but in this style of communication they are presented more as a conversational lecture than in a separate section of steps. This adds to the overall appreciation and understanding of the work as not what was done but why the method was used. Fig 4 provides the end results. As can be seen, from a complete absence of auditory response, a substantial recovery was obtained beginning 4 weeks after transplantation and stabilizing by 7 to 8 weeks. Additionally, the density of viable transplanted cells resulted in improved thresholds. Thus, not only do the cells survive, but they make meaningful neural

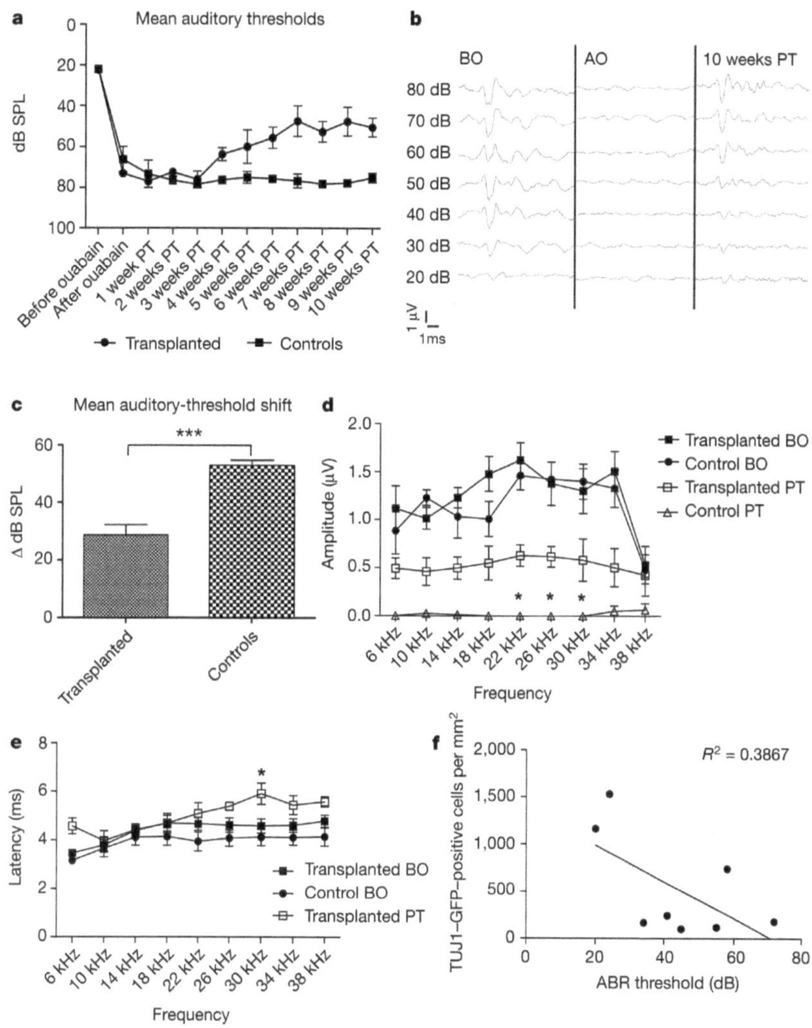

FIGURE 4.—Transplanted cells provide a recovery of ABR thresholds. **a**, Evolution of the mean ABR thresholds (click) obtained in the transplanted animals ($n = 518$; mean ± s.e.m.) compared to the controls ($n = 58$). **b**, Trace ABR showing the abolition of waves after ouabain (AO) treatment and the restoration of the complexes 10 weeks post transplanation (PT). **c**, Graph showing the mean auditory-threshold shift reduction obtained by the transplantation (transplanted 28.6 ± 3.6 dB; $n = 518$ versus 53 ± 1.7 dB; $n = 58$ in the control, $P = 0.0002$; mean + s.e.m). **d**, Comparison of the wave ii—wave iii amplitudes obtained by tone ABRs. A general trend of enhanced amplitudes was obtained across all frequencies tested, being significantly ($^*P < 0.05$) different from the untransplanted controls at 22, 26 and 30 kHz. Amplitudes before ouabain were equivalent between the transplanted ($n = 56$) and untransplanted animals ($n = 55$; mean ± s.e.m.). **e**, Latencies of wave ii—wave iii complexes were, in general, comparable before ouabain and after transplantation. Only at 30 kHz was a significant delay was observed (BO: 4.58 ± 0.2 ms, $n = 56$; PT: 5.9 ± 0.4 ms, $n = 55$; $P < 0.05$; mean ± s.e.m.). **f**, A significant correlation was observed between the mean density of TUJ1—GFP-positive cells and the ABR thresholds ($n = 58$; $P < 0.05$). $^*P < 0.05$; $^{***}P < 0.001$. (Reprinted by permission from Macmillan Publishers Ltd: Nature. Chen W, Jongkamonwiwat N, Abbas L, et al. Restoration of auditory evoked responses by human ES-cell-derived otic progenitors. *Nature*. 2012;490:278-282, Copyright 2012, with permission from Macmillan Publishers Limited.)

connections. Although not yet ready for human trials, this is a significant step along that path.

B. J. Balough, MD

The contribution of hearing to normal balance

Kanegaonkar RG, Amin K, Clarke M (Medway Maritime Hosp, Gillingham, UK)

J Laryngol Otol 126:984-988, 2012

Introduction.—Normal balance relies on three sensory inputs: vision, proprioception and the peripheral vestibular system. This study assessed hearing change and postural control in normal subjects.

Materials and Methods.—Postural control in 20 normal volunteers was assessed using a Nintendo Wii gaming console and balance board. Each subject was tested standing upright for 30 seconds in a clinic room and a soundproof room with their eyes open, eyes closed, whilst standing on and off foam, and with and without ear defenders.

Results.—There was significantly more postural sway in the following subjects: those standing with their eyes closed *vs* those with eyes open (normal room, $p = 0.0002$; soundproof room, $p = 0.0164$); those standing on foam with eyes open *vs* those standing normally with eyes open (in both rooms; $p < 0.05$); those standing with eyes open in a soundproof room *vs* a normal room ($p = 0.0164$); and those standing on foam in a soundproof room with eyes open and wearing ear defenders *vs* those in the same circumstances but without ear defenders.

Conclusion.—Our results suggest that this method provides a simple, inexpensive tool for assessing static postural control. Whilst it is recognised that visual input and proprioception play a central role in maintaining posture, our findings suggest that ambient sound and hearing may also have a significant influence (Table 3).

► Hearing provides not only communication but also a sense of place within our environment. Unlike vision, which is restricted to direct lines of sight, hearing can provide a 360° sense of the environment around us, which contributes to our sense of place and movement within that environment. To what extent this contributes to our postural stability is the subject of this study. An excellent

TABLE 3.—Postural Sway in Soundproof Room: Statistical Comparison

Comparison	Friedman's Statistic	*p*
Eyes open *vs* eyes closed	5.7619	0.0164
Eyes open *vs* eyes open with ear defenders	0.0476	0.8273
Eyes open *vs* eyes open on foam	3.8571	0.0495
Eyes open *vs* eyes open on foam with ear defenders	5.7619	0.0164
Eyes closed *vs* eyes closed with ear defenders	0.0476	0.8273
Eyes closed *vs* eyes closed on foam	0.4286	0.5127
Eyes closed on foam *vs* eyes closed on foam with ear defenders	3.8571	0.0495

summary of normal human balance function is provided in the first 3 paragraphs of the introduction. It is plainly written, easy to understand, and, with minor alterations, could be easily used to educate patients and others about how the balance system operates. It is worth reading. The next valuable piece from the study is their use of a video game console and accompanying balance board. This provides a simple and inexpensive method for performing balance assessment for those in need but with limited budgets or space for more dedicated vestibular testing equipment. Although used here for research data, this setup could easily be used to provide objective data at baseline and after treatment or a course of therapy. Although the design of the study is straightforward, the data presentation and discussion are a bit cumbersome, which detracts from the overall article value. But, as shown in Table 3, hearing does seem to play a role in positional awareness, but only a tertiary role after vision or postural stability are degraded. The implication here is important; namely, that in those with poor vision or postural control, such as the elderly, hearing rehabilitation becomes important to maintain balance and avoid falls.

B. J. Balough, MD

Gadolinium distribution in cochlear perilymph: differences between intratympanic and intravenous gadolinium injection

Yamazaki M, Naganawa S, Kawai H, et al (Nagoya Univ Graduate School of Medicine, Showa-ku, Japan)

Neuroradiology 54:1161-1169, 2012

Introduction.—Three-dimensional fluid-attenuated inversion recovery (3D-FLAIR) imaging 24 h after intratympanic gadolinium injection (IT method) or 4 h after intravenous injection (IV method) has been used to visualize endolymphatic hydrops in Ménière's disease. The aims of this study were to evaluate the difference in gadolinium distribution in cochlear perilymph between the two methods by comparing the enhancement of the basal and apical turns and clarify the pharmacokinetics in cochlear perilymph.

Methods.—A total of 24 ears of 22 patients who underwent the IT method (gadolinium-diethylene-triamine pentaacetic acid was diluted eightfold with saline) and 28 ears of 17 patients who underwent the IV method (double dose of gadoteridol (0.5 mmol/ml); 0.2 mmol/kg body weight in total amount) at 3 T was analyzed retrospectively. Regions of interest of the perilymph of the cochlear basal turn (B), of the apical turn (A), and the medulla oblongata (M) were determined on each patient. The signal intensity ratios between B and M (BMR), A and M (AMR), and A and B (ABR) were subsequently evaluated.

Results.—The IT-BMR (2.63 ± 1.22) was higher than the IV-BMR (1. 46 ± 0.45) ($p < 0.001$). There was no significant difference between the IT- (1.46 ± 0.76) and IV-AMRs (1.21 ± 0.48) ($p = 0.15$). The IT-ABR (0.58 ± 0.17) was lower than the IV-ABR (0. 84 ± 0.22) ($p < 0.001$).

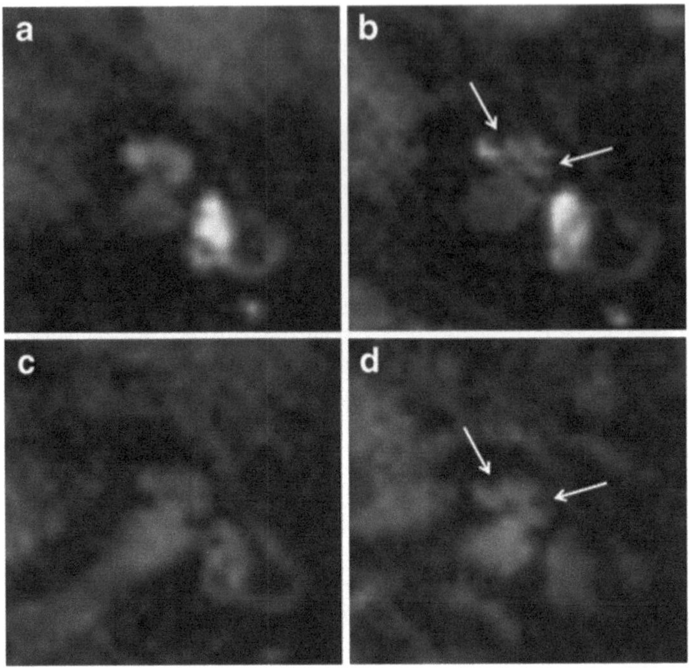

FIGURE 3.—3D-FLAIR images of the left cochlea at the level of the modiolus of a 67-year-old woman (**a**), a 68-year-old man (**b**), a 63-year-old woman (**c**), and a 28-year-old man (**d**) with suspected Ménière's disease are presented. Images **a** and **b** were obtained 24 h after intratympanic gadolinium injection and images **c** and **d** were obtained 4 h after intravenous gadolinium injection. On all images, the perilymph of the cochlea shows a high signal intensity. On images **b** and **d**, significant endolymphatic hydrops in the cochlea can be recognized as areas of low intensity (*arrows* on **b** and **d**) and the area of the endolymphatic space exceeds the area of the scala vestibule (endolymphatic hydrops grade 2). In contrast, on images **a** and **c**, there are no endolymphatic hydrops in the cochlea and the recognition of the endolymphatic space is difficult (endolymphatic hydrops grade 0). (With kind permission from Springer Science+Business Media. Yamazaki M, Naganawa S, Kawai H, et al. Gadolinium distribution in cochlear perilymph: differences between intratympanic and intravenous gadolinium injection. *Neuroradiology.* 2012;54:1161-1169, with permission from Springer-Verlag.)

Conclusion.—Gadolinium was predominantly distributed in the basal turn compared with the apical turn in the IT method, whereas it was more uniformly distributed in the IV method. These characteristics might reflect the distribution of therapeutic medications administered either intratympanically or systemically (Fig 3).

▶ Advances in imaging technology continue to rapidly evolve, allowing visualization of anatomic structures in greater detail. Among those structures of interest is the inner ear, given its protected location deep within the temporal bone. In this study, 2 of the methods that have been developed using intravenous or intratympanic administration of contrast are directly compared. The "introduction" and "methods" sections describe the contrast delivery and imaging process in good enough detail to allow others to readily repeat this or similar studies using these techniques. Each method has its advantages. Intravenous administration allows both ears to be visualized, potentially revealing silent disease in the nonsuspect ear or clarifying which ear has the disease when symptoms or other data may be conflicting. Additionally, intravenous administration is routine for radiology suites, avoiding a separate visit. However, intravenous administration requires imaging 4 hours later, leading to potential scheduling inconveniences for the patient. Additionally, the dose of contrast is double the usual amount, which may be problematic for some patients. On the other hand, intratympanic administration is performed the day before imaging and avoids systemic delivery of contrast. The intensity of contrast enhancement may also be greater but mostly in the basal turn and less in the apical turn because of diffusion. Each ear must also be injected separately. Fig 3 provides an example of the detail that can be obtained from each method. Although the purpose of this study was to evaluate for endolymphatic hydrops in groups of patients with suspected Ménière's disease, the 2 patient groups were different, making head-to-head comparisons for this application difficult. Additionally, the patients were not stratified into categories of confirmed, suspected, or probable of having Ménière's disease based on accepted criteria. Thus, there is limited utility in the article for this purpose. However, as these techniques develop and become more widely accepted, it is beneficial to understand their differences and limitations; therefore, it is included in this year's selections.

B. J. Balough, MD

External Ear, Middle Ear and Mastoid

Language and Behavioral Outcomes in Children With Developmental Disabilities Using Cochlear Implants

Cruz I, The CDaCI Investigative Team (Univ of Miami, FL; et al)

Otol Neurotol 33:751-760, 2012

Objective.—Over the past decade, the number of deaf children with developmental disabilities receiving cochlear implants has increased dramatically. However, little is known about the developmental outcomes of these children post-implantation. The current study evaluated oral language and behavioral outcomes over 3 years after implantation in a sample of typically developing deaf children and children with developmental disabilities.

Study Design.—A three year longitudinal study of the effects of cochlear implantation on language and behavioral outcomes in children with and without additional disabilities.

Setting.—Six cochlear implant centers in the United States.

Patients.—The study cohort consisted of 188 deaf children. Eighty-five percent of the sample (n = 157) had a single diagnosis of severe to profound hearing loss and 15% (n = 31) had an additional disability.

Main Outcome Measures.—Oral language was assessed using the Reynell Developmental Language Scales, and behavioral outcomes were assessed using the Child Behavior Checklist.

Results.—Results using multilevel modeling indicated that deaf children with and without additional disabilities improved significantly in oral language skills post-implantation. However, children with additional disabilities made slower progress. In terms of specific diagnoses, children with developmental disorders, such as autism, made the slowest progress over time. In addition, behavior problems increased significantly in this group, whereas behavior problems decreased over 3 years in the typically developing deaf sample.

Conclusion.—Overall, given the improvements in expressive and receptive language skills documented over 3 years, these findings support the use of cochlear implants for deaf children with developmental disabilities.

▶ Over time the criteria for cochlear implantation have expanded to include children younger in age. As the authors discuss in their introduction, these younger children are often implanted before the emergence of additional disabilities. As a result, more of these children with additional disabilities are available for study as to the effects on implant performance in this population. An interesting corollary to this discussion is that previously these children would not have been considered for candidacy, but that is outside the scope of this article. Two items were analyzed: language development and behavior. Not surprisingly, those with additional disability had lower initial scores for language initially and throughout the study period. However, despite the lower starting and finishing scores, significant progress was made in the groups regardless of disability type, although more slowly than in those with deafness alone. Additionally, those with attention deficit performed the same as those without any additional disability. Regarding the behavioral measures, for the deaf-only group these improved over time. For those with additional disabilities, the scores declined. Thus cochlear implantation did not provide appreciable benefit in behavior. This is shown in Fig 3 of the original article, although the captions do not reflect the findings. It is unclear why this comment is made based on the data, and it represents a criticism of the article. Thus, although language development is aided by cochlear implantation, the behavioral gains typically seen in the deaf child are not reproduced in those with additional disabilities. This information is important in shaping expectations for parents and caregivers alike. As one of the first studies of its kind and for these important findings, it is included in this year's list.

B. J. Balough, MD

Cochlear Implantation: A Personal and Societal Economic Perspective Examining the Effects of Cochlear Implantation on Personal Income

Monteiro E, Shipp D, Chen J, et al (Sunnybrook Health Sciences Centre, Toronto, Ontario, Canada)

J Otolaryngol Head Neck Surg 41:S43-S48, 2012

Objective.—Although cochlear implantation has been shown to improve quality of life, the socioeconomic benefit to the individual and society has not been thoroughly investigated. Our objective was to determine the economic impact of profound deafness and subsequent effects of unilateral cochlear implantation.

Design.—Retrospective analysis of a prospectively collected cochlear implantation database.

Setting.—An academic, tertiary care hospital.

Methods.—A prospectively collected cochlear implantation database of 702 patients was reviewed. Known Canadian economic surrogates were used to estimate the personal economic impact of both deafness and unilateral cochlear implantation.

Main Outcome Measures.—The main outcome measures included employment rates and personal income prior to and following cochlear implantation.

Results.—A total of 637 patients had sufficient occupational data for inclusion in the study; 36.7% suffered a negative economic impact as a result of their deafness. Cochlear implantation was associated with a significant increase in median yearly income compared to preimplantation ($42 672 vs $30 432; $p = .007$).

Conclusions.—Cochlear implantation not only improves quality of life but also translates into significant economic benefits for patients and the Canadian economy. These benefits appear to exceed the overall costs of cochlear implantation.

▶ Numerous prior studies have demonstrated the economic benefit of cochlear implantation for society and enhanced quality of life for the individual. Uniquely, this article studies the economic impact of implantation of the individual. For this reason, it has been added to this year's selections. Not surprisingly, the disability of deafness results in job loss, early retirement, and permanent removal from the workforce in significant numbers, as shown in Table 2 of the original article. The corresponding benefit is illustrated in Fig 2 of the original article. The references included provide an excellent background for those wishing to further explore this area. As with any study of this nature involving population data, self-reporting surveys, and estimates, the results are approximations. These limitations are acknowledged by the authors, mitigated by having a single cohort prospectively followed. The strength of the findings also supports their conclusions, despite the limitations of the design. In their discussion, the authors tie the individual economic benefit back to society. Namely, the increased personal income is in part returned to the government through increased tax revenue. As government becomes more important as a health care purchaser, this is an important consideration. One item not addressed by the study in this regard is that of implant device cost. Unlike most other sophisticated electronic devices that rapidly decline in cost after initial introduction, cochlear implants have not significantly declined in cost, thereby limiting their accessibility to many who would benefit around the world. Although some of this high cost may be explained by research and development budgets, the basic costs of circuitry and manufacturing should be low. Thus, although studies such as this prove the economic benefit is valuable, more studies are needed to examine and question the cost structure of implantation so that more may share in the benefits.

B. J. Balough, MD

The Importance of Ulceration of Cutaneous Melanoma of the Head and Neck: A Comparison of Ear (Pinna) and Nonear Sites

Augenstein AC, Capello ZJ, Little JA, et al (Univ of Louisville School of Medicine, KY)

Laryngoscope 122:2468-2472, 2012

Objectives/Hypothesis.—To compare clinicopathologic and prognostic factors associated with ear melanomas and nonear melanomas of the head and neck (H&N).

Study Design.—Post hoc analysis of the database from a multi-institutional, prospective, randomized study.

Methods.—Clinicopathologic factors were assessed and correlated with survival and recurrence. Univariate and multivariate analysis of prognostic factors affecting disease-free survival (DFS) and overall survival (OS) were performed.

Results.—Of 405 patients with H&N melanomas ≥ 1.0 mm Breslow thickness, 59 patients had melanomas of the ear. Most were Caucasian (96.6%) males (79.7%) with a mean age of 52 years. The mean Breslow thickness was 2.5 mm; 34.5% had signs of ulceration. Sentinel lymph node (SLN) positivity was seen in 7.1%. The incidence of locoregional and distant recurrence were similar. OS for ear melanoma was significantly impacted by ulceration status ($P = .013$), whereas both ulceration and SLN positivity predicted survival in nonear melanoma ($P < .001$ and $P = .015$, respectively). Thicker melanomas in the nonear group demonstrated significantly decreased DFS, whereas other factors in both groups lost their predictive value ($P = .035$).

Conclusions.—In the Sunbelt Melanoma Trial, ulceration was the strongest predictor of overall survival in melanoma of the ear. Ulceration and SLN status correlated with poorer OS in nonear melanoma of the H&N, whereas increasing depth correlated with poorer DFS in those same patients. Recurrence and survival were not impacted by anatomic site, but the prognostic significance of ulceration, thickness, and SLN status in the H&N may vary with the site of the melanoma (Tables 3 and 5).

▶ It is well known that basal cell and squamous cell cutaneous malignancies of the ears are potentially more dangerous than other head and neck locations. This article seeks to answer the same question for melanoma of the auricle. The data are taken from a large, multicenter study of melanoma. The authors discuss the limitations of the study, chiefly that the nonear head and neck melanomas outnumbered the ear melanomas by 6 to 1, thus dominating the calculations. The ear group was also a relatively small number of patients for this type of analysis. It is unlikely such large groups of patients could be collected in any other fashion. Tables 3 and 5 show the results in which ulceration was a significant factor in addition to the expected positive sentinel lymph node and Breslow thickness. Interestingly, the impact was larger for overall survival than for disease-free survival. However, there were no differences between ear and nonear sites in

TABLE 3.—Univariant and Multivariant Statistical Models of Overall Survival of Ear Melanoma

Variable	Log-Rank *P* Value	Hazard Ratio (95% CI)	Cox *P* Value
Ear	.569	0.9 (0.5-1.9)	.865
Breslow thickness, mm	<.001	—	.223
0.0–2.0	—	Reference	Reference
2.0–4.0	—	1.3 (0.8-2.3)	.307
>4.0	—	1.8 (0.9-3.4)	.089
SLN positive	<.001	1.9 (1.1-3.3)	.024
Ulceration	<.001	3.2 (1.9-5.2)	.000

CI = confidence interval; SLN = sentinel lymph node.

TABLE 5.—Univariate and Multivariate Statistical Models of Disease-Free Survival of Ear Melanoma

Variable	Log-Rank *P* Value	Hazard Ratio (95% CI)	Cox *P* Value
Age	NA	0.99 (0.97-1.01)	.378
Ear	.883	0.9 (0.4-2.0)	.834
Breslow thickness, mm	.001	—	.057
0.0–2.0	—	Reference	Reference
2.0–4.0	—	1.6 (0.9-2.9)	.124
>4.0	—	2.3 (1.1-4.8)	.021
SLN positive	.014	1.6 (0.8-3.1)	.190
Ulceration	.009	1.6 (0.9-2.8)	.084

CI = confidence interval; NA = not applicable; SLN = sentinel lymph node.

these factors, unlike what has been seen in other cutaneous malignancies of the ear, which is an important factor to have defined.

B. J. Balough, MD

How Long is Long Enough to Follow up Children After Cholesteatoma Surgery?: A 29-year Study

Kuo C-L, Shiao A-S, Liao W-H, et al (Taipei Veterans General Hosp and Natl Yang-Ming Univ School of Medicine, Taiwan)
Laryngoscope 122:2568-2573, 2012

Objectives/Hypothesis.—To identify an association between follow-up period and cholesteatoma recidivism.

Study Design.—Retrospective review.

Methods.—From 1982 to 2011, we retrospectively screened a consecutive series of children (≤18 years) with acquired cholesteatomas after primary surgery. The cumulative recidivism rates were calculated using standard calculation methods and Kaplan-Meier survival analysis.

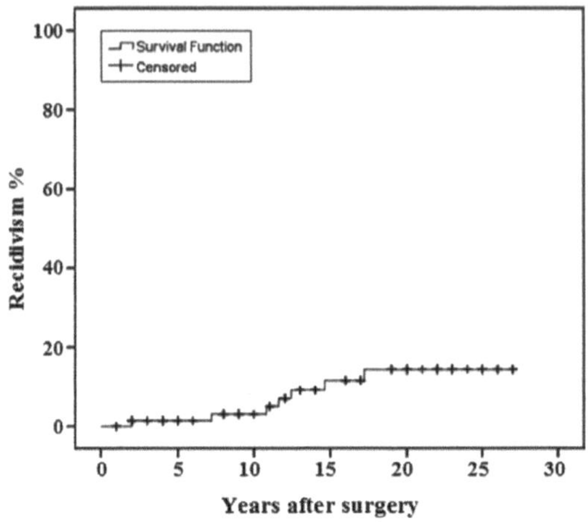

FIGURE 1.—Kaplan-Meier survival analysis of cholesteatoma recidivism. The risk of recidivism reached a stable level after 18 years. (Reprinted from Kuo C-L, Shiao A-S, Liao W-H, et al. How long is long enough to follow up children after cholesteatoma surgery?: a 29-year study. *Laryngoscope*. 2012;122:2568-2573, with permission from Laryngoscope and John Wiley and Sons, www.interscience.wiley.com.)

Results.—A total of 73 operations were performed on 71 patients. The mean age was 10.7 years, and the mean follow-up period was 15.4 years. The number of censored cases increased with the follow-up time. Sixty-four (88%) operations had a follow-up period of 5 years or longer, and 41 (56%) operations 15 years or longer. Cholesteatoma recidivism was observed in seven ears (five recurrent and two residual diseases). The mean detection time was 10.4 years (range 1.9–17.2 years). Five of the seven ears (71.4%) with recidivism were detected more than 10 years after surgery. The recidivism rate increased with the follow-up time. However, the rates at 5, 10, 15, 20, and 25 years as calculated by the standard calculation method (1.4%, 2.7%, 8.2%, 9.5% and 9.5%, respectively) were underestimated compared with that by Kaplan-Meier analysis (1.4%, 3.1%, 11.6%, 14.4% and 14.4%, respectively).

Conclusions.—The Kaplan-Meier survival analysis method should be used when discussing recidivism rates, because the number of censored cases inevitably increases with observation time. Due to the late occurrence of recidivism and because the recidivism rate increases as time goes on, children should be periodically followed up for as long as possible (Fig 1, Table 1).

▶ Rarely does a study provide more than a 25-year follow-up such as this one. Nor does one usually challenge conventional wisdom with such convincing data. Fig 1 provides the time course of cholesteatoma recurrence. As can be seen from the graph, after an initial jump there is a plateau out past 5 years, then another plateau to just past 10 years, and then a consistent, steady rise until a final plateau just before 20 years. This correlates to a recurrence rate of 1.4% at 5 years, 3.1% at 10 years, 11.6% at 15 years, and, finally, 14.4% at

TABLE 1.—CAO Staging System of Cholesteatoma[11]

Score	C (Cholesteatoma)*	A (Atelectasis)†	O (Ossicle)
1	1 area of middle ear cleft involved	Normal or grade I atelectasis	Normal or destruction of 1 ossicle
2	2 areas of middle ear cleft involved	Grade II or III atelectasis‡	Destruction of 2 ossicles
3	3, 4 or 5 areas of middle ear cleft involved	Grade IV atelectasis§	Destruction of 3 ossicles

Editor's Note: Please refer to original journal article for full references.
*The five areas of middle ear cleft are tympanic cavity, attic, aditus, antrum, and mastoid cavity.
†The degree of atelectasis is determined according to Sade[12] and Tos[13] classifications.
‡In cases of eardrum perforation, less than 50% of the middle ear mucosa is destroyed.
§In cases of eardrum perforation, more than 50% of the middle ear mucosa is destroyed.

20 years and beyond. Thus, there is a 10-fold higher rate at 20 years than at 5 years and a threefold higher rate at 15 years than at 10 years. As the authors discuss, based on these results, second-look surgery at 1 year may lead to a false sense of security and may be unnecessary. Further, the generally recommended 5-year period of follow-up is clearly not adequate. They favor regular visits for surveillance at least for 18 years or until adulthood based on their results. Another additional element is introduced in this article. The senior author has developed a grading system for cholesteatoma based on the extent of middle ear disease, the degree of tympanic membrane atelectasis, and the amount of ossicular erosion. Termed the CAO (cholesteatoma, atelectasis, ossicle) staging system, it is represented in Table 1. Interestingly, all but 1 of the recurrent cases were stage 3 (score of 7–9) on this system. Given the ease of use and should it prove to have true prognostic benefit as borne out in future studies, then this may be a very useful system. There are a few limitations in this study. First, despite the long duration of follow-up, the study population is relatively small, consisting of only 73 subjects. Second, although most underwent canal wall down operations, not all were treated in the same fashion, which may have affected the results. But given the other merits of the study, it is still a very worthwhile read with the potential to change practice patterns.

B. J. Balough, MD

Facial Nerve and Skull Base

Growth Characteristics of Vestibular Schwannomas

Moffat DA, Kasbekar A, Axon PR, et al (Cambridge Univ Teaching Hosps NHS Foundation Trust, UK; Monklands Hosp, Lanarkshire, UK; et al)
Otol Neurotol 33:1053-1058, 2012

Objective.—To assess the growth characteristics of small- to medium-sized vestibular schwannomas in patients undergoing watch, wait, and rescan management.

Study Design.—Cohort study using prospectively collected size and tumor morphology data.

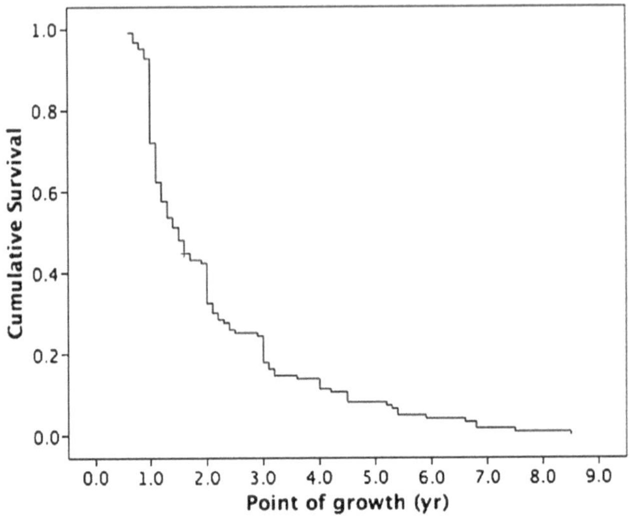

FIGURE 4.—Kaplan-Meier survival plot of growing tumors showing the point at which tumors first demonstrated radiologic evidence of growth after diagnosis. (Reprinted from Moffat DA, Kasbekar A, Axon PR, et al. Growth characteristics of vestibular schwannomas. *Otol Neurotol.* 2012;33:1053-1058, with permission from Otology & Neurotology, Inc.)

Setting.—Tertiary referral center for cranial base surgery.

Subjects and Methods.—Three hundred eighty-one patients with sporadic unilateral vestibular schwannomas and 2 or more magnetic resonance scans were included. Linear measurements were used to assess tumor size. The point of growth and pattern of growth progression were assessed. Factors influencing growth were investigated.

Results.—Approximately 33% of tumors demonstrated significant growth. Mean size at presentation was 9.9 mm (standard deviation [SD]. 4.8). For growing tumors, mean size at final review was 13.7 mm (SD, 4.8). This was a statistically significant increase in size ($p < 0.0001$). Mean annual change in size for growing tumors was 2.3 mm (SD, 2.3). 52.4% of growing tumors showed radiologically demonstrable first growth within 18 months of presentation. Approximately 7.2% of tumors showed radiologically demonstrable first growth after 5 years of follow-up. There were no demographic or morphologic predictors of growth.

Conclusion.—Tumor growth is usually slow and is most likely to occur within the first 3 years of observation. Growth may occur after five years of follow-up. A protocol for the scanning of patients is suggested based on the findings of the study (Fig 4).

▶ As the authors discuss in their introduction, although many studies have been published on the natural growth history of vestibular schwannomas, many are small series, use inconsistent measurements of size, or include a heterogeneous collection of tumors—large and neurofibromatosis types—all of which create problems interpreting the results. Thus, this study is significant in that it represents a single large cohort followed prospectively over many years and consisting of uniform reporting of size. This cohort was collected over a 20-year period in which in the last 15 years, observation became an increasingly popular treatment option. The most important data from the study are represented in Fig 4. For those tumors showing growth (nearly one-third of the entire cohort) most did so in the first 3 years, suggesting enhanced vigilance during this time. Equally important, however, is that some 7% of all growing tumors did so after 5 years, thus reinforcing the need for lifelong monitoring. This is perhaps the most significant finding from the study and supports their recommended scanning interval of 6 months, annually until 3 years, then every 2 years until 6 years, and every 3 years thereafter. Regarding the amount of growth, most grew between 2 and 4 mm/y. A few, however, grew at a rate faster than this with one showing an annual growth of more than 10 mm. Unfortunately, neither age, sex, nor size at presentation was predictive of future growth. Going forward, finding factors predictive of growth will be particularly valuable.

B. J. Balough, MD

The effect of the 2003 Consensus Reporting Standards on publications describing patients with vestibular schwannoma treated with stereotactic radiosurgery

Han SJ, Oh MC, Sughrue ME, et al (Univ of California at San Francisco)
J Clin Neurosci 19:1144-1147, 2012

In an effort to promote a uniform standard for reporting clinical results, the Consensus Meeting on Systems for Reporting Results in Acoustic Neuroma was convened in 2001, and the results of this meeting have been summarized by Kanzaki et al. in 2003. We describe publication compliance to these reporting parameters in a systematic analysis of publications obtained through a comprehensive literature search on patients with vestibular schwannoma (VS) treated with stereotactic radiosurgery (SRS). Each publication was scored based on whether it had properly reported each of eight elements described in the Consensus Meeting Reporting Guidelines (Guidelines). We compared the proportions of studies and cases that included each of the eight items prior to, and after, publication of the Guidelines. A significantly greater proportion of studies appropriately reported the size of the tumor after the release of the Guidelines (98% compared to 85%, $p = 0.04$). A significantly greater number of cases were reported properly adhering to the Guidelines in seven of the eight elements, with the exception of the cystic nature of the tumor. Report of post-treatment neurologic symptoms and complications saw the greatest degree of increase from before to after the publication of the Guidelines (47% to 68% of cases published, $p < 0.001$). Our findings suggest a potentially significant impact of the Guidelines on the quality of the information included in studies (Fig 2).

► This article provides a valuable reference for those wishing to review and critically compare studies on radiation treatment of vestibular schwannomas. Before

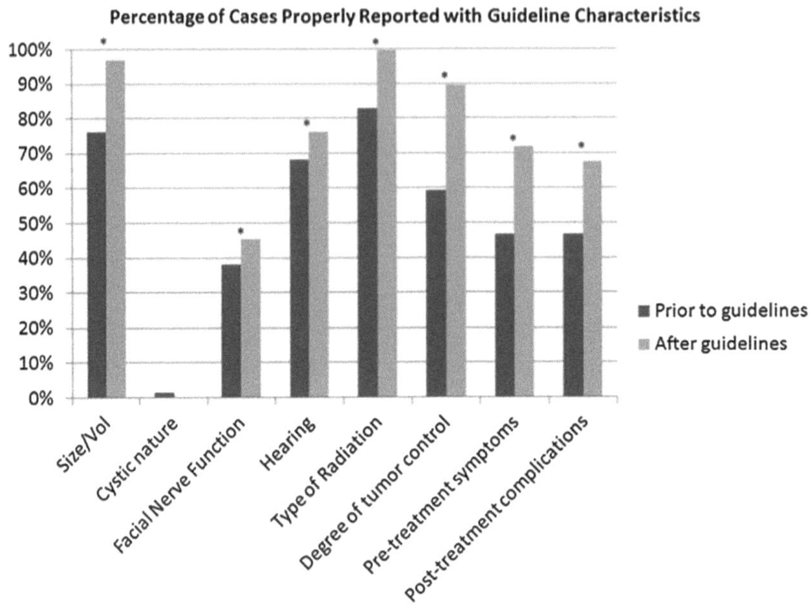

FIGURE 2.—Comparison of percentage of cases included in publications prior to, and after, publication of the Consensus Meeting Reporting Guidelines (Guidelines) that were properly reported with each of the Guideline characteristics. A significantly greater proportion of cases were reported properly adhering to the Guidelines in seven of the eight elements, including the size of the tumor, facial nerve function, hearing function, type and effect of radiosurgery, pre-treatment neurologic symptoms and post-treatment complications (* $= p < 0.05$). (Reprinted from Journal of Clinical Neuroscience. Han SJ, Oh MC, Sughrue ME, et al. The effect of the 2003 Consensus Reporting Standards on publications describing patients with vestibular schwannoma treated with stereotactic radiosurgery. *J Clin Neurosci.* 2012;19:1144-1147, Copyright 2012, with permission from Elsevier.)

2001, no consistent reporting standards existed, leading to great difficulty comparing results across institutions or among treatment modalities. Those reporting standards were published in 2003, and the 8 relevant for radiation are summarized in this article.[1] In the intervening near decade, overall quality and consistency have improved as demonstrated in Fig 2. Sadly, facial nerve reporting, which is critical in judging outcomes, remains less than 50%. This low percentage occurred despite a generous criterion in which even if House-Brackmann grading was not used, if similar descriptive terms were included the study, it was considered as meeting the guideline. Similarly, other critical elements, such as hearing, pretreatment symptoms, and posttreatment complications, remain reported less than 80% of the time. Thus, although the overall trends are improving, uniform quality data remain lacking in a substantial number of studies. In addition, the authors provide a thoughtful discussion regarding remaining elements in which the reporting guidelines fall short; namely, dose and fractionation regimen are not included, nor is cochlear dose for those studies reporting on hearing preservation.

B. J. Balough, MD

Reference

1. Kanzaki J, Tos M, Sanna M, Moffat DA, Monsell EM, Berliner KI. New and modified reporting systems from the consensus meeting on systems for reporting results in vestibular schwannoma. *Otol Neurotol.* 2003;24:642-648.

Utility Outcome Scores for Unilateral Facial Paralysis

Sinno H, Thibaudeau S, Izadpanah A, et al (McGill Univ, Montreal, Quebec, Canada; et al)

Ann Plast Surg 69:435-438, 2012

Background.—Facial paralysis is a debilitating condition. Dynamic and static facial reanimation remains a challenge for plastic surgeons and requires important resources. Our objective was to quantify the health state utility assessment (ie, utility score outcomes) of living with unilateral facial paralysis.

Methods.—Utility assessments using visual analog scale, time trade-off, and standard gamble were used to obtain utility outcome scores for unilateral facial paralysis from a prospective sample of the general population and medical students.

Results.—A total number of 123 individuals prospectively participated in the study. All measures (visual analog scale, time trade-off, and standard gamble) for unilateral facial paralysis [0.56 ± 0.18, 0.78 ± 0.21, and 0.79 ± 0.21 respectively] were significantly different ($P < 0.0001$) from the corresponding outcome scores for monocular blindness [0.61 ± 0.21, 0.83 ± 0.21, and 0.85 ± 0.18, respectively] and binocular blindness [0.33 ± 0.18, 0.65 ± 0.28, and 0.65 ± 0.29, respectively]. Linear regression analysis using age, race, income, and education as predictors of each of the utility scores for facial paralysis showed no statistical significance.

Conclusions.—In samples of the general population and medical students, all utility score outcome measures for facial paralysis were lower than those for monocular blindness. Our sample population, if faced with unilateral facial paralysis, would theoretically undergo facial reanimation procedures with a willingness to sacrifice 8 years of life and be willing to undergo a procedure with a 21% chance of mortality to attain perfect health, respectively.

▶ Here, the authors take a unique approach to facial paralysis to gauge its impact on the life of an individual so that it can be quantitatively compared with other significant morbidities and even mortality. To do this, the tool used is termed a *utility score*, which, in this case, combined 3 separate surveys, which included a time trade-off of years of life one is willing to sacrifice to restore normal facial function, standard gamble between remaining with facial paralysis or risking death from a restorative procedure, and visual analog score comparing facial paralysis with perfect health. The survey subjects rated a unilateral facial paralysis nearly midway between perfect health and death, and they would be willing to sacrifice one quarter of their expected remaining lifespan to have the facial paralysis reversed. Additionally, if a procedure existed to restore normal facial function, on average a 20% mortality rate would be acceptable to the group surveyed. These scores are on par with monocular blindness or end-stage renal disease. Far from being a theoretical exercise, those facing hand transplantation currently face 1 to 2 years of intensive daily rehabilitation after surgery. Additionally, the long-term immunosuppressant therapy is estimated to reduce expected lifespan by 10 years. Faced with unilateral or bilateral loss of hand, patients are accepting these risks. Although no current treatment to completely restore unilateral paralysis to normal function exists, this article highlights the severity of injury and the willingness of patients to sacrifice for rehabilitation. This has important ethical considerations when consulting patients and obtaining informed consent, especially for more involved procedures, such as free grafts with cross facial innervation. Lastly, it also underscores the severe and lasting impact a facial paralysis can have on a person. Obviously, utmost care should always be taken to avoid this devastating complication whenever possible. Articles such as this serve to remind us.

B. J. Balough, MD

Radiosurgery for Para-IAC Meningiomas: The Effect of Radiation Dose to the Cochlea on Hearing Outcome

Kim Y-H, Kim DG, Han JH, et al (Seoul Natl Univ Bundang Hosp, Seongnam-si, Korea; Seoul Natl Univ Hosp, Korea)

Int J Radiat Oncol Biol Phys 84:675-680, 2012

Purpose.—This study was performed to assess the radiosurgical results of meningiomas extending into the internal acoustic canal (para-IAC meningiomas), with a particular focus on the effect of radiation dose to the cochlea on hearing outcome.

Methods and Materials.—A total of 50 patients who underwent radiosurgery for para-IAC meningiomas between 1998 and 2009, which were followed for 2 years, were enrolled. The mean age was 55.8 years (range, 15–75). The mean tumor volume was 6.1 cm^3 (range, 1.0–19.0), the mean tumor length in the IAC was 6.9 mm (range, 1.3–13.3), and the mean prescribed marginal dose was 13.1 Gy (range, 10–15) at an isodose line of 50%. The mean follow-up duration was 46 months (range, 24–122).

Results.—Eight (16.0%) patients had nonserviceable hearing at the time of surgery. At the last follow-up, the tumor control rate was 94%; unchanged in 17 patients, decreased in 30 patients, and increased in 3 patients. Among 42 patients with serviceable hearing at the time of radiosurgery, it was preserved in 41 (97.6%) patients at the last follow-up. The maximal and mean radiation doses to the cochleae of these 41 patients were 5.8 Gy ± 0.3 (range, 3.1–11.5) and 4.3 Gy ± 0.2 (range, 2.2–7.5), respectively. The maximal dose to the cochlea of the patient who lost hearing after radiosurgery was 4.7 Gy.

Conclusions.—The radiation dose to the cochlea may have the minimal toxic effect on the hearing outcome in patients who undergo radiosurgery for para-IAC meningiomas.

▶ Similar to the article in this year's review on auditory brainstem response use for predicting hearing outcome, this article seeks to find predictive factors for hearing outcome. However, here the goal is to determine if modifying treatment can be used to improve outcome. As a unique element, the authors chose to examine meningiomas of the cerebellopontine angle rather than vestibular schwannomas. Although not specifically discussed, this approach potentially eliminates any factors related to the tumor arising from the auditory nerve itself. However, no effect was found relative to cochlear dose of radiation. Two main factors may account for this. First, although the cochlear doses are similar for both hearing-preserved and hearing-loss groups, the dosage is very low at 4.3 to 4.4 Gy. This is essentially the same maximal dose shown in other studies to benefit hearing. Thus, for those who lost hearing after treatment, factors other than cochlear dose likely predominated. Second, the length of follow-up is relatively short at 2 years. Thus, any late effects will not be seen, which may help separate out impact of cochlear dose. Therefore, although essentially a negative study with some limitations in design, it provides a good discussion and review of the topic and takes an interesting approach, making it worth including for this year's review.

B. J. Balough, MD

Influence of Age on Postural Compensation After Unilateral Deafferentation Due to Vestibular Schwannoma Surgery

Gauchard GC, Lion A, Perrin PP, et al (Univ of Lorraine, Villers-lès-Nancy, France; Natl Inst for Health and Med Res—Inserm U 954, Vandoeuvre-lès-Nancy, France)

Laryngoscope 122:2285-2290, 2012

Objectives/Hypothesis.—To evaluate the age-related effects of vestibular schwannoma (VS) on postural control and whether the postoperative postural strategies differ according to age.

Study Design.—Longitudinal, transversal study.

Methods.—Forty-seven VS patients were split into three groups according to age (group I, 14 patients aged from 30 to 44 years; group II, 21 patients aged from 45 to 59 years; and group III, 12 patients aged from 60 to 75 years). All patients underwent vestibular and posturographic testing shortly before as well as 8 days and 3 months after surgical tumor removal.

Results.—Vestibular and postural performance followed a classical time course with degradation just after surgery and recovery 3 months after surgery, whatever the age group. However, in the elderly the improvement of postural performances compared to preoperatively was more important, especially in conflicting situations.

Conclusions.—Despite of age-related decline in postural control and cognitive processes, neuroplasticity allowed not only a recovery but even an improvement of balance after surgical VS removal in the elderly. This study highlights the interest of VS surgery even at a more advanced age.

▶ The decision to surgically treat vestibular schwannoma can be complex, particularly in the elderly, in whom general health and ability to recover may be of greater concern than in younger patients. In this study, the issue of balance recovery after surgery was explored. As outlined in the introduction, age-related reduction in cognitive function and ability for central compensation might give the assumption that older patients will recover more poorly from vestibular loss after surgery. However, as this study details, it is precisely because of this reduced ability to compensate that surgical removal provides greater benefit in the elderly, as they appear to be unable to overcome the abnormal inputs generated by the tumor. This raises the interesting possibility that the same benefit may be gained by chemical or surgical ablation of the involved labyrinth without the surgical risks of tumor removal. Although the study provides this important finding, its design is overly complex with the involvement of additional vestibular tests that do not contribute to the overall result. Quality-of-life measures may have been of more benefit to assess functional ability before and after surgery. However, the posturography data alone are compelling enough that age alone in those that are otherwise healthy should not preclude surgery for vestibular schwannoma.

B. J. Balough, MD

Hearing Preservation in Patients With Unilateral Vestibular Schwannoma Who Undergo Stereotactic Radiosurgery: Reinterpretation of the Auditory Brainstem Response

Han JH, Kim DG, Chung H-T, et al (Seoul Natl Univ Bundang Hosp, Gyeonggi-do, Korea; Seoul Natl Univ Hosp, Korea)

Cancer 118:5441-5447, 2012

Background.—The objective of this study was to identify the prognostic factors for hearing preservation that would allow the more accurate stratification of patients who undergo stereotactic radiosurgery (SRS) for unilateral, sporadic vestibular schwannoma (VS).

Methods.—In total, 119 patients with VS who had serviceable hearing underwent SRS as primary treatment. The mean (±standard deviation) patient age was 48 ± 11 years, and the mean (±standard deviation) follow-up duration was 55.2 ± 35.7 months. The median marginal radiotherapy dose was 12.0 grays (Gy), and the mean (±standard deviation) tumor volume was 1.95 ± 2.24 cm^3. The mean (±standard deviation) pure tone average (PTA) score was 26 ± 12 decibels (dB) (range, 4-50 dB), and the mean (±standard deviation) maximum speech discrimination score was 91 ± 12% (range, 52-100%). The mean (±standard deviation) baseline values for the interlatency (IL) of waves I and III (IL I-III) and the IL of waves I through V (IL I-V) on auditory brainstem response were

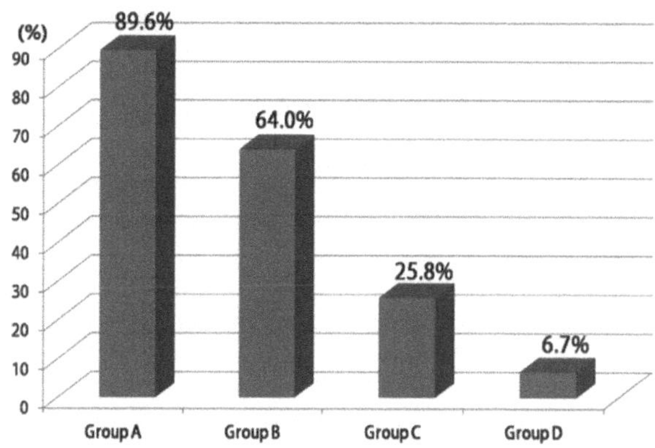

FIGURE 4.—This chart illustrates the rates of serviceable hearing in the 4 groups based on a classification and regression tree analysis of the groups. (Reprinted from Cancer. Han JH, Kim DG, Chung H-T, et al. Hearing preservation in patients with unilateral vestibular schwannoma who undergo stereotactic radiosurgery: reinterpretation of the auditory brainstem response. *Cancer.* 2012;118:5441-5447, Copyright 2012, American Cancer Society. This material is reproduced with permission of Wiley-Liss, Inc., a subsidiary of John Wiley & Sons, Inc., www.interscience.wiley.com.)

TABLE 3.—Risk Group Splits Based on the Results From Classification and Regression Tree Analysis

Risk Group	No. of Patients	No. With Hearing Preservation	Hearing Preservation, %
Group A: PTA≤20	48	43	89.6
Group B: IL I-V<5.225 mS and 21≤PTA≤30	25	16	64
Group C: IL I-V<5.225 mS and 31≤PTA≤50	31	8	25.8
Group D: IL I-V≥5.225 mS and PTA≤50	15	1	6.7

Abbreviations: IL I-V, the interlatency between wave I and V on the auditory brainstem response; mS, milliseconds; PTA, pure tone average score.

2.58 ± 0.60 milliseconds (mS) (range, 1.92-4.30 mS) and 4.80 ± 0.61 mS (range, 3.80-6.40 mS), respectively.

Results.—In multivariate analysis, the PTA score and IL I-V were significant and independent prognostic factors (hazard ratio, 1.072; 95% confidence interval, 1.046-1.098; $P < .001$; and hazard ratio, 1.534; 95% confidence interval, 1.008-2.336; $P = .046$, respectively). By using the PTA score and IL I-V, the patients were classified into 4 groups. The ratios of patients with serviceable hearing after SRS were 89.6%, 64.0%, 25.8%, and 6.7%, respectively, in Groups A through D ($P < .001$).

Conclusions.—The current results indicated that the classification system based on using the PTA score and the IL I-V of the auditory brainstem response may be useful and specific for predicting the rate of hearing preservation in each individual (Fig 4, Table 3).

▶ Regardless of pathology, the goal of treatment is to eliminate disease and preserve function. When that is not possible, then there is value in identifying prognosis. For vestibular schwannoma and stereotactic radiation, this goal translates to prevention of further tumor growth, maintaining facial nerve function, and preservation of remaining hearing. While the first 2 goals are obtained reliably, it is that last one that can prove elusive. In this study, the authors examine a large cohort of patients treated with stereotactic radiation who had excellent hearing before treatment to see what prognostic factors could be identified to predict hearing outcome. More than 40% of those with pretreatment hearing will lose that hearing within 5 years after treatment. The study is well designed with sound methodology. Table 3 provides the risk factors assigned to categories, which are represented graphically in Fig 4. What emerges in these data is the value of auditory brainstem response (ABR) in outcome prediction for those with less-than-perfect hearing. It is the key predictive determinant for those with any degree of loss beyond normal hearing. If the ABR is prolonged, the outcome will be poor regardless of remaining hearing. It is also surprising that speech discrimination was not found to be a significant predictive factor despite its important role in determining serviceable hearing. The explanation for this is discussed by the authors as is the theory behind the ABR as a surrogate measure for nerve compression and disruption. In the future, because of articles such as this, the ABR will become an increasingly important part of the pretreatment evaluation of vestibular schwannomas.

B. J. Balough, MD

3D-FIESTA MRI at 3 T demonstrating branches of the intraparotid facial nerve, parotid ducts and relation with benign parotid tumours

Li C, Li Y, Zhang D, et al (Shandong Univ, Jinan, China; Shandong Provincial Hosp of Shandong Univ, Jinan, China)

Clin Radiol 67:1078-1082, 2012

Aim.—To investigate the usefulness of three-dimensional (3D) fast imaging employing steady state precession (FIESTA) magnetic resonance imaging (MRI) at 3 T in evaluating the intraparotid components of the facial nerve and parotid ducts, and to compare the MRI images with surgical findings.

Materials and Methods.—Thirty-one cases of benign parotid tumours were studied with conventional and 3D FIESTA MRI sequences at 3T using a head coil. The most clinically useful 3D FIESTA images were acquired at parameters of 4.9 ms repetition time (TR); 1.5 effective echo time (TEeff); a flip of 55°, a field of view of 18 to 20 cm, a matrix of 512 × 320, an axial plane, no gaps, and a section thickness of 1 mm. Post-processed multiplanar images were obtained with an Advantage Windows (AW sdc 4.3) workstation. Parotid ducts, facial nerves, and tumours were identified on these images. The relationship of the tumours to the facial nerves and parotid ducts was confirmed at surgery.

Results.—The facial nerves appeared as linear structures of low intensity. The main trunk of the facial nerve was identified bilaterally in 93.5% of the 3D-FIESTA sequence images. Parotid ducts appeared as structures of high

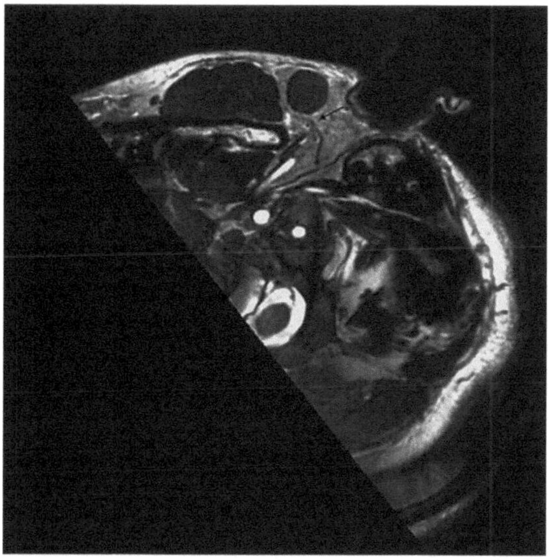

FIGURE 2.—A 50-year-old woman with pleomorphic adenomas. The relationship of the tumour with the cervicofacial division is shown in the 3D-FIESTA image (arrow). (Reprinted from Clinical Radiology. Li C, Li Y, Zhang D, et al. 3D-FIESTA MRI at 3 T demonstrating branches of the intraparotid facial nerve, parotid ducts and relation with benign parotid tumours. *Clin Radiol.* 2012;67:1078-1082, Copyright 2012, with permission from the Royal College of Radiologists.)

intensity on multiplanar 3D-FIESTA images (100%). The relationships of the tumours with the cervicofacial and temporofacial divisions of the facial nerve were correctly diagnosed in 26 of 31 cases (83.9%) using 3D-FIESTA sequence images.

Conclusion.—3D-FIESTA MRI at 3 T depicted the main trunk, cervicofacial and temporofacial divisions of the facial nerve, and the main parotid duct. It is useful for preoperative evaluation of parotid gland tumours (Fig 2).

▶ Preservation of nerve function is critical in most surgeries of the head and neck. Preservation of the facial nerve in particular is of paramount importance given its functional and aesthetic role and our limited abilities for satisfactory reconstruction. Typically, imaging modalities are of limited use because the nerves are not directly visible. Here a relatively standard modality is used with impressive ability to identify and track not only the main trunk but also branches of the facial nerve. Fig 2 shows an example of this where the lower division of the facial nerve can be seen clearly with a small rim of normal parotid tissue between it and the tumor. The 3-dimensional capabilities allow for reconstruction in multiple planes to enable tracking of the nerve course. Although clearly useful in parotid surgery, many other applications can be envisioned, such as tracking the recurrent and superior laryngeal nerves in thyroid surgery or multiple different cranial nerves in tumors of the skull base. As stronger 3-T magnets become more widely available, this imaging may become routine in preoperative evaluations should it prove useful in altering surgical approach or outcomes.

B. J. Balough, MD

Surgical Removal of Giant Acoustic Neuromas

Silva J, Cerejo A, Duarte F, et al (Univ of Porto, Portugal)

World Neurosurg 77:731-735, 2012

Objective.—The authors present the outcome of radical surgical removal of giant acoustic neuromas.

Methods.—Twenty-nine patients with acoustic neuroma with maximum diameter greater than 40 mm, submitted to surgery between the years 2005 and 2010, were reviewed by a retrospective study. The extension of tumor removal, surgical morbidity, facial nerve function, hearing, and evolution after surgery of preoperative neurologic conditions were the studied parameters.

Results.—All tumors were completely removed by a retrosigmoid approach, without perioperative mortality. As complications related to the surgery, there were three cases of local cerebrospinal fluid leak, one case of nasal cerebrospinal fluid leak, two cases of meningitis, one pseudomeningocele, and one case of transient lower cranial nerve dysfunction. The anatomic integrity of the facial nerve was preserved in 86% and facial function in 72%. In the 21 patients who did not need hypoglossal–facial anastomosis (72%), facial function was excellent or good (HB I-II) in 13 cases (45%), fair (HB III) in 5 cases (17%), and poor (HB IV) in 3 cases (10%). Before surgery, 12 patients (41%) had useful (H2) or moderate (H3) hearing. In 7 of these 12 patients (58%), it was possible to preserve some hearing function (with moderate hearing), after surgical removal of the tumors. Six patients presented with radiologic signs of hydrocephalus, two of them with visual disturbances. Two patients presented with trigeminal neuralgia (one contralateral), three with facial sensory loss and one with swallowing problems, that disappeared after surgery.

Conclusions.—Total removal of large acoustic neuroma can be achieved by retrosigmoid approach with acceptable morbidity and no mortality. Preoperative neurologic symptoms recovered after surgery in most cases. Facial function preservation was possible in the majority of cases. Even in large tumors, hearing preservation should be attempted if the patient has useful hearing preoperatively.

► Most recent discussions regarding acoustic neuroma treatment have centered on observation or stereotactic radiation.[1] But for giant tumors such as those reviewed in this article, surgery remains the only treatment option. Here the authors review their experience with gross total tumor removal in these challenging cases. Their overall facial nerve outcomes of < 50% good preservation are consistent with those published by Wiet a decade ago in his large series. What sets the article apart, however, is the excellent accompanying commentary articles by 3 world-renowned neurosurgeons.[2-4] What emerges from this discussion is that although complete tumor removal can safely be done for this size tumor, acceptable results for the surgeon may not be acceptable for the patient, especially in terms of preservation of facial nerve function. Though one might consider tumors of this size rare with increased emphasis on screening and wide availability of magnetic resonance imaging, referral centers still see these commonly. In this series, they averaged 6 per year. This is reflected in the commentary as well. So although complete tumor removal can be done, what should be done in these challenging cases? Both the authors and commentary reflect on subtotal or staged removal. This is described in the article by Patni and Kartush and what I follow in my own practice. The goals of surgery here are to significantly reduce the tumor volume, relieving brainstem compression and effects on the trigeminal and lower cranial nerves. As the tumor volume is reduced, careful attention is paid to the nerve monitoring, and as much tumor is removed as the facial nerve function will allow. A key element is to ensure tumor along the brainstem is removed. Staging in this fashion achieves much higher good (House-Brackmann 1 or 2) facial nerve outcome and converts a situation from where only surgery is an option to one where observation, radiation, or additional surgery can be offered; in essence, resetting the clock to a smaller-sized tumor. Given the option, most patients will accept the possibility of a second surgery for improved facial function.

B. J. Balough, MD

References

1. Wiet RJ, Mamikoglu B, Odom L, Hoistad DL. Long-term results of the first 500 cases of acoustic neuroma surgery. *Otolaryngol Head Neck Surg.* 2001;124: 645-651.
2. Gerganov VM, Samii M. Giant vestibular schwannomas. *World Neurosurg.* 2012; 77:627-628.
3. Sekhar LN, Tariq F, Ferreira M. Giant acoustic neuromas and their treatment. *World Neurosurg.* 2012;77:629-630.
4. Misra BK. Surgery for giant acoustic neuroma: total excision at what cost. *World Neurosurg.* 2012;77:625-626.

Vestibular Schwannoma Surgical Volume and Short-term Outcomes in Maryland

Ward BK, Gourin CG, Francis HW (The Johns Hopkins Med Institutions, Baltimore, MD)
Arch Otolaryngol Head Neck Surg 138:577-583, 2012

Objective.—To characterize contemporary practice patterns and outcomes of vestibular schwannoma surgery.

Design.—Cross-sectional analysis.

Setting.—Maryland Health Service Cost Review Commission database.

Patients.—The study included patients who underwent surgery for vestibular schwannoma between 1990 and 2009.

Main Outcome Measures.—Temporal trends and relationships between volume and in-hospital deaths, central nervous system (CNS) complications, length of hospitalization, and costs.

Results.—A total of 1177 surgical procedures were performed by 57 surgeons at 12 hospitals. Most cases were performed by high-volume surgeons (47%) at high-volume hospitals (79%). The number of cases increased from 474 in 1999-2000 to 703 in 2000-2009. Vestibular schwannoma surgery in 2000-2009 was associated with a decrease in CNS complications (odds ratio [OR] 0.4; $P < .001$) and an increase in cases performed by intermediate-volume (OR, 4.2; $P = .002$) and high-volume (OR, 3.2; $P = .005$) hospitals and intermediate-volume (OR, 1.9; $P = .004$) and high-volume (OR, 1.8; $P = .006$) surgeons. High-volume care was inversely related to the odds of urgent and emergent surgery (OR, 0.2; $P < .001$) and readmissions (OR, 0.1; $P = .02$). Surgeon volume accounted for 59% of the effect of hospital volume for urgent and emergent admissions and 20% for readmissions. After all other variables were controlled for, there was no significant association between hospital or surgeon volume and in-hospital mortality or CNS complications; however, surgery at high-volume hospitals was associated with significantly lower hospital-related costs ($P < .001$).

Conclusions.—These data suggest increased centralization of vestibular schwannoma surgery, with an increase in cases performed by intermediate- and high-volume providers and meaningful differences in high-volume surgical care that are mediated by surgeon volume and are associated with reduced hospital-related costs. Further investigation is warranted.

▶ With the coming changes in health care financing, increased emphasis will continue to be placed on consolidating care for complex and uncommon conditions, such as vestibular schwannoma, into specialized centers. In the data presented here, this consolidation has already been occurring over the last 20 years, regardless of a nearly 50% increase in overall surgical case numbers from the first 10-year study period to the second, despite emphasis on observation and stereotactic radiation for treatment. Increases in surveillance and earlier diagnosis likely led to this increased volume. Unfortunately, data on overall numbers of tumors evaluated are not presented, so this is an implied assumption. Figs 2 and 3 in the original article illustrate the increases for the intermediate- and high-volume groups across the 2 time periods as well as the declines for those with low volumes. It is interesting to note the relatively constant ratio among high- and intermediate-volume surgeons but the large relative increase in cases at the high-volume centers. Despite the lack of data to support improved quality of outcome, it is very likely that Fig 1 in the original article will be referenced in the future and possibly used to classify centers and surgeons by volume and, thus, is worth reviewing. A few significant limitations with this study are worth mentioning. First, numerous prior studies have shown that for surgeons, overall experience, particularly at the 100- and 500-case number, is a useful predictors of improved outcomes. No mention is made here of the surgeon's overall experience, and this may have been a significant confounding variable. Higher-volume centers may have relatively newer surgeons compared with lower-volume centers that have more experienced surgeons. Case frequency is likely a more important variable for hospitals, whereas overall experience is more important for surgeons. Second, and more importantly, neither facial nerve nor hearing outcomes were measured as central nervous system complications. Because these standard measures of quality outcomes for vestibular schwannoma treatment are missing, the conclusions derived from this study need to be judged from that perspective. Despite these shortcomings, the increasing emphasis on cost containment and quality will make studies such as this worth reviewing.

B. J. Balough, MD

General

Can uHear Me Now? Validation of an iPod-Based Hearing Loss Screening Test

Szudek J, Ostevik A, Dziegielewski P, et al (Univ of Alberta, Edmonton, Canada)
J Otolaryngol Head Neck Surg 41:S78-S84, 2012

Objective.—To evaluate the uHear iPod-based application as a test for hearing loss.

Methods.—We recruited 100 adult participants through a single otology practice. Patients with otorrhea and cognitive impairment were excluded. All patients completed the uHear test in the clinic and in the sound booth and underwent a standard audiogram by the same audiologist. We compared the results of the uHear test to the standard audiogram.

Results.—The uHear was able to correctly diagnose the presence of hearing loss (pure-tone average [PTA] > 40 dB) with a sensitivity of 98% (95% CI = 89–100), a specificity of 82% (95% CI = 75–88), and a positive likelihood ratio of 9 (95% CI = 6.0–16). Compared to the audiogram, the uHear overestimated the PTA among all ears by 14 dB in the clinic and by 8 dB in the sound booth ($p < .0001$). Compared to the audiogram, the uHear overestimated the PTA among ears with hearing loss by 6 dB in the clinic and by 4 dB in the sound booth.

Conclusions.—The uHear application is a reasonable screening test to rule out moderate hearing loss (PTA > 40 dB) and is valid at quantifying the degree of hearing loss in patients known to have abnormal hearing.

▶ In this article, the authors provide the first evaluation in the usefulness of a simple iPod application for use as a hearing screening tool in several environments. The results for all participants are illustrated in Fig 1 of the original article with an overestimation of the average hearing loss in the low frequencies but improving in the higher range. However, in Fig 2 of the original article, where only those with a demonstrated hearing loss were compared, the application becomes much more accurate. Although better in the quiet of a hearing booth, even when used in the clinic setting, the sensitivity and specificity are both extremely good, supporting the use of this application as a screening test when an audiogram is not practical, such as in remote clinics, in emergency rooms, and with hospital patients. It is important to remember that this is not a self-administered test by the patient, and, for best accuracy, the test must be administered by a person knowledgeable in its use. The authors review a few of the drawbacks of this application, the chief being that because of the limitations in the dynamic range of the iPod device itself, it may not be sensitive enough to detect mild hearing losses, as these may fall within the lower end of this range. Test-retest accuracy is also unknown and has not been studied. This may limit the usefulness for following hearing losses but should not interfere with its use as a screening test.

B. J. Balough, MD

Outcome of bone-anchored hearing aids for single-sided deafness: A prospective study

Pai I, Kelleher C, Nunn T, et al (St Thomas' Hosp, London, UK)

Acta Otolaryngol 132:751-755, 2012

Conclusion.—The bone-anchored hearing aid (BAHA) system can offer significant benefits to patients with single-sided deafness (SSD), primarily by lifting the head shadow effect.

Objective.—To evaluate the efficacy of BAHA for SSD by comparing pre- and postoperative speech, spatial and qualities of hearing scale (SSQ) scores.

Methods.—This was a prospective study conducted within a tertiary auditory implant department. The inclusion criteria were unilateral profound hearing loss with normal or mild high frequency hearing loss in the

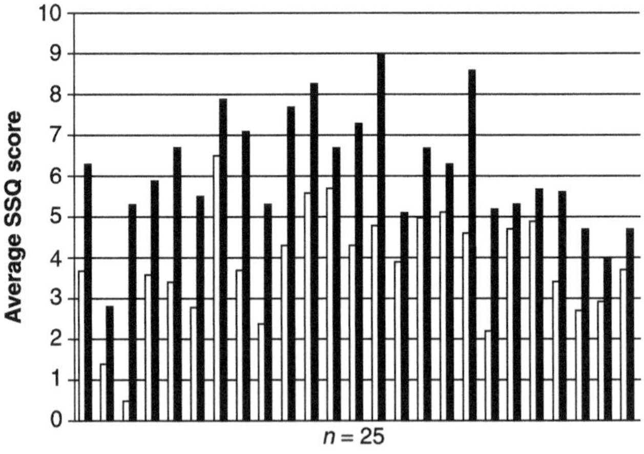

FIGURE 1.—Individual scores for the speech, spatial and qualities of hearing scale (SSQ): preoperative and postoperative scores for section 1 (speech hearing). □, preoperative; ■, postoperative. (Reprinted from Pai I, Kelleher C, Nunn T, et al. Outcome of bone-anchored hearing aids for single-sided deafness: a prospective study. *Acta Otolaryngol.* 2012;132:751-755, reprinted by permission of Taylor & Francis Ltd, _http://www.informaworld.com.)

hearing ear (pure tone average better than or equal to 25 dBHL measured at 0.5, 1, 2 and 3 kHz) and subjective benefits reported by patients following a home trial with a BAHA Softband. Patients who met the above criteria and opted for surgery were asked to complete the SSQ questionnaire. The post-operative SSQ response was collected after at least 6 months of consistent BAHA usage.

Results.—This study included 25 adult patients (mean age at implantation 57.5 years). There was a statistically significant improvement in the average SSQ score in all three sections of the questionnaire with the use of the BAHA. Our patients experienced most marked benefits in speech hearing in challenging listening situations. All patients remain consistent users and there has been no explantation to date (Fig 1).

▶ In this article, the authors bring into focus one of the most important items during the last decade since the bone-anchored hearing devices came to market: the increasing awareness and consideration of the impact of single-sided deafness. Previously, even though hearing aid options existed for rehabilitation, little emphasis was placed on the functional impact from the loss of binaural hearing. To some extent, this is because of the limitations of standard audiologic methods to assess the functional loss encountered by only one hearing ear. To overcome this limitation, the authors have uniquely turned to a quality-of-life instrument, the speech, spatial, and qualities of hearing scale (SSQ), to quantify the impact of single-sided deafness on communication in noise and sound localization. As illustrated in Fig 1, every patient showed overall improvement after rehabilitation. Interestingly, as the results are broken down into specific components, individual patients will vary in which aspects show the greatest improvement. The authors acknowledge the limitations of the study, chief of which is that patients have self-selected having a disability from their unilateral deafness. Though not specifically mentioned, the duration of deafness seems to be important. Those more remote in time from the onset of their loss often are less interested in rehabilitation than those more acutely affected. This remains an unexplained aspect of this disorder, although the authors hint at mechanisms in their discussion. Use of tools such as the SSQ provides an important new way to examine this and other questions.

B. J. Balough, MD

Does Tinnitus Affect the Sound Localization Ability?

An Y-H, Lee LH, Yoon SW (Eulji Univ School of Medicine, Seoul, Republic of Korea)

Otol Neurotol 33:692-698, 2012

Objective.—To investigate whether tinnitus affects sound localization ability.

Study Design.—Prospective controlled study.

Setting.—Tertiary referral center.

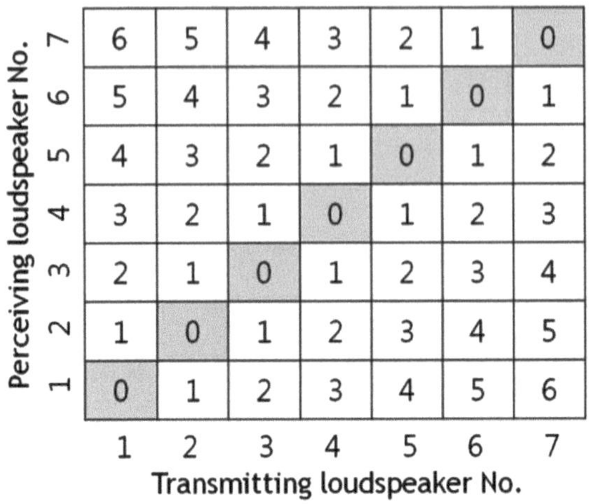

FIGURE 1.—Calculation protocol for the ES resulting from the sound localization test. ES was calculated by scoring 1 point for each 30 degrees of difference between the stimulus-presenting speaker and the perceiving loudspeaker. The numbers indicate ES. (Reprinted from An Y-H, Lee LH, Yoon SW. Does tinnitus affect the sound localization ability? *Otol Neurotol.* 2012;33:692-698, with permission from Otology & Neurotology, Inc.)

TABLE 2.—Comparisons of Mean Values of Error Score Resulting From Sound Localization Test Between Tinnitus Group and Control Group (Mean ± Standard Deviation)

Stimulus (kHz)	Mean Error Score of Tinnitus Group	Mean Error Score of Control Group	*p*
0.25	3.6 ± 3.3	2.0 ± 1.9	<0.05
1	5.1 ± 3.8	2.9 ± 2.3	<0.05
4	5.4 ± 2.8	4.1 ± 2.4	<0.05
8	4.8 ± 2.5	4.1 ± 2.4	>0.05
Total	18.8 ± 9.2	13.1 ± 7.5	<0.05

Patients.—Forty tinnitus patients (mean age, 36.7 ± 14.3 yr; hearing threshold, < 20 dB HL; tinnitus group) and 40 controls (mean age, 39.3 ± 12.9 yr; hearing threshold, < 20 dB HL; control group).

Methods.—We performed a sound localization test (SLT) with 7 speakers positioned in a semicircle on the horizontal plane at a distance of 1 m from the subject, at 30-degree intervals. Subjects were asked to identify the stimulus-presenting speaker, through a forced-choice procedure. The error score was calculated by scoring 1 point for each 30 degrees of difference between the stimulus-presenting speaker and the speaker identified by the subject.

Results.—The mean SLT total error score (TES) of the tinnitus group (18.8 ± 9.2) was significantly higher than that of the control group (13.1 ± 7.5) ($p < 0.05$). Regarding SLT responses for stimulation from speakers located at each side of the listener, mean TES in patients with tinnitus on the same side as the speaker was higher than that in patients with opposite side or bilateral tinnitus. Age showed a positive correlation with TES in the tinnitus ($r = 0.44$, $p < 0.05$) and control groups ($r = 0.35$, $p < 0.05$).

Conclusion.—We consider that tinnitus interferes with sound localization ability and that interference is worse for sound originating from the same side as the tinnitus. Age is a worsening factor in sound localization ability (Fig 1, Table 2).

▶ Most studies on tinnitus focus on treatment outcomes. Here, the authors examine the impact of tinnitus on auditory function. They use an interesting forced-choice methodology to determine accuracy scores for spatial localization. This scoring system is shown in Fig 1 with the table to calculate the overall error score. In the background, a very good synopsis is presented on the auditory mechanisms for spatial localization and how they are influenced by frequency. Additionally, the rationale for using spatial localization as a measure of the central auditory effects of tinnitus is presented. This is compelling and may have relevance if further developed for other tinnitus studies as a way to more objectively calculate tinnitus disability or response to treatment. The results are demonstrated in Table 2 and, as expected, show that the measure is more sensitive for sounds presented at lower frequency. This was independent of the tinnitus-matched frequency and supports the underlying hypothesis of the study. The main limitation of the study is that it is weighed down with numerous additional audiologic measures and the discussion of those measures, which adds little to what is already known. The other main limitation is that no mention or stratification regarding duration or severity of the tinnitus in the study group is provided. Although this is a significant limitation, it is common with the majority of tinnitus literature. Despite these limitations, the unique nature of this study, the excellent background reference information on sound localization, and the deeper impact of the results make it worth review.

B. J. Balough, MD

The New Baha Implant: A Prospective Osseointegration Study

D'Eredità R, Caroncini M, Saetti R (Vicenza Civil Hosp, Italy)

Otolaryngol Head Neck Surg 146:979-983, 2012

Objectives.—To assess stability of a new-design titanium implant (Cochlear Baha BAI300) in bone-anchored hearing aid (Baha) recipients over time.

Study Design and Setting.—Prospective case series with planned data collection at a tertiary care institution. Twelve patients who underwent Baha surgery over 12 months were analyzed.

Subjects.—All patients (3 children, age range 6-10 years, mean 7.7 years, median 7.3 years; 9 adults, age range 34-73 years, mean 52.8 years, median 48 years) underwent the 1-stage procedure following the standard Brånemark technique. In all procedures, the single-skin incision was applied.

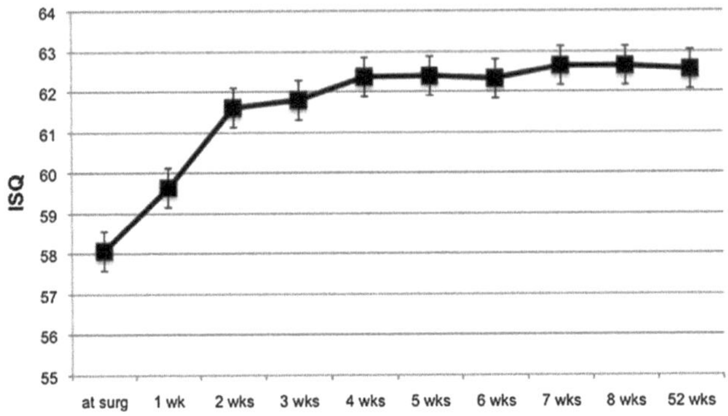

FIGURE.—Mean implant stability quotient (ISQ) values are reported over time. A steep increase in ISQ values was obtained during the first 2 weeks after implantation, reaching a plateau at the third week. No significant ISQ changes were observed over the 1-year follow-up. (Reprinted from Otolaryngology - Head and Neck Surgery. D'Eredità R, Caroncini M, Saetti R. The new Baha Implant: a prospective osseointegration study. *Otolaryngol Head Neck Surg* 2012;146:979-983, Copyright 2012, with permission from the American Academy of Otolaryngology-Head and Neck Surgery Foundation.)

Methods.—The stability of the implant was measured with implant stability quotient (ISQ) measurement tests. All patients were tested at surgery and every week after for 1 year. Wound-healing time, degree of soft tissue reactions around the abutment, and need for revision surgery were examined. Two-tailed Student t test and χ^2 for all comparisons were calculated; $P < .05$ values were considered significant.

Results.—The new implant showed a steep increase of ISQ values over the first 2 weeks and reached stable ISQ values 3 weeks after surgery. Complete skin healing time was obtained in 8 days on average (range, 7-12 days; median 7.6 days). Neither implant extrusion nor skin revision surgery was observed in our patients during the first year of follow-up.

Conclusions.—This new implant revealed stability and fast integration. The data from the present study suggest the new implant may be suitable for early loading protocols (Fig).

▶ One of the main limitations of bone-anchored hearing devices has been the long delay between surgery and device use to allow for bone integration. Although limited in numbers, this study examines implant integration time using an implant stability quotient (ISQ). The authors describe this methodology in detail, and it appears to be a standard engineering method for judging bone integration. As seen in Fig, the implants within 3 weeks rapidly reach a level of long-term stability in the measured ISQ. Although no comment is made regarding the absolute measured values obtained (between 62 and 63), whether these were satisfactory or expected, references are provided suggesting that these numbers are indeed adequate. More importantly, in the 1-year follow-up there were no adverse implant effects despite the early loading. Some discussion is provided regarding the similarity between the values for children and adults. Although this is true, some caution should be exercised given the small number of children, 3, in the study. The authors acknowledge this point. It is assumed that this more rapid integration is caused by changes made in the implant design, a wider base, and changes in the thread design and coating. Another limitation is that no comparable ISQ measures are provided for standard implants. Despite this and the other mentioned limitations, these data support a potentially significant change in clinical protocol to allow much earlier implant loading, leading to improved patient satisfaction.

B. J. Balough, MD

Intratympanic Steroid Treatment for Sudden Deafness: A Meta-analysis of Randomized Controlled Trials

Garavello W, Galluzzi F, Gaini RM, et al (Univ of Milano-Bicocca, Monza, Italy)
Otol Neurotol 33:724-729, 2012

Background.—The efficacy of intratympanic steroid (ITS) treatment in sudden deafness (SD) remains controversial. To shed light on this issue, we performed a systematic review of randomized controlled trials to assess the overall efficacy of ITS therapy and to clarify whether it is more suitable as a first-line approach (primary treatment) or as a salvage treatment when traditional systemic agents have failed.

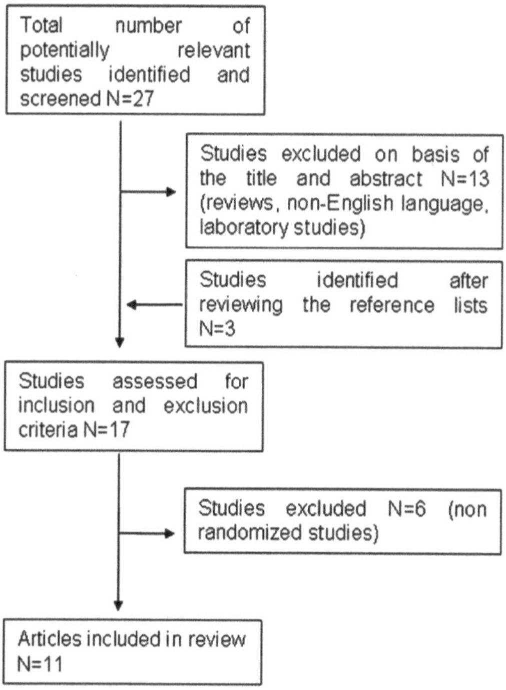

FIGURE 1.—Flowchart of the reviewing process. (Reprinted from Garavello W, Galluzzi F, Gaini RM, et al. Intratympanic steroid treatment for sudden deafness: a meta-analysis of randomized controlled trials. *Otol Neurotol*. 2012;33:724-729, with permission from Otology & Neurotology, Inc.)

TABLE 1.—Randomized Studies Assessing the Efficacy of Intratympanic Steroid for Sudden Hearing Loss

Author	Year	Country	No. Subjects Cases/Controls	Protocol Therapy Cases	Additional Therapy Cases	Protocol Therapy Controls	Criteria of Improvement PTA	Criteria of Improvement WDS
Primary								
Battaglia et al. (10)	2008	United States	21/39	DEX 12 mg/ml × 0.5–0.7 ml once per week for 3 wk	Placebo taper or IT	PD p.o. 60 mg/d for 7 d 50 mg/d for 2 d 40 mg/d for 2 d <10 mg/d for 3 d	15 dB	SDS
Ahn et al. (11)	2008	Korea	60/60	DEX 5 mg/ml × 0.3–0.4 ml of 3 injections (days 1, 3, and 5)	Protocol therapy controls	MP p.o. 48 mg/d for 14 d Vitamins Lipoprostaglandin E_1 Low-salt diet	Siegel's criteria	NR
Hong et al. (12)	2009	Korea	32/31	DEX 5 mg/ml × 0.3–0.4 ml once per day for 8 d	ND	PD p.o. 60 mg/d for 4 d 40 mg/d for 2 d 20 mg/d for 2 d	Siegel's criteria	NR
Rauch et al. (14)	2011	United States	113/108	MP 40 mg/ml × 1 ml once every 3–4 d for 2 wk	ND	PD 60 mg/d for 14 d gradually tapered for 5 d	10 dB	WRS
Salvage								
Ho et al. (20)	2004	China	15/14	DEX 4 mg/ml × 0.4–0.7 ml once per week for 3 wk	Protocol therapy controls	MP p.o. 1 mg/kg per day for 5 d tapering to 10 mg/d for 5 d Fludiazepam 0.25 mg 3× a day for 10 d Nicametate citrate 3× a day for 10 d Vitamin B complex for 10 d Carbogen inhalation therapy for 5 d (95% O_2 and 5% CO_2)	30 dB	NR
Xenellis et al. (21)	2006	Greece	19/18	MP 40 mg/ml × 1.5–2 ml 4 injections for 15 d	Protocol therapy controls	PD i.v. 1 mg/kg per day for 10 d gradually tapered for 5 d Acyclovir 4 g/d for 5 d Buflomedil hydrochloride 300 mg 3× a day for 10 d	10 dB	NR
Plontke et al. (13)	2009	Germany	11/10	DEX 4 mg/ml-rate × 6 μl/h 1× a day for 14 d	Protocol therapy controls	PD i.v. 250 mg/d for 3 d Reduction 50% every 2× a day for 5 d Pentoxifylline 400 mg 3× a day for 8 d α-Liponic acid 600 mg/d for 8 d	30 dB or recovery 50% of loss	SRT SDS SD_{max}

Zhou et al. (15)	2011	United States	37/39	MP 40 mg/ml × 0.5 ml 1× a day for 4 d	Protocol therapy controls	MP i.v. 125 mg/d for 1 d p.o. 32 mg/d for 5 d 16 mg/d for 2vd 8 mg/d for 2 d Nafthydrofuryl 200 mg 3× a day Diazepam 5 mg 3× a day Low-molecular-weight heparin s.c. 0.4 ml 2× a day	15 dB	SDS > 15%
Li et al. (18)	2011	China	24/41	MP 40 mg/ml × 1 ml once every 3 d for 15 d	Protocol therapy controls	PD i.v. 1 mg/kg per day for 5 d gradually tapered for 9 d	10 dB	NR
Arslan et al. (16)	2011	Turkey	85/73	MP 125 mg/ml × 0.5 ml once on alternate days for 5 d	Protocol therapy controls	MP i.v. 100 mg/d for 1 d p.o. 80 mg/d for 2 d tapered to 20 mg/d every 2 d Dextran 40000 i.v. 5 ml/kg per day for 5 d	10 dB	NR
Wu et al. (17)	2011	China	27/28	DEX 4 mg/ml × 0.5 ml 4 for 2 wk	Protocol therapy controls	MP i.v. 40 mg/12 h × 5 d PD p.o. 1 mg/kg gradually tapered for 5 d	10 dB	NR

Siegel's criteria (22).

DEX indicates dexamethasone; MP, methylprednisolone; ND, not delivered; NR, not reported; PD, prednisone; SD_{max}, maximum speech discrimination; SDS, speech discrimination score; SRT, speech recognition threshold; WRS, word recognition score.

Editor's Note: Please refer to original journal article for full references.

Methods.—An electronic database search (MEDLINE and PubMed) was performed with the objective of identifying all studies published in the English language between January 1980 and November 2011 on the efficacy of ITS in the treatment of SD. All relevant articles were retrieved, and the related reference lists were reviewed systematically to identify other reports that could be included. Data were synthesized using the Mantel-Haenszel model. Results are expressed as odds ratio (OR) with 95% confidence interval (CI).

Results.—A total of 11 randomized studies including 472 subjects allocated to ITS and 453 controls were selected. Intratympanic steroid regimens used and treatments administered to controls varied widely across studies. When considering together trials investigating ITS therapy as a primary (n = 4) or salvage (n = 7) treatment, the common OR for recovery was 1.7 (95% CI, 1.3–2.3). When considering them separately, the common ORs for recovery were 0.9 (95% CI, 0.7–1.6) for primary and 2.9 (95% CI, 1.9–4.5) for salvage therapy.

Conclusion.—Intratympanic steroid therapy seems to confer a certain degree of benefit as a salvage but not as a primary treatment of SD. However, further evidence is needed to clarify some yet uncertain aspects, such as the optimal protocol of therapy (Fig 1, Table 1).

▶ Unlike more common disorders, sudden deafness is a relatively rare and sporadic condition, making detailed study difficult unless through large and lengthy multicenter trials. Thus, a meta-analysis such as this becomes very valuable. Fortunately, despite the rare nature of the condition, Fig 1 shows some 40% of the studies available for review were worthy of inclusion to evaluate the effectiveness of intratympanic steroid administration for the treatment of sudden deafness. These are provided in Table 1 and divided into primary and salvage treatment with relevant details regarding each protocol. This listing provides an important resource for those interested in further study of the topic. The data here support the conclusions of the consensus panel recently published by the American Academy of Otolaryngology-Head and Neck Surgery, namely, that for use as a primary treatment modality, there is little support for additional benefit. However, for salvage there is good evidence for its use. The authors provide an excellent discussion of the results of these studies and their analysis to include a hypothesis as to the differences in effects seen between primary and salvage therapy. Additionally, as can be seen in Fig 1, there is wide variation between the steroid used and the dosage and administration protocols as well as the criteria to determine success. Thus, although this analysis supports the use of intratympanic steroid for salvage and not as a primary modality, numerous further studies are needed to better define these additional details.

B. J. Balough, MD

Auditory Abilities After Cochlear Implantation in Adults With Unilateral Deafness: A Pilot Study

Firszt JB, Holden LK, Reeder RM, et al (Washington Univ School of Medicine, St Louis, MO; et al)

Otol Neurotol 33:1339-1346, 2012

Objective.—This pilot study examined speech recognition, localization, temporal and spectral discrimination, and subjective reports of cochlear implant (CI) recipients with unilateral deafness.

Study Design.—Three adult male participants with short-term unilateral deafness (< 5 yr) participated. All had sudden onset of severe-to-profound hearing loss in 1 ear, which then received a CI, and normal or near normal hearing in the other ear. Speech recognition in quiet and noise, localization, discrimination of temporal and spectral cues, and a subjective questionnaire were obtained over several days. Listening conditions were CI, normal hearing (NH) ear, and bilaterally (CI and NH).

Results.—All participants had open-set speech recognition and excellent audibility (250–6,000 Hz) with the CI. Localization improved bilaterally compared with the NH ear alone. Word recognition in noise was significantly better bilaterally than with the NH ear for 2 participants. Sentence recognition in various noise conditions did not show significant bilateral improvement; however, the CI did not hinder performance in noise even when noise was toward the CI side. The addition of the CI improved temporal difference discrimination for 2 participants and spectral difference discrimination for all participants. Participants wore the CI full time, and subjective reports were positive.

Conclusion.—Overall, the CI recipients with unilateral deafness obtained open-set speech recognition, improved localization, improved word recognition in noise, and improved perception of their ability to hear in everyday life. A larger study is warranted to further quantify the benefits and limitations of cochlear implantation in individuals with unilateral deafness.

▶ Over the last several years, a variety of articles has begun to appear, such as this one, in which cochlear implantation has been performed in unilaterally deafened patients. Several rehabilitative options currently exist for unilateral deafness—contralateral routing of signals, bone-anchored hearing aids, SoundBite—but none of these truly restore binaural hearing. This study examines the capability of unilateral cochlear implantation with a contralateral normal hearing (NH) ear to provide binaural hearing. Several standard measures of localization and speech understanding were used to test bilateral hearing capability. In all cases, bilateral stimulation outperformed NH ear alone. Equally as important, the cochlear implant signal does not appear to interfere with perception in the NH ear. As evidence of this and perhaps most importantly, all 3 participants consistently wear their implant full time, which highly suggests benefit to which the data provides objective supporting evidence. Despite the benefits shown in this article as well as others, several questions remain. Among these are patient selection and optimal aural rehabilitation. Additionally, conclusions are limited by the small numbers of patients. Undoubtedly, many more studies will appear in coming years to further clarify the role of cochlear implantation in unilateral deafness.

B. J. Balough, MD

Fractionated Stereotactic Radiotherapy of Vestibular Schwannomas Accelerates Hearing Loss

Rasmussen R, Claesson M, Stangerup S-E, et al (Rigshospitalet, Copenhagen, Denmark)

Int J Radiat Oncol Biol Phys 83:e607-e611, 2012

Objective.—To evaluate long-term tumor control and hearing preservation rates in patients with vestibular schwannoma treated with fractionated stereotactic radiotherapy (FSRT), comparing hearing preservation rates to an untreated control group. The relationship between radiation dose to the cochlea and hearing preservation was also investigated.

Methods and Materials.—Forty-two patients receiving FSRT between 1997 and 2008 with a minimum follow-up of 2 years were included. All patients received 54 Gy in 27-30 fractions during 5.5-6.0 weeks. Clinical and audiometry data were collected prospectively. From a "wait and-scan" group, 409 patients were selected as control subjects, matched by initial audiometric parameters. Radiation dose to the cochlea was measured using the original treatment plan and then related to changes in acoustic parameters.

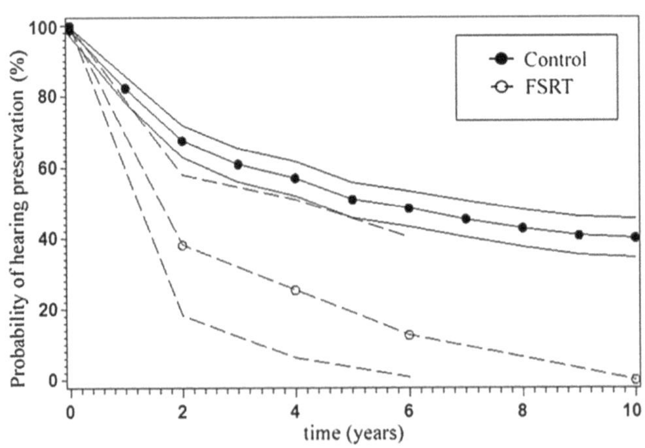

FIGURE 3.—Hearing preservation rates after fractionated stereotactic radiotherapy (FSRT) compared with a "wait-and-scan" control group with 95% confidence interval. The *P* value for log-rank test comparing the 2 curves was .008. (Reprinted from the International Journal of Radiation Oncology Biology Physics. Rasmussen R, Claesson M, Stangerup S-E, et al. Fractionated stereotactic radiotherapy of vestibular schwannomas accelerates hearing loss. *Int J Radiat Oncol Biol Phys*. 2012;83:e607-e611, Copyright 2012, with permission from Elsevier.)

Results.—Actuarial 2-, 4-, and 10-year tumor control rates were 100%, 91.5%, and 85.0%, respectively. Twenty-one patients had serviceable hearing before FSRT, 8 of whom (38%) retained serviceable hearing at 2 years after FSRT. No patients retained serviceable hearing after 10 years. At 2 years, hearing preservation rates in the control group were 1.8 times higher compared with the group receiving FSRT ($P = .007$). Radiation dose to the cochlea was significantly correlated to deterioration of the speech reception threshold ($P = .03$) but not to discrimination loss.

Conclusion.—FSRT accelerates the naturally occurring hearing loss in patients with vestibular schwannoma. Our findings, using fractionation of radiotherapy, parallel results using single-dose radiation. The radiation dose to the cochlea is correlated to hearing loss measured as the speech reception threshold (Fig 3).

▶ Stereotactic radiation varies in device used and dosage provided. Among these modalities is fractionated radiation. The operative theory behind fractionation is that higher tumor doses can be delivered over time with less potential toxicity to normal tissue; this study seeks to validate this theory. Several strengths are present in this report: data from a single center with a homogenous treatment algorithm, long-term follow-up averaging 5 years with data out to 10 years, prospective audiologic data to include both pure tone average and discrimination scores, and a large control cohort from the same patient population. Fig 3 shows the hearing data over time comparing the treatment and control groups. The graph clearly shows poor preservation of Garner-Robertson class 1 hearing in the treatment group with a rapid decline in the first 2 years. Additionally, the resection-free survival rate was 80% out through 10 years then decreasing to 50%. Just as with the hearing data, this fares poorly with other prior studies. However, this may be because of the higher-quality data and longer terms of follow-up in this study. It is important to remember, however, that the treated tumors were biologically more aggressive in that they all showed growth, whereas the tumors in the control group by definition had no growth and were biologically quiet. Not all other studies will show such a distinction, as some nongrowing tumors will be in the treatment arm. For example, other published studies will quote treatment-free survival rates in the high 90% range, but when growth is used as a determinant of failure, some 40% will continue to grow. Those numbers and that of this study are thus very similar. Regarding the poor hearing preservation rate, the authors discuss cochlear dose, and, as has been found in other studies, a high cochlear dose correlated to higher rates of hearing loss. Thus, if cochlear dose can be limited, radiation may lead to improved hearing preservation rates. Additionally, stratification based on tumor size, auditory brainstem response morphology, filling of the internal auditory canal, and other factors may help better define which tumors will fare well from radiation for hearing preservation vs surgery or observation.

B. J. Balough, MD

Outcomes of Intratympanic Gentamicin Injection to Treat Ménière's Disease

Huon L-K, Fang T-Y, Wang P-C (Cathay General Hosp, New Taipei City, Taiwan, Republic of China)

Otol Neurotol 33:706-714, 2012

Objective.—To investigate the outcomes of intratympanic (IT) gentamicin sulfate injection to treat intractable Ménière's disease (MD) using evidence-based methods.

Data Source.—Data were retrieved from a MEDLINE search (January 1995 through January 2011).

Study Selection.—Selected were English-language articles presenting outcomes of IT gentamicin injection to treat MD that had a prospective study design and an evidence level of II or higher.

Data Extraction.—The database was searched using Boolean combinations of the keywords *intratympanic, gentamicin*, and *Ménière's disease.*

Data Synthesis.—Dichotomous outcomes (success rate and total deafness) were expressed using a Mantel-Haenszel fixed-effects model. Pretreatment and posttreatment pure-tone audiometry results, and word discrimination scores were summarized using data synthesis techniques.

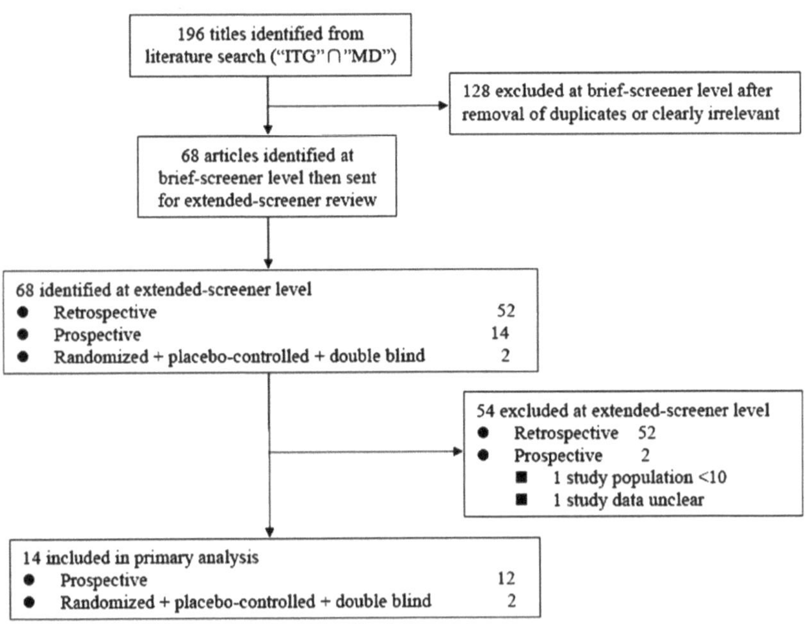

FIGURE 1.—Article selection algorithm showing that the MEDLINE search revealed 14 original articles dealing with intratympanic gentamicin sulfate injection for MD between January 1995 and January 2011. (Reprinted from Huon L-K, Fang T-Y, Wang P-C. Outcomes of intratympanic gentamicin injection to treat Ménière's disease. *Otol Neurotol.* 2012;33:706-714, with permission from Otology & Neurotology, Inc.)

TABLE 1.—Summary of Major Study Treatment Protocols

Study	Design	Patients	Age	Concentration (mg/ml)	Treatment Protocol	Treatment Content	Total Injections
Casani et al. (2005) (13)	Prospective	26	58	20	Fixed	Low dose	1.2 ± 0.6
Horii et al. (2006) (14)	Prospective	28	51.4	26	Fixed	Low dose	3
Helling et al. (2009) (15)	Prospective	19	53.7	12	Fixed	Low dose	1.4 ± 0.6
Harner et al. (2001) (16)	Prospective	56	57	40	Fixed	Low dose	1.6 ± 0.9
Postema et al. (2008) (17)	Prospective, double blinded, randomized	16	53	30	Fixed	Weekly	4
Quaranta et al. (1999) (18)	Prospective	11	52.9	80	Fixed	High dose	2.3 ± 0.4
Quaranta et al. (2001) (19)	Prospective	15	46.1	20	Fixed	Low dose	2.7 ± 6.8
Boleas-Aguirre et al. (2007) (5)	Prospective	127	53	26.7	Titration	Titration weekly	3 ± 2
Kaasinen et al. (1998) (6)	Prospective	93	50.9	30	Titration	Titration weekly	2.4 ± 1
Lange et al. (2004) (7)	Prospective	57	54	12	Titration	Titration weekly	1.5 ± 0.8
Martin et al. (2003) (8)	Prospective	71	53.6	26.7	Titration	Titration weekly	2.5
Minor et al. (1999) (9)	Prospective	34	53	26.7	Titration	Titration weekly	2.8 ± 1.3
Stokroos et al. (2004) (10)	Prospective, double blinded, randomized	12	59	30	Titration	Titration weekly	1.5 ± 0.5
Wu et al. (1999) (11)	Prospective	34	52.3	26.7	Titration	Titration weekly	2.7 ± 1.5
Casani et al. (2005) (13)	Prospective	26	58	20	Fixed	Low dose	1.2 ± 0.6

Editor's Note: Please refer to original journal article for full references.

Conclusion.—A critical literature appraisal and meta-analysis shows that IT gentamicin injection can control vertigo in patients with MD who have limited hearing injury. The quality of research in this field has improved remarkably over the years. However, a large-scale randomized controlled trial is warranted to confirm the predictive factors for the effectiveness of IT gentamicin injection in treating MD (Fig 1, Table 1).

▶ Intratympanic gentamicin remains a popular ablative nonsurgical choice for the treatment of Ménière's disease. Despite its popularity, numerous questions remain regarding dose and treatment protocol. This is not much different than more than a decade ago in spite of numerous publications on the subject. This is because of the often poor quality of the publications, which is very well illustrated in Fig 1. Of 196 articles found, only 14, a mere 7%, were of sufficient merit to be included in the analysis. In itself, the collection of these 14 high-quality studies, which are outlined in Table 1, makes this a worthy study for review and reference. However, several other items are valuable as well. First is the impact on auditory function. Traditionally, use of gentamicin can reduce hearing in as many as 20%. That is not borne out in this analysis, in which overall hearing levels did not change and only a small percentage experienced complete loss of hearing. Thus, gentamicin from this study would have a similar rate of hearing preservation as vestibular nerve section. Additionally, gentamicin has some beneficial effect on tinnitus as well in slightly more than 10% but no benefit for aural fullness. Second, success is independent of protocol whether fixed or titration with an overall class A and B control rate of more than 87%. Hearing preservation is a bit worse with titration, but, interestingly, tinnitus relief was better under titration protocols opposite of the hearing result. Third, although protocol does not seem to make a difference in result, total delivered dose does seem to matter, with success to be expected if more than 13 mg is delivered. What this analysis seems to reveal is that much of what is commented on regarding gentamicin therapy is wisdom gleaned from poor studies repeated over time. As the authors conclude, large prospective and well-controlled trials are needed to include quality-of-life measures to assess chronic disequilibrium and vertigo control.

B. J. Balough, MD

The Role of Obesity in Spontaneous Temporal Bone Encephaloceles and CSF Leak

Stucken EZ, Selesnick SH, Brown KD (Weill Cornell Med College and New York Presbyterian Hosp)

Otol Neurotol 33:1412-1417, 2012

Objective.—Temporal bone encephaloceles and cerebrospinal fluid (CSF) otorrhea can lead to life-threatening sequelae such as meningitis and cerebritis. Obesity has been associated with spontaneous CSF leaks. We wished to determine if there were differences in the body mass index (BMI) of patients

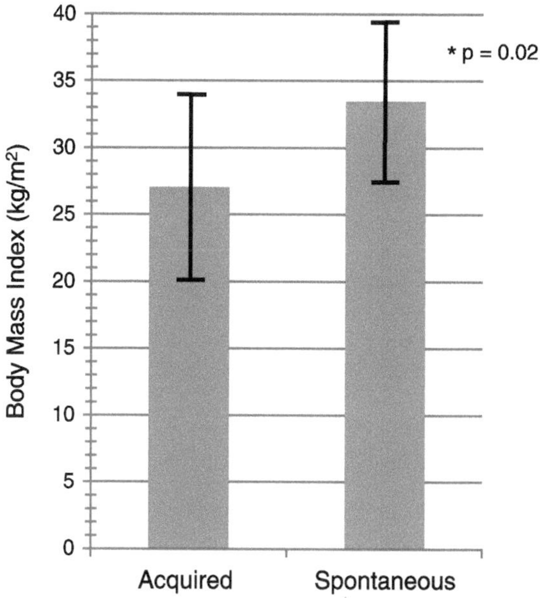

FIGURE 2.—Average BMI in acquired and spontaneous encephaloceles. (Reprinted from Stucken EZ, Selesnick SH, Brown KD. The role of obesity in spontaneous temporal bone encephaloceles and CSF leak. *Otol Neurotol.* 2012;33:1412-1417, with permission from Otology & Neurotology, Inc.)

with spontaneous temporal bone encephaloceles/CSF leaks and nonspontaneous temporal bone encephaloceles/CSF leaks to help determine if obesity may be associated with their development.

Study Design.—Single institution retrospective comparison.

Methods.—Demographic and clinical information was obtained from 20 patients treated for surgically confirmed temporal bone dehiscence leading to encephalocele and/or CSF otorrhea. Statistical analysis was performed on patients with spontaneous and nonspontaneous encephaloceles/CSF leaks to determine if there were differences in the degree of obesity between these groups.

Results.—Temporal bone dehiscence was spontaneous in 11 patients, related to chronic infection in 4 patients, posttraumatic in 3 patients, postsurgical in 1 patient, and because of massive hydrocephalus in a final patient. The average BMI for patients with spontaneous encephalocele was 33.4 kg/m^2. The average BMI for patients with nonspontaneous encephaloceles was 27.0 kg/m^2. This difference was statistically significant ($p = 0.02$).

Conclusion.—Although several previous studies have demonstrated an association of obesity with spontaneous encephaloceles or CSF leaks, this study is one of the first to demonstrate a statistically significant increase in BMI for patients with spontaneous encephaloceles and CSF leaks as compared with patients developing them for other reasons. This suggests a potential etiologic role of obesity in the development of spontaneous encephaloceles and CSF leaks.

Level of Evidence.—4 (Fig 2).

▶ In the United States and other countries, as obesity rates increase, particularly childhood obesity rates, many diseases are increasing in prevalence or are seen earlier in life. Spontaneous cerebrospinal fluid (CSF) leak to the middle ear with or without encephalocele can lead to many serious complications including meningitis. This study was undertaken to determine if average body mass index (BMI) was elevated in spontaneous cases as opposed to those with other known etiologies, such as trauma, infection, or after prior surgery. Although the ranges overlap, Fig 2 illustrates a clear and statistically significant elevation in BMI between the spontaneous and acquired cases of encephaloceles. The bar graph, however, is a bit misleading in that the lowest BMI value for an acquired case was 13.4 and for the spontaneous cases 22. The study also suffers from small numbers of patients and the terms *CSF*, *tegmen dehiscence*, and *encephalocele* are used interchangeably. Despite these limitations, the data provide valuable evidence of the impact of obesity. Because spontaneous CSF leak may be difficult to distinguish from ordinary middle ear effusion and imaging studies are not definitive, a high index of suspicion should exist in those with elevated BMI.

B. J. Balough, MD

Third-Generation Bisphosphonates for Treatment of Sensorineural Hearing Loss in Otosclerosis

Quesnel AM, Seton M, Merchant SN, et al (Massachusetts Eye and Ear Infirmary, Boston, MA; Massachusetts General Hosp, Boston; et al)

Otol Neurotol 33:1308-1314, 2012

Objective.—To evaluate hearing outcomes in patients treated with third generation bisphosphonates for otosclerosis-related sensorineural hearing loss (SNHL).

Hypothesis.—Otosclerosis is a disease of abnormal bone remodeling in the otic capsule. In recent years, third generation bisphosphonates, with more powerful anti-resorptive properties and increased bone affinity, have demonstrated effectiveness in the treatment of osteoporosis and other metabolic bone diseases. We hypothesized that newer generation bisphosphonates, such as risedronate and zoledronate, would be effective in slowing the progression of SNHL in patients with otosclerosis.

Study Design.—Retrospective review.

Setting.—Tertiary referral center, ambulatory care.

Interventions.—Risedronate or zoledronate administration.

Main Outcome Measures.—Bone conduction pure tone threshold averages (PTAs) and word recognition (WR) scores were examined for each ear before and after bisphosphonate treatment. Criteria for significant

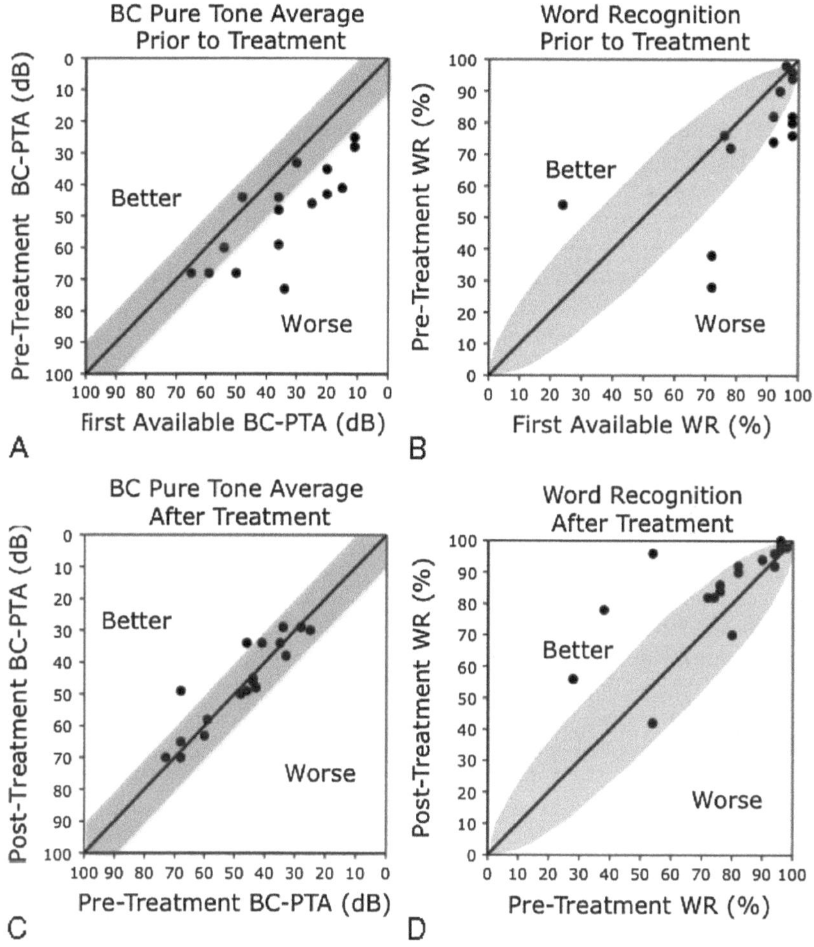

FIGURE.—*A* and *B*, BC-PTA and WR score in the pretreatment interval. *C* and *D*, BC-PTA and WR in the posttreatment interval. Each point on the graph represents 1 ear. The *black line* is a reference line that marks no change between the first available and the immediate pretreatment audiograms in *A* and *B* and between the immediate pretreatment and posttreatment audiograms in C and *D*. Change is not considered significant within the shaded area, with significance defined by more than 10 dB change in PTA (*A* and *C*) or by the binomial model of variance for WR (*B* and *D*). The majority of the ears are below the line in *A* and *B*. In contrast, most ears after treatment, as shown in C and *D*, are close to the line or above the line. (Reprinted from Quesnel AM, Seton M, Merchant SN, et al. Third-generation bisphosphonates for treatment of sensorineural hearing loss in otosclerosis. *Otol Neurotol*. 2012;33:1308-1314, with permission ffom Otology & Neurotology, Inc.)

change were defined as greater than 10 decibels in PTA or between 4% and 18% in WR based on binomial variance.

Results.—All 10 patients had audiometric progression of SNHL in the pretreatment monitoring interval and 12 ears met criteria for significant progression. All 10 patients (19 ears) showed at least no significant progression of SNHL (i.e., stabilization) at an average follow-up of 13 months. Two patients (3 ears) showed improvement by defined audiometric criteria. There were no major complications.

Conclusion.—Treatment with zoledronate or risedronate stabilized progressive SNHL related to otosclerosis in this small group of patients. Further evaluation of third-generation bisphosphonate treatments is warranted (Fig).

▶ Although the conductive component of otosclerosis is easy to remedy with surgery, the sensorineural component that often accompanies it is relatively resistant to treatment. Historically, fluoride supplementation was used in an attempt to stabilize hearing with the thought that this would strengthen the bone and prevent resorption. Results, however, are uncertain. The reasoning behind bisphosphonate use and the advantages of the latest generation of these drugs are discussed. The authors also review a significant challenge in addressing this problem, namely, that although sensorineural loss can be common, only a small percentage of patients with otosclerosis will have progressive declines. They approach this issue by identifying a small group of patients with progressive declines in word recognition (WR) or bone thresholds. Fig shows the before and after treatment relative changes. The goal of treatment here is to hold the line and prevent further declines. It is interesting to note that in some cases, the WR scores actually seemed to improve. Translated to an average, WR improved by 5.5% after treatment (average decline before treatment, 3.7%) and bone conduction rate of declined slowed from 4.3 dB before treatment to 1 dB after treatment. The authors are careful to mention that there was high variability in these results. However, the trend is for improvement in WR with stabilization of bone threshold. Given the short duration of study, it is unclear if these results will be lasting or temporary. Given the potential systemic toxicity and side effects of bisphosphonates, further study is needed, and any treated patients require close follow-up. However, for selected patients, this treatment shows promise.

B. J. Balough, MD

Traumatic Tympanic Membrane Perforations: Clinical and Audiometric Findings in 198 Patients

Hempel JM, Becker A, Müller J, et al (Ludwig Maximilian Univ, Munich, Germany)

Otol Neurotol 33:1357-1362, 2012

Objective.—To obtain clinical and audiometric findings in traumatic tympanic membrane perforations from a typical patient collective in a Western industrial nation because the appropriate data have an important relevance in medicolegal questions.

Study Design.—Retrospective data collection.

Setting.—Germany's largest university clinic for otorhinolaryngology, head and neck surgery.

Subject and Methods.—From the medical records of 198 patients with traumatic tympanic membrane perforations, the following data were collected: demographic data, date and mechanism of the trauma, otoscopic findings and collateral injuries, kind of therapy and its results, pure tone audiometry, and statement of tinnitus or vertigo in the course.

Results.—Most patients were young (mean age, 29.2 yr) and male (62%). Men and women are equally represented in perforations resulting from a physical blow to the ear (44.7% vs 46.7%); a collision was more often the cause in men (23.6% vs 14.7%), whereas an accidental perforation by insertion of a cotton bud was approximately 2 times more common on women (13.8% vs 25.3%). The left ear was more often affected than the right ear (58.5% vs 41.5%). Collateral damage was found in only 1% of the cases. In blows, collisions, barotraumas, and the insertion of sharp objects, the inferior parts of the tympanic membrane were most often affected; the most severe (subtotal) perforations were caused by explosions, weld beads, and insertion of cotton buds. For therapy, myringoplasty had an overall success rate of 88.9%; splinting with silicon foils, 51.6%; and "no therapy," 53.3%. Bone conduction thresholds for the affected ear were higher in low, middle, and high frequencies compared with the contralateral ear by trend, but a statistical difference was only found in the high frequencies. In follow-up examinations, the hearing thresholds in the high frequencies were no longer significantly different. A "c^5 dip" or "fis^5 dip" was found in 18.0% and 9.2%. Tinnitus and vertigo were reported in 30.8 and 8.1%, respectively, but only in 2.0% and 0% during follow-up.

Conclusion.—High-frequency hearing loss, tinnitus, and vertigo in traumatic tympanic membrane perforations have a good prognosis.

► Patterns of trauma can vary depending on locale and development. In more industrialized and urban environments, rates and types of otologic trauma should be expected to reflect these surroundings. In this 10-year review of their tympanic membrane perforations, the authors discuss the source of injury and rates among men and women as well as other related otologic symptoms of hearing loss, tinnitus, and vertigo. One of their most important findings is that although vertigo (8%) and tinnitus (30%) are common at initial presentation, they rarely if ever persist (0% vertigo, 2% tinnitus). Similarly, except for frequencies greater than 3000 Hz, hearing loss from traumatic perforation is also unlikely to persist. Unfortunately, the hearing results are not broken down by source of injury; thus, it is unknown if these high frequency losses were seen from predominantly one type of cause (blast, concussive, barotrauma) as might be expected. Another interesting finding is that observation, fat graft, and patch all had similar levels of poor rates of success in closure at roughly 50%. Traditionally, spontaneous closure of perforation is thought to be 90% within the first few months after injury, which has been my experience. Here the authors opted to treat 75% of the perforations in some fashion within a day of injury. It would seem then that active intervention may lead to worse results, yet their observation-only numbers were similarly poor. However, a plausible explanation is that only more severe cases were referred to the Ear, Nose, and Throat Clinic. Yet, this aspect of the data is a bit puzzling and may be worth additional investigations. Despite this curiosity, the remainder of the report provides a valuable update on the topic and is worth reading.

B. J. Balough, MD

Randomized clinical trial for geotropic horizontal canal benign paroxysmal positional vertigo

Kim JS, Oh S-Y, Lee S-H, et al (Seoul Natl Univ Bundang Hosp, Korea; Chonbuk Natl Univ Hosp, Jeonju, South Korea; Chonnam Natl Univ Med School, Gwangju, Republic of Korea; et al)

Neurology 79:700-707, 2012

Objectives.—To determine the immediate and long-term therapeutic efficacies of barbecue rotation and Gufoni maneuvers, a randomized,

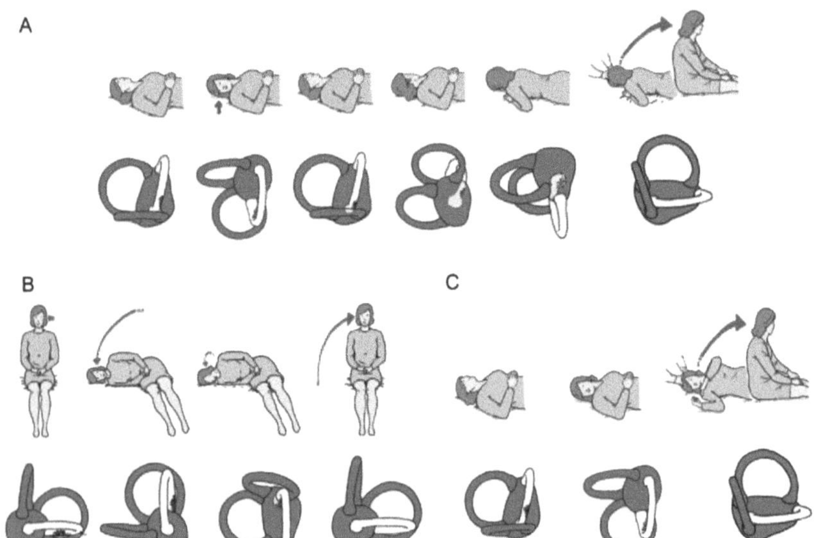

FIGURE 2.—Illustrations of barbecue rotation (A), Gufoni (B), and sham (C) maneuvers for the geotropic type of benign paroxysmal positional vertigo involving the horizontal canal (HC) (arrow: affected ear). (A) For the barbecue rotation maneuver, the head and trunk are rotated 90° at each step in the direction of the healthy ear while the patient is supine. Each step is maintained for 30–60 seconds until the induced nystagmus dissipated. After 270° of rotation, the patient is brought to the sitting position. (B) In the sitting position, the debris are located in the dependent posterior arm of the left HC. Side-lying to the healthy side causes the particles to move further toward the posterior part of the HC and could produce an utriculopetal (ampullofugal) flow and intense horizontal nystagmus beating toward the ground. After the head is rotated toward the ground, particles move further toward the posterior part and fall into the vestibule, causing an ampullofugal flow and nystagmus beating toward the healthy side. Each position is maintained for 2 minutes. Then the patient is returned to the upright position. (C) For the sham maneuver, patients lie down from the sitting position. After 30 seconds, the head is rotated 90° in the direction of the affected ear, which would cause ampullopetal (utriculofugal) migration of the debris. After another 60 seconds, patients are brought to the sitting position. (Reprinted from Kim JS, Oh S-Y, Lee S-H, et al. Randomized clinical trial for geotropic horizontal canal benign paroxysmal positional vertigo. *Neurology.* 2012;79:700-707, with permission from AAN Enterprises, Inc.)

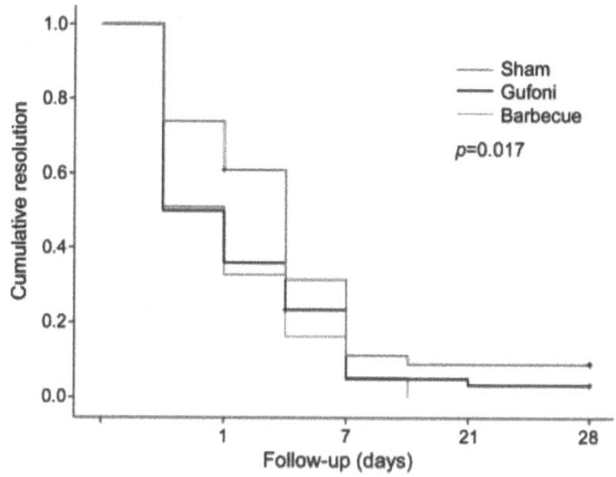

FIGURE 3.—Kaplan-Meier survival curve. The Kaplan-Meier survival curve with a log-rank test for cumulative therapeutic effects shows a better outcome with the barbecue rotation ($p = 0.005$) and Gufoni ($p = 0.044$) maneuvers than with the sham maneuver. However, the therapeutic effects are not different between the barbecue rotation and Gufoni groups ($p = 0.399$). (Reprinted from Kim JS, Oh S-Y, Lee S-H, et al. Randomized clinical trial for geotropic horizontal canal benign paroxysmal positional vertigo. *Neurology*. 2012;79:700-707, with permission from AAN Enterprises, Inc.)

prospective, and sham-controlled study was conducted in patients with the geotropic type of benign paroxysmal positional vertigo involving the horizontal semicircular canal (HC-BPPV).

Methods.—In 10 nationwide dizziness clinics in Korea, 170 consecutive patients (107 women, age range 11–97 years, mean age ± SD 61 ± 15 years, median = 61 years) with geotropic HC-BPPV were randomly assigned to barbecue rotation (n = 56), Gufoni (n = 64), or sham maneuver (n = 50). An immediate response was determined within 1 hour after a maximum of 2 trials of each maneuver on the visit day. We also assessed the cumulative results of each maneuver by following up the patients for 1 month.

Results.—After a maximum of 2 maneuvers on the initial visit day, barbecue rotation (38 of 55 [69.1%]) and Gufoni (39 of 64 [60.9%]) maneuvers showed better responses than the sham maneuver (17 of 48 [35.4%]). The cumulative therapeutic effects were also better with barbecue rotation ($p = 0.006$) and Gufoni ($p = 0.031$) maneuvers than with the sham maneuver. However, therapeutic efficacies did not differ between the barbecue rotation and Gufoni groups in terms of both immediate ($p = 0.46$) and long-term ($p = 0.10$) outcomes.

Conclusion.—Using a prospective randomized trial, we demonstrated that barbecue rotation and Gufoni maneuvers are effective in treating geotropic HC-BPPV.

Classification of Evidence.—This study provides Class I evidence that barbecue rotation and Gufoni maneuvers are effective in the treatment of geotropic HC-BPPV (Figs 2 and 3).

▶ Horizontal semicircular canal benign paroxysmal positional vertigo (BPPV) is less common than posterior canal vertigo but still accounts for one-quarter to one-third of all cases. Here the authors do a head-to-head comparison between 2 methods of treatment and a sham control. Fig 2 illustrates these 3 methods. The method they term *barbeque rotation* is also known by the name *log roll*. Interestingly, although both active treatment protocols are statistically significantly better than control (60%–70% resolution), neither has the high efficacy associated with repositioning for posterior canalithiasis (> 80%). One explanation that the authors explore is canal conversion, but this rate was extremely small (< 2%). Thus, patients with horizontal canal BPPV should be counseled regarding the lower efficacy regardless of treatment than that of posterior canal BPPV. This may be because of a higher proportion of cupulolithiasis than canalithiasis in horizontal canal BPPV. Lastly, even in the sham treatment group, a high proportion of symptoms is resolved by 1 week (some 80%) and remain so for the 4-week duration of study (Fig 3). This suggests that horizontal BPPV is inherently unstable and in most cases resolves quickly without treatment. There remains, however, a persistent symptomatic population that is similar in number regardless of treatment.

B. J. Balough, MD

Spectrum of Immune-Mediated Inner Ear Disease and Cochlear Implant Results

Malik MU, Pandian V, Masood H, et al (Johns Hopkins Univ, Baltimore, MD; Johns Hopkins Hosp, Baltimore, MD)
Laryngoscope 122:2557-2562, 2012

Objectives/Hypothesis.—To characterize the progression of hearing loss in patients with immune-mediated inner ear disease (IMIED), and to identify disease- and patient-specific factors associated with cochlear implant (CI) performance.

Study Design.—Retrospective cohort study.

Methods.—Subjects consisted of CI patients suspected to have lost their hearing due to IMIED. The primary dependent variable for functional decline was time to deafness, whereas for CI benefit it was post-CI speech perception scores. Independent variables included presence or absence of systemic autoimmune disease, age at CI, and insertion depth of the cochlear electrode.

Results.—A transient favorable response to immunosuppressive therapy was reported in 16 of 26 patients (66.67%). The time to deafness differed between an organ (ear)-specific immune-mediated group, a systemic immune-mediated group including Cogan syndrome and relapsing polychondritis (subgroup A), and a systemic immune-mediated group associated with other autoimmune diseases (subgroup B; $P = .001$). Disease group (-15.52; $P = .04$), insertion depth of the CI electrode (40.71; $P = .01$), and the age at CI (-0.48, $P = .05$) were associated with speech perception results.

Conclusions.—Triaging IMIED cases based on presence and type of systemic autoimmune disease may aid in selecting a management strategy.

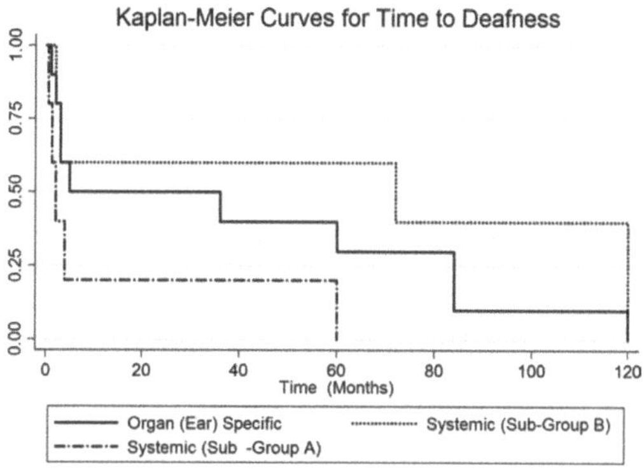

FIGURE 1.—This figure compares time to deafness between three immune-mediated inner ear disease (IMIED) groups: 1) organ (ear) specific immune-mediated (OS-IMIED), 2) a systemic immunemediated group consisting of relapsing polychondritis and Cogan syndrome (subgroup A), and 3) other systemic autoimmune diseases (subgroup B). Systemic subgroup A demonstrated the fastest deterioration in hearing function, followed by the OS-IMIED group and systemic subgroup B. (Reprinted from Malik MU, Pandian V, Masood H, et al. Spectrum of immune-mediated inner ear disease and cochlear implant results. *Laryngoscope*. 2012;122:2557-2562, with permission from Laryngoscope and John Wiley and Sons, www.interscience.wiley.com.)

Knowledge about the predictors of CI outcome will help clinicians select appropriate patients for CIs. In the setting of significant and irreversible hearing deficit, the restoration of hearing using a cochlear prosthesis may be appropriate earlier rather than later (Fig 1).

► Although only at best representing 1% of acquired deafness, autoimmune-related ear disorders are an interesting subset explored in this study. Often grouped together, the authors here have divided them into organ-specific and systemic groups with the systemic group further divided into 2 subgroups. As shown in Fig 1, some interesting differences emerge when the groups are separated in this way. Chief among these is that the systemic diseases can be much more aggressive than ear-mediated disease in the cases of Cogan syndrome and relapsing polychondritis, whereas the other systemic causes are less aggressive. This information can be useful in counseling patients regarding prognosis and expectations. Unfortunately, the small numbers in the study limit the impact of other findings. The most important of these being that the organ-specific disease had a better response to pharmacotherapy than did the systemic disease. It is also important to remember that in this study all patients progressed to deafness and received a cochlear implant. Thus, they are more severe forms of their respective disorders. Despite these limitations, interesting differences have been identified that are worth further study.

B. J. Balough, MD

Quality of Life of Patients With Bilateral Vestibulopathy

Guinand N, Boselie F, Guyot J-P, et al (Univ Hosp Maastricht, the Netherlands; Univ Hosps of Geneva, Switzerland)

Ann Otol Rhinol Laryngol 121:471-477, 2012

Objectives.—Currently, there is no evidence of an effective treatment for patients with bilateral vestibulopathy (BV). Their main complaints are oscillopsia and imbalance. Opinions about the impact of BV on their quality of life are controversial, and their handicap is not always recognized, even among otoneurologists. The aim of this study was to objectively assess the health status of BV patients in order to evaluate the need for pursuing efforts toward the development of new treatments.

Methods.—The Short-Form Health Survey (SF-36), the Dizziness Handicap Inventory (DHI), the Short Falls Efficacy Scale–International (Short FES-I), and an oscillopsia severity questionnaire were submitted to 39 BV patients. The SF-36 scores were compared to the scores of a general Dutch population. The DHI scores were correlated to the oscillopsia severity scores. The Short FES-I scores were compared to scores in an elderly population. Residual otolithic function was correlated to all scores, and hearing to SF-36 scores.

Results.—Compared to the general Dutch population, the BV patients scored significantly worse on the "physical functioning," "role physical," "general health," "vitality," and "social functioning" SF-36 variables ($p < 0.05$). The DHI scores were strongly correlated with the oscillopsia severity scores ($r = 0.75$; $p < 0.000001$). The Short FES-I scores indicated a slight to moderate increase in the patients' fear of falling. No significant score differences were found between BV patients with residual otolithic function and patients with complete BV. There was no correlation between hearing status and SF-36 scores.

Conclusions.—The results correlate with our clinical impression that BV has a strong negative impact on physical and social functioning, leading to a quality-of-life deterioration. There is a clear need for a therapeutic

TABLE 2.—Oscillopsia Severity questionnaire

Oscillopsia Severity Questionnaire
1. Do you have the sensation that the visual environment is moving when it's not?
2. By dim light, do you have the sensation that what you see is not stable?
3. Is it difficult for you to recognize known faces when you are walking?
4. When you are reading, do you have the sensation that the text is not stable?
5. When you are watching television, do you have the sensation that the image is not stable?
6. When you are driving your car, do you have the sensation that what you see is not stable?
7. As a car passenger, do you have the sensation that what you see is not stable?
8. When you are riding a bicycle, do you have the sensation that what you see is not stable?
9. When you are walking on uneven ground, do you have the sensation that what you see is not stable?

always = 5, often = 4, sometimes = 3, seldom = 2, never = 1.

solution. Efforts toward the development of a vestibular implant are justified (Table 2).

▶ It is well recognized that a complete loss of vestibular function is severely disabling. Here a variety of quality-of-life instruments were used to gauge the degree and nature of this disability. Two of these, the Short Form-36 and Dizziness Handicap Inventory (DHI), are widely used. A unique oscillopsia questionnaire was developed as well and is represented in Table 2. Consisting of only 9 questions, this scale may be useful for screening for oscillopsia as well as for grading the severity of its impact on the individual. The latter may be useful to measure the benefit of therapeutic interventions or as the patient accommodates over time. The oscillopsia questionnaire also demonstrated high internal validity and correlated well to the DHI. Another item of interest from this article is that in the study population, in nearly 50% of the 39 patients no cause for the bilateral vestibular hypofunction was identified. As frustrating as this diagnosis is to patient and physician alike, not being able to determine (or prevent) a cause is more so. The high rate of unknown causes suggests an opportunity for further work in this area. Interestingly, despite similar inclusion criteria in terms of physiologic testing, not all patients were similarly handicapped by their condition and showed a range from mild to severe handicap. In addition, when otolithic function was measured, just over 50% of the subjects had measurable cervical vestibular evoked myogenic potentials. Unfortunately, perhaps because of insufficient numbers, this was not further analyzed as a subset to see if this retention of otolithic function indeed mitigated the severity of handicap. This also may be a useful future study.

B. J. Balough, MD

Transmastoid Semicircular Canal Occlusion: A Safe and Highly Effective Treatment for Benign Paroxysmal Positional Vertigo and Superior Canal Dehiscence

Beyea JA, Agrawal SK, Parnes LS (The Univ of Western Ontario, London, Canada)

Laryngoscope 122:1862-1866, 2012

Objectives/Hypothesis.—Transmastoid occlusion of the superior semicircular canal in superior semicircular canal dehiscence (SSCD) syndrome and the posterior semicircular canal in intractable benign paroxysmal positional vertigo (BPPV) will produce resolution of preoperative symptoms.

Study Design.—Retrospective review, quality assurance.

Methods.—Sixteen patients with SSCD and 61 patients (65 ears) with intractable BPPV who underwent canal occlusion were reviewed. All patients underwent occlusion of the affected semicircular canal through a transmastoid approach.

Results.—Preoperative symptoms (vestibular, 13 patients; pulsatile tinnitus, 2 patients; or hyperacusis, 1 patient) were greatly improved or completely resolved in 15 of the 16 SSCD patients who underwent

TABLE 1.—Preoperative Superior Semicircular Canal Dehiscence Syndrome Patient Characteristics (N = 16)

Patient Characteristic	No. Positive
Aural fullness	6
Autophony	7
Hyperacusis as sole complaint	1
Pulsatile tinnitus	8
Pulsatile tinnitus as sole complaint	2
Tullio phenomenon	10
Positive fistula test (subjective or objective)	5
Audiogram—conductive hearing loss	7
VEMP—low threshold	6*
High-resolution CT scan—SSC dehiscence	16

VEMP = vestibular evoked myogenic potential response; CT = computed tomography; SSC = superior semicircular canal.
*Only 11 patients were tested with VEMP. If a patient was referred to our center with prior CT confirmation of a superior semicircular canal dehiscence, a VEMP was not performed. All VEMP testing was cervical VEMP.

TABLE 3.—Postoperative Superior Semicircular Canal Dehiscence Syndrome Patient Characteristics (N = 16)

Patient Characteristic	No.
Vestibular symptoms resolved	6
Vestibular symptoms improved	6
Vestibular symptoms not improved	1
Pulsatile tinnitus improved	8
Pulsatile tinnitus as sole complaint improved	2
Hyperacusis as sole complaint improved	1
Hearing improved	2
Hearing preserved	14
Hearing worsened	0
Postoperative oral steroids for sterile labyrinthitis	3

transmastoid occlusion of the superior canal. Hearing was preserved in 14 patients and improved in two patients. Vestibular symptoms were resolved in all intractable BPPV patients who underwent transmastoid occlusion of the posterior canal. One patient had a late recurrence of atypical BPPV. Almost all BPPV patients with normal preoperative hearing have an initial transient postoperative hearing loss, which when tested for is usually a mild to moderate mixed loss. Delayed sensorineural hearing loss was noted in three patients; one loss was profound whereas two were mild.

Conclusions.—The transmastoid approach to canal plugging is successful in the treatment of symptoms in both SSCD and intractable BPPV, and is a familiar approach for the otologist. This is a viable alternative to the middle fossa approach for SSCD, thereby avoiding a craniotomy. Transmastoid is the definitive approach for posterior canal occlusion (Tables 1 and 3).

▶ This article represents the senior author's experience with canal occlusion for superior canal dehiscence and intractable benign positional vertigo. It also discusses his methods for performing these procedures in good detail. The preoperative characteristics for the superior canal dehiscence series are shown in Table 1, and the postoperative results are shown in Table 3. These results demonstrate that transmastoid canal occlusion can be a very effective method of treatment and should be considered as an option to the middle fossa approach. Although effective, the data could have been better presented by using the same categories in the pre- and postoperative tables. It is interesting to note that for this series, computed tomography—verified presence of dehiscence with appropriate symptoms was used to make the diagnosis, and a vestibular evoked myogenic potential (VEMP) was not used for confirmation in all cases. The authors acknowledge this point. In my experience, the value of having a positive VEMP preoperatively is that it provides an objective measure for successful surgical closure postoperatively when it is shown to be normal. Despite these small criticisms, this is a very important reference study demonstrating the role of canal occlusion for this disorder.

B. J. Balough, MD

Particle Repositioning Maneuver Versus Brandt-Daroff Exercise for Treatment of Unilateral Idiopathic BPPV of the Posterior Semicircular Canal: A Randomized Prospective Clinical Trial With Short- and Long-Term Outcome

Amor-Dorado JC, Barreira-Fernández MP, Aran-Gonzalez I, et al (Univ Hosp Lucus Augusti, Lugo, Spain; Complexo Hospitalario de Pontevedra, Spain; et al)
Otol Neurotol 33:1401-1407, 2012

Objective.—To compare the outcome and probability of recurrence in a series of patients with unilateral idiopathic benign paroxysmal positional vertigo of the posterior canal (PC-BPPV) that were randomly treated by Brandt-Daroff exercise (B-D exercise) or by particle repositioning maneuver (PRM).

Study Design.—Randomized prospective clinical trial.

Setting.—Tertiary referral center.

Patients.—Patients were included in this study if they complained of vertigo and had been diagnosed as having unilateral idiopathic PC-BPPV for at least 1 week before Dix-Hallpike maneuver (DHM), remained for 30 days in the randomly assigned treatment, and had at least 48 months' follow-up.

Intervention.—Forty-one patients were treated with a single PRM and 40 patients by B-D exercise.

Main Outcome Measure.—Resolution of benign paroxysmal positional nystagmus on the DHM. The probability of recurrence was also studied.

Results.—At Day 7, DHM was negative in 80.5% of the PRM-treated patients and in 25% of those treated by B-D exercise ($p < 0.001$). At Month 1, the differences between both treatment groups remained statistically significant (92.7% in PRM versus 42.5% in the B-D exercise had a negative DHM; $p < 0.001$). The variable that influenced that DHM became negative was the PRM (RR = 4.8; 95% confidence interval, 2.5–9.2;

$p < 0.001$). The number of recurrences in PRM and B-D exercise were 0.56 ± 0.8 and 0.48 ± 0.8, respectively ($p = 0.48$). The recurrence rate at 48 months was 35.5% (15/41) in B-D exercise and 36.6% (9/31) in the PRM group ($p = 0.62$). Although the time interval until the first recurrence was similar ($p = 0.44$), patients included in the PRM group showed a significantly longer time interval between the first and second recurrence ($p = 0.04$).

Conclusion.—PRM is more effective treatment and as safe as B-D exercise in the short term for unilateral and idiopathic PC-BPPV, and although it does not reduce the probability of recurrence in the 4-year follow-up period compared with B-D exercise, it may delay the second recurrence's onset in those patients who had already experienced a single recurrence. Our study supports the use of PRM as the treatment of choice in unilateral and idiopathic PC-BPPV, although exercise may be also considered as an alternative treatment in selected cases.

▶ This is a well-designed and executed study that provides valuable insight into the treatment of the most common cause of inner ear vertigo. Not surprisingly, canalith repositioning was more immediately effective than Brandt-Daroff exercises as a primary modality of treatment. The success rate of initial repositioning is consistent with prior studies at 80%. Surprisingly, however, symptom resolution averaged more than 8 days, which is a bit long in my experience and from other similar studies. This study also provides a time course for those patients managed by exercises alone. Based on the data, patients can expect 1 to 2 months for their symptoms to fully resolve. The other valuable findings are the recurrence data. The long follow-up of 4 years allows for accurate estimation of recurrence. As would be expected, neither treatment influenced the rate of recurrence, with both groups having slighty more than one-third of patients experiencing a return of positional vertigo. In my own practice, a positive Dix-Hallpike or modified Dix-Hallpike maneuver confirming posterior canal benign positional vertigo will lead to canalith repositioning on that visit, with a return visit or call in 1 week to ensure resolution. If, on the other hand, the Dix-Hallpike is negative but the symptoms are highly suggestive of benign positional vertigo, then Brandt-Daroff exercises are given with follow-up in 6 to 8 weeks. This study supports that practice.

B. J. Balough, MD

Surgical Technique

Prosthetic Reconstruction from the Tympanic Membrane to the Stapes Head or to the Stapes Footplate? A Laser Doppler Study

Alian WA, Majdalawieh OF, Van Wijhe RG, et al (Dalhousie Univ, Halifax, NS; et al)

J Otolaryngol Head Neck Surg 41:84-93, 2012

Background.—In the absence of the incus, many surgeons believe that reconstruction from the tympanic membrane to the stapes head is more effective than reconstruction to the stapes footplate. This has rarely been tested empirically. Published better clinical results with reconstruction to the stapes head might simply reflect less underlying disease in ears with an intact stapes superstructure.

Objective.—To compare vibration transmission of these two forms of prosthetic reconstruction.

Methods.—A fresh human cadaveric temporal bone model was used. Round window vibrations in response to sound in the ear canal were measured with a laser Doppler vibrometer. After incus removal, the discontinuity was repaired using a titanium prosthesis. Reconstruction from the tympanic membrane to the stapes head was compared to reconstruction to the stapes footplate.

Results.—Reconstruction of both types decreased round window vibrations by 10 to 15 dB between 500 and 3000 Hz compared to the intact middle ear. Reconstruction to the stapes head performed 5 to 10 dB better at lower frequencies (500–2000 Hz), but this was only statistically significant at 1 and 2 kHz.

Conclusions.—There is only a 5 to 10 dB mechanical advantage gained by reconstruction from the tympanic membrane to the stapes head compared to reconstruction to the footplate for frequencies between 1 and 2 kHz.

▶ In this article, the senior author continues a series of experiments to better provide empirical data to support our concepts behind ossicular reconstruction rather than rely on traditional perception. In this specific case, the tradition under scrutiny is that the presence of an intact stapes provides a better reconstructive hearing result than the footplate alone. The results are demonstrated in Fig 4 of the original article. What can be seen is the stapes head reconstruction does indeed perform better in most of the typical speech frequencies from 500 Hz through 2000 Hz. However, more importantly, neither provides a natural response with an overall trend in poorer sound transmission as the frequency increases compared with the intact chain. Our own work in this area has focused on the dynamic nature of the ossicular chain with active involvement of the malleus-incus joint, which can be seen to uncouple the sound transmission as frequency is changed. Thus, there are inherent limitations in static reconstruction of the ossicular chain regardless of method used. Yet there is value in having these limitations studied and our understanding refined; hence, the value of this article. Additionally, these laboratory measurements do not take into account the effects of healing. Even if the results can be similar in the laboratory, the greater stability of the stapes head in the reconstruction can prevent slipped prostheses, resulting in much better individual results. Similarly, using the remaining crura or a footplate shoe to center and stabilize the prosthesis can also avoid these failures. Here is where well-controlled clinical studies can be used to complement the knowledge gained from basic science experiments such as this.

B. J. Balough, MD

From incus bypass to malleostapedotomy: technical improvements and results

Rambousek A, Schlegel CH, Linder TE (Kantonsspital Luzern, Lucerne, Switzerland)
J Laryngol Otol 126:995-1002, 2012

Objective.—To assess results of malleostapedotomy using a Fisch Storz titanium piston with at least 10 months' follow up.

Methods.—Using a prospective database, the indications, surgical technique, and pre- and post-operative audiometric data for 60 patients undergoing malleostapedotomy between 2002 and 2010 were evaluated. Diagnoses and primary and revision surgeries were compared with reference to the literature.

Results.—Sixty endaural malleostapedotomies were performed, 28 as a primary intervention and 32 as revision surgery. In 68 per cent, the underlying pathology was otosclerosis. The most common reason for revision surgery (i.e. in 59 per cent) was prosthesis dysfunction. Overall, the mean air–bone gap (0.5–3 kHz) for the primary intervention and revision surgery groups was 9.4 and 11.3 dB, respectively; an air–bone gap of less than 20 dB was obtained in 100 and 81 per cent of patients, respectively. There was no significant audiological difference between the primary and revision surgeries groups, and no deafness.

Conclusion.—Malleostapedotomy shows comparable results to standard incus-stapedotomy and may be preferable in the presented situations (Table 3).

▶ This article presents a variation in surgical technique for malleus to vestibule reconstruction on a relatively large series of 60 patients. The details of the method are presented in very good detail and includes commentary on why this variation was developed and the advantages the authors feel it provides. There are 3 key components to this technique that are emphasized and can be visualized in Fig

TABLE 3.—Pre- and Post-Malleostapedotomy ABG Results

Parameter	0.5–3 kHz	0.5–4 kHz	0.5 kHz	1 kHz	2 kHz	3 kHz	4 kHz
Primary surgery							
Pre-op ABG (mean; dB)	26.3	28.8	40	30	15	15	25
Post-op ABG (mean; dB)	9.4	10.6	10	12.5	5	5	15
Pts with ABG closure							
– <10 dB (%)	61	50	64	50	86	43	43
– <20 dB (%)	100	93	93	93	100	68	71
Revision surgery							
Pre-op ABG (mean; dB)	27.5	30	30	30	20	20	32.5
Post-op ABG (mean; dB)	11.3	13.8	15	15	5	10	20
Pts with ABG closure							
– <10 dB (%)	38	34	47	47	75	63	34
– <20 dB (%)	81	78	66	84	88	88	69

ABG = air–bone gap; Pre-op = pre-operative; Post-op = post-operative.

1 of the original article. First, an endaural approach provides better visualization and greater elevation of the tympanomeatal flap superiorly. Second, removal of the incus provides better visualization of the stapes footplate. This is particularly helpful if a prior prosthesis is still in place so that work can be accomplished prior to removing the previous prosthesis. Third, the prosthesis is attached just inferior to the lateral process of the malleus. This provides a more consistent size and limits excursion with tympanic membrane movement. The chief advantage of this technique is that, from the data presented, it can be used to address a variety of middle ear pathologies and not just problematic revision otosclerosis cases in which the incus is not useable. Although the basic components of the technique can be easily performed, the disadvantage seems to lie in the fashioning and bending of the prosthesis to conform to the shape required. This may entail some degree of learning curve and could limit widespread adoption of this method. Practice in the temporal bone lab may be needed. However, as can be seen in Table 3, the results are quite good for both primary and revision cases. Thus, this technique warrants consideration as a method worth developing.

B. J. Balough, MD

Advantages of Hyaluronic Acid Fat Graft Myringoplasty Over Fat Graft Myringoplasty

Saliba I, Knapik M, Froehlich P, et al (Univ of Montreal, Quebec, Canada)
Arch Otolaryngol Head Neck Surg 138:950-955, 2012

Objectives.—To compare hyaluronic acid fat graft myringoplasty (HAFGM) with fat graft myringoplasty (FGM) on grade I tympanic membrane perforations (TMPs) (<25% of the tympanic membrane surface) and to assess 12-month postoperative hearing outcomes in a pediatric population.

Design.—Prospective study.

Setting.—Tertiary care pediatric center.

Patients.—Ninety-two children with a TMP were included in the study and were operated on using either the HAFGM (n = 50) or FGM (n = 42) technique. Age at surgery ranged from 4 to 17 years (mean age, 11.52 years).

Interventions.—Hyaluronic acid fat graft myringoplasty is a new technique for TMP repair in a pediatric population and is performed using local anesthesia at the outpatient office.

Main Outcome Measures.—Postoperative status of the tympanic membrane, hearing improvement, and incidence of complications.

Results.—Successful closure of the tympanic membrane was achieved in 90% of the HAFGM group and in 57.1% of the FGM group ($P = .004$). The mean (SD) postoperative air-bone gap in the HAFGM (6.86 [8.52] dB) group was significantly lower than in the FGM (18.32 [13.44] dB) group ($P < .002$). The mean postoperative follow-up time was 31.5 and 34.7 months for HAFGM and FGM groups, respectively. No difference was observed between children 10 years or younger and children older than 10 years. In the 2 groups, no postoperative complications were observed. The location of the perforation was not found to be a factor indicative of failure.

Conclusions.—The success rate of HAFGM is superior to that of FGM alone. Hyaluronic acid fat graft myringoplasty can be performed as an office-based procedure using local anesthesia and requires no hospitalization. Because of its substantial advantages, HAFGM could be considered as the first choice for the reconstruction of a dry TMP in the pediatric population.

▶ This is a continuation of a series of articles[1-3] by the first author on this technique: the hyaluronic acid fat graft myringoplasty (HAFGM). In this article, a head-to-head comparison is made between the modified fat graft myringoplasty and standard myringoplasty. Because it is not specifically stated in the methods section, it is unclear if the patients were randomized into the 2 groups. In this study, only small (< 25%) perforations were included, although in prior studies larger perforations were treated with similarly favorable results. The success rate reported for fat graft alone (57%) is similar to my own experience and why I do not favor its use. As discussed, this may be because the fat graft is pushed through the perforation with substance of the fat rising above the plane of the tympanic membrane. In HAFGM, the fat is pushed into the middle ear so that the surface is level with the plane of the tympanic membrane. This difference may be partially responsible for the increased success, separate from the hyaluronic acid membrane. The remainder of the article provides 1-year follow-up data to support the high success rate (90%) with excellent audiometric outcomes. Surprisingly, despite the placement of the fat into the middle ear, the photos provided demonstrate that the fat resorbs over time and no residual remains within the middle ear as adhesions. One final point is worth noting from this article: A comparison is made in the outcomes between age groups; no difference was found. This adds to a growing body of evidence that age in and of itself is not a determinant for success in tympanoplasty in children. Although I remain skeptical that this procedure can be performed in the office on young children as stated by the authors, the data presented support its use in older children who will tolerate local anesthesia alone, saving a trip to the operating room. For younger children, it is worth trying to reduce the need for a more extensive formal tympanoplasty.

B. J. Balough, MD

References

1. Saliba I. Hyaluronic acid fat graft myringoplasty: how we do it. *Clin Otolaryngol.* 2008;33:610-614.
2. Saliba I, Froehlich P. Hyaluronic acid fat graft myringoplasty: an office-based technique adapted to children. *Arch Otolaryngol Head Neck Surg.* 2011;137:1203-1209.
3. Saliba I, Woods O. Hyaluronic acid fat graft myringoplasty: a minimally invasive technique. *Laryngoscope.* 2011;121:375-380.

5 Pediatric Otolaryngology

Airway

Drug-Induced Sleep Endoscopy in Persistent Pediatric Sleep-Disordered Breathing After Adenotonsillectomy

Durr ML, Meyer AK, Kezirian EJ, et al (Univ of California, San Francisco)
Arch Otolaryngol Head Neck Surg 138:638-643, 2012

Objectives.—To demonstrate the feasibility of drug-induced sleep endoscopy (DISE) in the pediatric population and to examine DISE results in children with persistent sleep-disordered breathing (SDB) after tonsillectomy and adenoidectomy (T&A).

Design.—Retrospective case series with medical chart review.

Setting.—Tertiary pediatric medical center.

Patients.—Thirteen pediatric subjects with persistent SDB after T&A are included in the study.

Intervention.—Drug-induced sleep endoscopy was performed on all patients with documentation of all sites of persistent airway obstruction.

Results.—Multilevel upper-airway obstruction was identified in the majority of patients, most commonly related to tongue base obstruction, adenoid regrowth, and/or inferior turbinate hypertrophy. There were no differences among the 4 subgroups.

Conclusions.—Findings from DISE suggest that multiple factors contribute to airway obstruction in persistent SDB after T&A. Further research can address the extent to which directed surgical treatment can improve outcomes in these patients.

▶ Successful treatment of persistent sleep-disordered breathing (SDB) after tonsillectomy and adenoidectomy (T&A) in children is challenging given the difficulty of obtaining a comprehensive airway examination. Drug-induced sleep endoscopy (DISE) is a technique of upper-airway fiberoptic endoscopic examination during conditions of sedation that was first described in adults. The objectives of this study were to demonstrate the feasibility of DISE in a pediatric population in the operating room and to examine DISE findings in children with persistent SDB after T&A. DISE findings in 13 children were compared across 4 subgroups: subjects with cerebral palsy, subjects with trisomy 21 syndrome, overweight or obese subjects, and otherwise healthy subjects. All subjects tolerated DISE, and there were no complications. Multilevel obstruction occurred in all subjects except 2 with obstruction located at the tongue base only. The mean number of obstructive pathologic conditions per subject was 2.8 (1.6). Tongue base obstruction was the most common diagnosis and was present in 11 subjects (85%). This was followed by adenoid regrowth (69%) and inferior turbinate hypertrophy (54%). The study population was too small to study the subgroups in detail. This study did not compare the findings with those of office-based nasendoscopy, but it showed that DISE is possible, is safe, and may have an important role in identifying the causes of obstructive sleep apnea after T&A in children.

R. B. Mitchell, MD

Balloon Dilation Laryngoplasty for Subglottic Stenosis in Children: Eight Years' Experience

Hautefort C, Teissier N, Viala P, et al (Univ Paris VII Denis-Diderot, France)
Arch Otolaryngol Head Neck Surg 138:235-240, 2012

Objective.—To evaluate outcomes of balloon dilation laryngoplasty for laryngeal stenosis in children.

Design.—Retrospective study.

Setting.—Academic tertiary care department of pediatric otolaryngology.

Patients.—All children treated with laryngeal balloon dilation (primarily or secondarily following laryngeal surgery) from 2002 to 2010.

Main Outcome Measures.—Stenosis severity, measured using the Cotton and Myer classification.

Results.—A total of 44 children ranging in age from 1 month to 10 years (14 [32%] with grade II stenosis, 25 [59%] with grade III stenosis, and 4 [9%] with grade IV stenosis) were included. Twelve children [27%] had congenital laryngeal stenoses, and the in other 32 [73%], stenosis was acquired. A total of 52 balloon dilation laryngoplasties were performed, and 37 (71%) were deemed successful. Twenty of the 31 patients undergoing primary dilation (65%) had successful outcomes, and in the other 11 [35%], outcomes were unsuccessful (4 had grade II stenosis and 7 had grade III stenosis) and required either laryngotracheal reconstruction or tracheotomy. Twenty-one balloon dilations were performed as a secondary procedure after recent open surgery; 17 of the procedures (81%) were successful, and thus surgical revision was avoided.

Conclusion.—Balloon dilation laryngoplasty is an efficient and safe technique for the treatment of both primary and secondary pediatric laryngotracheal stenosis.

▶ Balloon dilation laryngoplasty is a minimally invasive approach to treating subglottic stenosis both as a primary treatment and as secondary treatment after open surgical procedures. Two groups of children were compared (primary vs secondary dilations, and successful vs failed cases) in this retrospective review.

Forty-four patients were included who underwent a total of 98 balloon dilation procedures. In this series, secondary dilations succeeded and avoided revision surgery in about 80% of cases, with a mean number of 2 dilation sessions. They report similar results, though with smaller numbers, for primary dilations. The authors conclude that balloon dilations are safe and efficient in the treatment of subglottic stenosis in children and reduce the need for open laryngeal surgery by 70% to 80%. Good indications include primary or secondary treatment of acquired stenosis of all grades, secondary treatment of congenital stenosis, and primary treatment of some congenital cases. They also opine that open surgery remains the best choice in cases of severe congenital stenosis, glottis immobility, or after 2 to 3 dilation procedures without significant improvement. This study adds to the body of literature that has reported success with balloon dilation for selected cases of subglottic stenosis in children.

R. B. Mitchell, MD

General

A Review of Beta Antagonist Treatment for Infantile Hemangioma

Phillips CB, Pacha O, Biliciler-Denkta G, et al (Univ of Texas Health Science Ctr, Houston)

J Drugs Dermatol 11:826-829, 2012

Infantile hemangiomas are benign vascular neoplasms of childhood that often have implications on development, cosmesis, and comfort. Traditional therapy has involved either observation or corticosteroids, depending on location and size. Recent studies have reported the successful use of beta-adrenergic antagonists in treating infantile hemangiomas. This succinct review discusses the properties and current applications of beta-adrenergic antagonists as well as the established treatments for infantile hemangioma.

▶ The majority of the available literature on beta receptor antagonists and infantile hemangiomas pertains to propranolol. Propranolol's efficacy is most probably attributable to its inhibition of vasodilation and angiogenesis functions associated with beta-2 blockade. Recently there has been an interest in the role of other more selective beta receptors antagonists in the management of infantile hemangiomas. A recent publication reported the successful resolution of infantile hemangioma when atenolol was substituted for propranolol after an adverse reaction.[1] In light of the current promising literature on propranolol, timolol, and atenolol, the role of beta-blockers in managing infantile hemangioma is likely to expand. This article discusses the individual properties of available beta antagonists and is helpful for otolaryngologists who manage infantile hemangiomas. Further studies are needed to establish pediatric safety and efficacy for many beta-blockers, but in light of the current promising literature on propranolol, timolol, and atenolol, the role of beta-blockers in managing infantile hemangioma is likely to expand.

R. B. Mitchell, MD

Reference

1. Raphaël MF, de Graaf M, Breugem CC, Pasmans SG, Breur JM. Atenolol: a promising alternative to propranolol for the treatment of hemangiomas. *J Am Acad Dermatol.* 2011;65:420-421.

Reducing Disposable Equipment Waste for Tonsillectomy and Adenotonsillectomy Cases

Penn E, Yasso SF, Wei JL (Children's Memorial Hosp, Chicago, IL; Children's Mercy Hosp and Clinics, Kansas City, MO; Univ of Kansas Med Ctr, Kansas City)
Otolaryngol Head Neck Surg 147:615-618, 2012

Large amounts of waste in hospitals are generated in the operating rooms from disposable surgical supplies. Tonsillectomy/adenotonsillectomy (T&A) cases use many disposable supplies that are not recyclable. It is critical to reduce disposable waste, as such waste directly affects the environment and increases health care costs. The authors noticed a difference between the number of disposable items prepared, available, but almost never used, for each tonsillectomy case between a children's hospital setting and a university ambulatory surgery center setting. The aims were the following: (1) identify what disposable medical supplies were unnecessarily opened for each case, (2) eliminate all disposable medical waste that was not critical to the case in both settings, and (3) determine the cost reduction at both hospital and surgery center facilities by revising the current disposable instruments/supplies pulled for tonsillectomy cases. The authors report projected cost savings and reduction in waste for one children's hospital and nationally based on their waste reduction.

▶ This is a thoughtful study that highlights the enormous potential for savings in hospitals across the United States. It is no surprise that the waste in most operating rooms is enormous. The goal of this study was to help eliminate unnecessary disposable medical waste and reduce cost to the facilities by revising the current disposable supplies pulled for all tonsillectomy/adenotonsillectomy cases. The figures are staggering. They were able to eliminate 12 of the 40 disposable items from the prepared tonsil packs and, thus, reduce costs from $77.29 to $66.04 with a projected cost savings to the hospital of $17 149.50 for the following year by simply utilizing the new packs. The authors extrapolate this to an annual national saving of about $5 million. However, this is only part of the equation because much of this waste is not recycled. The authors address this issue in a thoughtful way. They make a convincing argument for all surgeons to make a conscious effort to decrease unnecessary disposable medical waste produced by the most common procedures in each specialty. In this way, costs decrease, the environment is protected, and quality and outcomes are maintained. I recommend that this article is read by otolaryngologists and shared with our non-otolaryngology colleagues.

R. B. Mitchell, MD

Diagnosis and treatment of tracheobronchial foreign bodies in 1024 children

Wang G, Pan Z, Li H, et al (Children's Hosp of Chongqing Med Univ, China)

J Pediatr Surg 47:2004-2010, 2012

Objective.—This study sought to summarize the experience of diagnosis and treatment of tracheobronchial foreign bodies in children to effectively reduce complications and mortality.

Methods.—The medical records of 1024 pediatric patients admitted to our hospital from January 1997 to September 2011 and diagnosed with clinically suspected tracheobronchial foreign body aspiration were retrospectively analyzed.

Results.—Of the 1024 children patients, 674 were boys (65.8%) and 350 girls (34.2%). Two died of respiratory and circulatory failure (foreign bodies detected upon bronchoscopy but not retrieved) before surgery, 65 patients underwent direct bronchoscopic removal of foreign bodies due to their critical status, and 957 received chest radiographs and chest fluoroscopy or multidetector spiral computed tomographic scans (941 positive). Foreign bodies were expectorated before surgery in 3 cases. There were 953 cases of bronchoscopically proven airway foreign body aspiration, with a diagnostic accuracy of 94.5%. Ninety-eight foreign bodies were lodged in the main bronchus and/or bilateral bronchi, 506 in the right main bronchus, and 349 in the left main bronchus. Atelectasis was noted in 42 patients, including 11 with pulmonary consolidation, whose lungs were re-expanded by endobronchial lavage and sputum aspiration. In 3 patients with bronchiectasis, conservative treatment following foreign body removal was followed by no improvement, and pulmonary lobectomy was performed. Foreign bodies were successfully extracted at the first bronchoscopic attempt in 948 cases, accounting for 99.7% of the total. However, 3 patients had to undergo another bronchoscopy to remove the foreign bodies. The most common types of foreign bodies were peanuts, melon seeds, and beans.

Conclusions.—Timely accurate diagnosis and treatment of tracheobronchial foreign bodies in children can avoid delay in treatment and effectively reduce complications and mortality.

► This report is interesting for the large patient population that was analyzed retrospectively. The medical records of 1024 children with suspected tracheobronchial foreign bodies treated at the Department of Cardiothoracic Surgery of the Children's Hospital of Chongqing Medical University from January 1997 to September 2011 were included. One hundred ninety-seven cases (20.1%) were misdiagnosed as pneumonia, tracheobronchitis, laryngitis or asthma, with the duration of misdiagnosis lasting from 3 days to 2 years. Of the misdiagnosed cases, 65 (29.7%) were misdiagnosed for more than 6 months. Foreign body removal was performed successfully in 951 cases (including 948 removed successfully at the first attempt; 9 patients who underwent another bronchoscopy because of abnormalities upon reexamination; and 3 patients found to still harbor the foreign body, which was successfully removed at the second attempt). The authors argue for the use of multidetector spiral computed tomography as a supplementary test for unremarkable radiographic examinations or before bronchoscopy. This study details the presentation, investigation, and complications of airway foreign bodies. It concludes that "timely and accurate diagnosis and treatment of tracheobronchial foreign bodies in children can avoid delay in treatment and effectively reduce the complications and mortality." We certainly agree with the conclusions.

R. B. Mitchell, MD

Head and Neck Lymphatic Malformation Treatment: A Systematic Review

Adams MT, Saltzman B, Perkins JA (Madigan Army Med Ctr, Tacoma, WA; Seattle Children's Res Inst, WA; Univ of Washington School of Medicine, Seattle)

Otolaryngol Head Neck Surg 147:627-639, 2012

Objective.—To systematically review literature pertaining to head and neck lymphatic malformation treatment and to use individual-level data presented in qualifying case series to describe the reported efficacy, complications, and functional impact of surgery and sclerotherapy. The authors evaluated whether treatment modalities differ by lymphatic malformation stage.

Data Sources.—The terms *lymphangioendothelioma, lymphangioma, cystic hygroma*, and *malformation* were used to perform an Ovid literature search yielding 6292 references. The authors excluded references that did not involve head and neck lymphatic malformation treatment, include at least 5 patients, follow patients 1 year, define treatment modality, and state complications.

Review Methods.—The authors summarized data from 1205 patients reported in 41 articles. Individual-level data, in the 29 articles reporting these data, were pooled and tabulated.

Results.—The absence of within-study comparisons of treatment success, as well as the range of reporting methods, precluded a formal meta-analysis. Most reports were case series (37; 90%). The primary treatment modality was sclerotherapy in 17 (41%), surgery in 16 (39%), or surgery combined with other modalities in 9 (20%). Individual-level data were captured for 283 patients. No treatment modality clearly resulted in superior treatment outcome. Complications were more frequent in surgical series but were reported inconsistently in sclerotherapy studies.

Conclusion.—There is evidence that lymphatic malformation treatment can be done effectively with surgery or sclerotherapy, but further study is necessary to determine which is superior. Standardized guidelines for reporting lymphatic malformation case series do not currently exist, making comparison of treatment outcomes of differing treatment modalities difficult.

▶ This review was conducted to evaluate the medical literature on lymphatic malformation (LM) treatment and determine evidence to support either surgical therapy or sclerotherapy for LM treatment. This review provides a useful overview for otolaryngologists who treat children who have neck masses. The limitations of the current literature on LM preclude a formal meta-analysis because most publications are retrospective case series in which within-publication comparisons between treatments are not done. Several themes can be summarized. Similar numbers of reports describe sclerotherapy and surgery. Most European reports described surgical therapy. Lower-staged macrocystic LMs are most common and most effectively treated. Most reported first LM treatments occurred in patients younger than 5 years. Lymphatic malformation persistence, as judged clinically and radiographically, is very common, especially in higher-staged LMs. Data available in published literature are neither sufficiently consistent nor complete to determine if surgical treatment is associated with more complications than sclerotherapy treatment. Death associated with LM treatment occurs infrequently and was reported only before 1995. The number of reported treatments of primary sclerotherapy was double the reported number of surgeries per patient. There was no consistent method of assessing and reporting treatment outcomes. So overall, the literature does not support one modality over another, more research is needed, and more standardization of reported data would be helpful. The authors recommend that institutional protocols become commonplace based on the expertise and experience of the clinicians.

R. B. Mitchell, MD

Comparison of tonsillar biofilms between patients with recurrent tonsillitis and a control group

Woo JH, Kim ST, Kang IG, et al (Gachon Univ, Incheon, Korea)
Acta Otolaryngol 132:1115-1120, 2012

Conclusion.—The results of the study suggest that biofilms play a causative role in recurrent tonsillitis.

Objective.—To analyze the association between tonsillar biofilms and recurrent tonsillitis.

Methods.—The recurrent tonsillitis group comprised patients with a history of at least five episodes of tonsillitis per year over the previous 2 years. The control group comprised volunteers scheduled for laryngeal microsurgery with no history of tonsillitis over the previous 2 years. Between October 2009 and August 2010, specimens were obtained from 20 patients with recurrent tonsillitis and 20 volunteers (controls). Scanning electron microscopy (SEM) was used to confirm the presence of biofilms. Biofilms were graded at a magnification of $\times 500$ by SEM and classified into five grades. The percentages of subjects affected and biofilm grades were compared between the recurrent tonsillitis and control groups.

Results.—The two groups were matched for age and sex. SEM revealed that biofilms were significantly more prevalent in the recurrent tonsillitis group than in the control group. Furthermore, the biofilms in the recurrent tonsillitis group were of significantly higher grade than those in the control group.

▶ The aim of this study was to analyze the association between recurrent tonsillitis and the presence of biofilms. The authors reference previous studies but argue that this is the first study to include a control population. The results of this study showed that the presence, rate, and grade of biofilms were significantly higher in the recurrent tonsillitis group than the control group. The results do not rule out other patient factors that might have contributed to the development of tonsillitis, and it does not conclude that biofilms are causal for tonsillitis. There is a large "so what?" element to this study. Identifying children with tonsillitis and high-grade biofilms may help in identifying surgical candidates that are unlikely to resolve with time. However, this study does not look specifically at this. Nonetheless, the results support the view that biofilms in the tonsils can play a pathogenically important role in recurrent tonsillitis.

R. B. Mitchell, MD

Complications of Adenotonsillectomy in Patients Younger Than 3 Years

Spencer DJ, Jones JE (Weill Cornell Med College and The Rockefeller Univ, NY; New York–Presbyterian Hosp/Weill Cornell Med Ctr)

Arch Otolaryngol Head Neck Surg 138:335-339, 2012

Objective.—To evaluate the complication rate for adenotonsillectomy in children younger than 3 years, without a diagnosis of severe obstructive sleep apnea, to assess the necessity for postoperative inpatient admission.

Design.—Retrospective medical record review (January 1, 2003, through October 31, 2009).

Setting.—Tertiary care academic medical center.

Patients.—Retrospective medical record review of 105 patients younger than 3 years who underwent adenotonsillectomy performed by a single surgeon. Nineteen patients were excluded from our review because of incomplete medical records or severe underlying disease, leaving a total of 86 patients with medical records available for inclusion in our study. Patient medical records were deidentified and reviewed for age, sex, indications for surgery, intraoperative and perioperative interventions, and postoperative complications. One child with a diagnosis of severe obstructive sleep apnea was excluded from the study.

Main Outcome Measures.—Complications, including bleeding, dehydration requiring admission, and airway intervention, during the intraoperative or perioperative period were recorded.

Results.—The mean age of the study population was approximately 27.5 months (range, 13-35 months), with most children (76.5%) between 23 and 31 months of age. Among the patients whose records were reviewed,

80 (93.0%) did not experience any intraoperative or postoperative complications. Dehydration was the most common complication and was the cause of all documented readmissions (4.7%) in our patients who ranged in age from 14 to 30 months. Two patients had other complications, reactive airway disease (n = 1) and postoperative fever (n = 1), which were identified and treated in the post-anesthesia care unit, resulting in same-day discharge. No airway complications were noted in our study.

Conclusions.—Our study reveals a low complication rate in children younger than 3 years. The recommendations for mandatory admission for children younger than 3 years should be reexamined. Criteria for inpatient admission for children younger than 3 years should be based on preoperative and postoperative clinical evaluation of the patient and an evaluation of the family resources for adequately caring for young children at home in the postoperative period. These recommendations apply only to otherwise healthy children (American Society of Anesthesiologists classifications I and II) without a diagnosis of severe obstructive sleep apnea syndrome.

▶ The American Academy of Pediatrics and American Academy of Otolaryngology/Head and Neck Surgery guidelines state that all children younger than 3 years who were undergoing adenotonsillectomy should be admitted overnight for postoperative observation. This retrospective review challenges this requirement.

The authors recommend admitting all children 24 months or younger and reevaluating them 6 hours after admission for possible discharge. Children older than 24 months can be scheduled for ambulatory admission and admitted only if postoperative complications arise. The results show a low risk of complications from adenotonsillectomy in very young children. Previous findings have agreed with these findings, although they have had equally poor quality of evidence with significant bias. The authors recognize that this change in practice will require careful selection of patients preoperatively, a dedicated pediatric team of nurses and anesthesiologists, and communication with families during the postoperative period. The positive side is more efficient use of health care resources and providing young children with a more comfortable home setting for recovery after adenotonsillectomy.

R. B. Mitchell, MD

Comparison of Imaging Modalities in Pediatric Thyroglossal Duct Cysts

Huoh KC, Durr ML, Meyer AK, et al (Univ of California, San Francisco)

Laryngoscope 122:1405-1408, 2012

Objectives/Hypothesis.—To determine and compare the accuracy of different imaging modalities including ultrasound (US), magnetic resonance imaging (MRI), and computed tomography (CT) in the diagnosis of thyroglossal duct cysts (TGDC) in children.

Study Design.—Retrospective chart review.

Methods.—A retrospective chart review was performed on patients under the age of 18 years who had undergone surgical excision of midline neck masses between January 2002 and June 2011. All patients had preoperative imaging. Data including age at surgery, preoperative imaging results, and postoperative pathology results were recorded. Preoperative imaging diagnoses were then compared to postoperative pathologic diagnoses. Diagnostic test statistics were performed.

Results.—A total of 44 patients met the study criteria. There were 15 patients who underwent more than one modality of imaging study. US had a sensitivity of 75% in diagnosis of TGDC. MRI sensitivity was 60% and CT was 82%. None of the tests had high specificity for TGDC; US was the highest at 80%. All three modalities had positive predictive values higher than 90%. US had the highest positive likelihood ratio (3.8), although the 95% confidence interval was not statistically significant.

Conclusions.—In a comparison of the three most commonly used imaging modalities for pediatric TGDC, US was the preferred exam given its comparable accuracy, ease of administration, and lower cost. In addition, the added risks of general anesthesia with MRI and ionizing radiation with CT are not justified in this setting given their equivalent or inferior performance when compared to US in this cohort.

▶ This study aimed to determine whether magnetic resonance imaging (MRI) or computed tomography (CT) offers improved diagnostic accuracy over ultrasound (US) by correlating preoperative imaging diagnoses to final pathologic diagnoses. All patients underwent preoperative imaging with US, MRI, or CT and some patients had more than 1 modality of imaging. Charts were reviewed for preoperative imaging diagnosis and postoperative pathologic diagnosis. CT was the most sensitive diagnostic test (82%), followed by US (75%) and MRI (60%). All 3 modalities had high positive predictive values (90%). MRI and CT were not significantly more accurate in the diagnosis of thyroglossal duct cysts (TGDC) than US. MRI had lower sensitivity and specificity than US, and CT had only a slight advantage in sensitivity over US. A positive imaging diagnosis of TGDC with any modality is predictive of the real diagnosis. This study supports the use of US as equally accurate compared with MRI and CT with superiority over the other 2 modalities in cost and safety. This study has many limitations but supports current thinking and usage of US as the investigation of choice for a midline neck mass in a child.

R. B. Mitchell, MD

Asthma: The Great Imitator in Foreign Body Aspiration?

Saliba J, Mijovic T, Daniel S, et al (Montreal Children's Hosp, Quebec, Canada)
J Otolaryngol Head Neck Surg 41:200-206, 2012

Objective.—To determine the prevalence of underlying lower airway inflammatory conditions in children who underwent rigid bronchoscopy (RB) for a suspected foreign body aspiration (FBA) in the tracheobronchial tree and to identify the characteristics of patients who could benefit from a trial of antiasthma treatment prior to undergoing a diagnostic bronchoscopy.

Design.—Retrospective chart review.

Setting.—Children with suspected FBA in the tracheobronchial tree who underwent RB at the Montreal Children's Hospital (2001–2009).

Methods.—Patient characteristics such as clinical, radiologic, and bronchoscopic findings on presentation, as well as prior use of inhaled bronchodilators or corticosteroids, were analyzed. A p value $< .05$ was considered significant.

Main Outcome Measures.—Use of inhaled bronchodilators or corticosteroids, signs, symptoms, and radiologic and bronchoscopic findings on presentation.

Results.—Fifty-five children underwent an RB for suspected FBA. Foreign bodies were found in 36 subjects. Asthmatics were significantly more likely to have a negative bronchoscopy than nonasthmatics (80.0% vs 30.0%, $p < .05$). Otherwise, clinical and radiologic findings were not significantly different in these two groups. The median time between the suspected choking event and the first otolaryngology evaluation was 14 days in asthmatics (range 5 hours–90 days), whereas it was 16 hours in nonasthmatics (range 0.5 hours–120 days).

Conclusion.—A conservative approach cannot be justified in suspected asthmatic children with possible FBA, in whom the indications for diagnostic bronchoscopy must be tailored to each patient to ensure a timely diagnosis.

▶ The decision to proceed with rigid bronchoscopy (RB) for a suspected foreign body aspiration (FBA) can be challenging. This is particularly true in patients with asthma, a very common entity that tends to mimic FBA and confuses clinicians in their decision making.

The goal of this study was to determine the prevalence of suspected asthma in children who undergo RB for a suspected FBA and to identify the characteristics of patients who could benefit from a trial of antiasthma treatment prior to undergoing a diagnostic bronchoscopy. Patients with positive FBA were significantly more likely to have focally decreased breath sounds on physical examination and lower oxygen saturation compared with those without. There were no significant differences in all recorded elements on the history and physical examination between suspected asthmatic and nonasthmatic children. All suspected asthmatic patients had at least 1 prior visit to the emergency department related to wheezing (mean, 2.2 visits) compared with only 4 patients (8%) in the nonasthmatic subjects. The most clinically relevant finding is in the delay in presentation in asthmatic patients. The median time from the suspected initial choking event to the first otolaryngology evaluation was 14 days in suspected asthmatics (mean, 27 days; range, 5 hours to 90 days) compared with 16 hours in nonasthmatics (mean, 7.2 days; range, 0.5 hours to 120 days). Very few studies have specifically evaluated the significance of asthma in patients who underwent RB for a suspected FBA.

This is an important study in that it highlights the need to avoid a conservative approach in asthmatic patients. In suspected FBS in asthmatic patients, RB is justified earlier rather than later, and the clinician's judgment should always prevail in doubtful situations to ensure a timely diagnostic bronchoscopy.

R. B. Mitchell, MD

Annual temperature and the prevalence of frequent ear infections in childhood

Miller ME, Shapiro NL, Bhattacharyya N (David Geffen School of Medicine at UCLA; Brigham and Women's Hosp, Boston, MA)

Am J Otolaryngol 33:51-55, 2012

Objectives.—The aim of this study was to determine if changes in annual temperature influence the prevalence of frequent otitis media (FOM) and respiratory allergy in children.

Methods.—Annual prevalence data for FOM (defined as 3 or more ear infections per year), respiratory allergy, and seizures (nonrespiratory, control condition) in children were extracted from the National Health Interview Survey for 1998 to 2006. Average US annual temperatures for the same period were recorded from the Environmental Protection Agency. Complex samples logistic regression analyses were performed to identify possible correlations between annual temperature and each of the 3 disease conditions, controlling for age and sex.

Results.—A total of 113 067 children were studied (mean age, 8.6 years; 51.1% girls). Overall prevalences (±95% confidence interval) were 6.3% ± 0.2%, 11.8% ± 0.2%, and 0.7% ± 0.1% for FOM, respiratory allergy, and seizures (nonrespiratory, control condition), respectively. Average annual temperatures ranged from 53.64°F to 55.09°F. Regression analysis found that annual temperature did not influence the prevalence of FOM ($P = .681$); male sex and younger age were associated with a higher prevalence of FOM ($P = .025$ and $P < .001$, respectively). Similarly, annual temperature did not influence prevalence of respiratory allergy ($P = .883$); male sex and increasing age were associated with a higher prevalence of respiratory allergy (both $P < .001$). Annual temperature and sex did not influence seizure prevalence; however, increasing age was negatively associated.

Conclusions.—Changes in average annual temperature do not appear to influence the prevalence of otitis media or respiratory allergy. This negative finding suggests that although global warming continues to affect our environment, childhood otolaryngologic disease prevalence may not be directly influenced.

▶ Few studies have investigated the possible correlation of average annual temperatures and otolaryngologic disease prevalence, especially in children. The authors argue that increasing temperatures with global warming may increase these common infections.

They argue that among respiratory diseases that may be impacted by global warming, otitis media deserves special consideration because of its tremendous disease burden. Logistic regression analyses found that annual temperature did not influence the prevalence of otitis media, whereas male sex and younger age were associated with a higher prevalence. Similarly, annual temperature did not influence prevalence of respiratory allergy, but male sex and increasing age were associated with a higher prevalence. The current negative finding may demonstrate that average temperature is not likely to be the dominant cause of the increase in allergy burden or that larger changes in temperatures over a longer period are needed to observe this association more accurately. Based on this study, it appears that in the absence of more dramatic annual temperature changes, we do not expect prevalence of otitis media to change significantly as global warming may continue to affect our environment.

R. B. Mitchell, MD

Outcomes

Children with severe or moderate obstructive sleep apnoea syndrome show a high incidence of persistence after adenotonsillectomy

Tagaya M, Nakata S, Yasuma F, et al (Nagoya Univ, Japan; Natl Hosp Organization Suzuka Hosp, Mie, Japan; et al)
Acta Otolaryngol 132:1208-1214, 2012

Conclusion.—Persistent obstructive sleep apnoea syndrome (OSAS) occurs in approximately 20% of normal-weight children after adenotonsillectomy (T&A) and, in nearly 70% of them, it is caused by adenoid regrowth. Patients with severe or moderate OSAS showed a high incidence of persistent disease even after T&A. Allergic disease, severity and large adenoid size are associated with adenoid regrowth and persistent disease.

Objectives.—To investigate factors contributing to persistent OSAS and adenoid regrowth after T&A in normal-weight children.

Methods.—This was a prospective, observational study at a single institute and involved 49 normal-weight children with severe or moderate OSAS (apnoea–hypopnoea index, AHI, ≥ 5) who underwent T&A. Background information, nasal endoscopic data and pre- and postoperative polysomnographic data were collected. A third polysomnography (PSG) was performed 1.5 year postoperatively in children who subsequently developed symptoms of sleep disturbance.

Results.—Thirteen children (27%, 13/49) were symptomatic 1.5 years after T&A. Allergic rhinitis (38.5% vs 11.1%, $p = 0.03$) and allergic disease (69.2% vs 30.6%, $p = 0.02$) were seen more frequently in these children. A third PSG confirmed persistent disease (AHI ≥ 5) in nine children (18.4%, 9/49). Six children (12.2%, 6/49) were diagnosed as having adenoid regrowth and three (6.1%, 3/49) underwent revision adenoidectomy.

▶ This study investigated factors contributing to persistent obstructive sleep apnea syndrome (OSAS) after adenotonsillectomy (T&A) in normal-weight children. The strength of this study was in the extensive follow-up that these children received. Postoperative polysomnography was performed routinely 2 to 4 months after surgery and all children were followed up with nasal endoscopy every 3 months for 1.5 years after surgery. All children that remained symptomatic underwent a third polysomnography at 1.5 years after T&A. Adenoid regrowth was diagnosed when the adenoid size increased by at least 1 grade between the early postoperative visit and the one at 1.5 years. A total of 27% (13/49) of normal-weight healthy children after T&A were subsequently symptomatic at the 1.5-year follow-up, 12% (12/49) still had severe or moderate persistent OSAS 3 months postoperatively, and 18% (9/49) had it at the 1.5-year follow-up. Twelve percent (6/49) of children were diagnosed with adenoid regrowth. Apneahypopnea index and adenoid size were higher in subsequently symptomatic than in asymptomatic children preoperatively and postoperatively. This study suggests that severe or moderate persistent OSAS is relatively common in normal-weight healthy children after T&A and that symptomatic children will benefit from postoperative endoscopy and a repeat adenoidectomy.

R. B. Mitchell, MD

Outcomes of Adenotonsillectomy in Patients With Prader-Willi Syndrome

Meyer SL, Splaingard M, Repaske DR, et al (Nationwide Children's Hosp, Columbus, OH; et al)
Arch Otolaryngol Head Neck Surg 138:1047-1051, 2012

Objective.—To assess the efficacy of upper airway surgical intervention in patients with Prader-Willi syndrome (PWS). Due to reports of sudden death in children undergoing treatment with growth hormone for PWS, detection of sleep-disordered breathing by polysomnography (PSG) has been recommended.

Design.—Retrospective study.

Setting.—Multidisciplinary PWS Center at a tertiary care children's hospital.

Patients.—Thirteen pediatric patients with PWS who underwent adenotonsillectomy (T&A) with pre-PSG and post-PSG.

Main Outcome Measures.—Comparison of PSG results before and after T&A.

Results.—Six of our patients were girls (46%); 8 had genetic characteristics consistent with deletion (61%), and the remaining 5 had genetic characteristics consistent with uniparental disomy (39%). The median age at T&A was 3 years (age range, 6 months to 11 years), and the median age at start of growth hormone treatment was 8.5 months (range, 2 months to 6 years). Nine of the 13 patients had mild to moderate obstructive sleep apnea (OSA) or obstructive hypoventilation (69%); in 8 of these 9, breathing normalized after T&A. Four children had severe OSA prior to surgery (31%). Breathing normalized in 2 of these after surgery, but 2 had PSG findings of residual combined obstructive and central apneas postoperatively.

Conclusions.—Adenotonsillectomy, while effective in most children with PWS who demonstrate mild to moderate OSA, may not be curative in children with severe OSA. An increase in central apneas can occur in some children with PWS postoperatively, and it is important to repeat PSG after surgery. Further studies are necessary to determine optimal treatment for some children with PWS and sleep-disordered breathing.

▶ Prader-Willi syndrome (PWS) is a genetic disorder resulting from absence of expression of the paternally derived PWS/Angelman syndrome region (q11-q13) of chromosome. Patients with PWS are at risk for sleep-disordered breathing with central and obstructive components. Obstructive sleep-disordered breathing is multifactorial and related to poor muscle tone in the upper and lower airway, obesity, and adenoid and/or tonsil hypertrophy. Growth hormone therapy, commonly used in children with PWS, can contribute to obstructive sleep-disordered breathing as a known cause of tonsillar and adenoid hypertrophy. Unfortunately, there are limited and conflicting data regarding adenotonsillectomy (T&A) in children with PWS, with the largest previous study consisting of 5 patients. This study reports that T&A is generally effective in most children with PWS who demonstrate mild to moderate obstructive sleep apnea (OSA) but is less likely to be curative in those with severe OSA (similar results to that seen in non-PWS children). Half of the children with severe OSA before surgery continued to have severe sleep-disordered breathing postoperatively. This is a small study population and has the limitations of retrospective studies, namely, bias. It is hard, based on these data, to make recommendations about the role of polysomnography (PSG) or growth hormone in children with PSG but, nonetheless, it adds data to the current body of knowledge.

R. B. Mitchell, MD

Impact of Adenotonsillectomy on High-Sensitivity C-Reactive Protein Levels in Obese Children with Obstructive Sleep Apnea

Chu L, Yao H, Wang B (Chongqing Med Univ, China; Dept of Children's Hosp of Chongqing Med Univ, China)

Otolaryngol Head Neck Surg 147:538-543, 2012

Objective.—To evaluate the effect of adenotonsillectomy (T&A) in obese children with obstructive sleep apnea (OSA) and to compare changes in high-sensitivity C-reactive protein (hs-CRP) levels before and 6 months after T&A in obese children with OSA.

Study Design.—Before and after study with planned data collection.

Setting.—Tertiary care, university-based pediatric hospital.

Subjects and Methods.—Seventy-five obese children with OSA were included. Clinical information such as the apneahypopnea index (AHI), nadir oxyhemoglobin saturation (SaO_2), and body mass index (BMI) were recorded. The hs-CRP level was determined before T&A and at the 6-month follow-up examination.

Results.—Reductions in AHI (21.96 ± 9.277 before T&A vs 8.64 ± 5.997 after 6 months of T&A) and higher levels of nadir SaO_2 (74.08 ± 7.860 before T&A vs 86.87 ± 5.586 after 6 months of T&A)

were observed. The hs-CRP levels were obviously correlated with BMI ($r = 0.7948$, $P < .001$). Other than AHI ($r = 0.0579$, $P = .6217$) in obese children, however, hs-CRP levels showed no changes 6 months after T&A therapy.

Conclusion.—T&A treatment improves clinical signs and symptoms in obese children but does not reduce chronic inflammation as reflected by hs-CRP. To lower the risks of cardiovascular disease and diabetes mellitus morbidity, other treatments should be taken into account.

▶ This study looks at the role of adenotonsillectomy (T&A) for obstructive sleep apnea (OSA) in obese children. The polysomnography data they report are well-known, namely that OSA after T&A improves but does not resolve. The question is whether T&A is effective at reducing C-reactive protein (CRP) levels. CRP is an important circulating marker of inflammation and is one of the proposed links between OSA and inflammation. This protein, which is synthesized in the liver in response to upstream inflammatory signaling pathways, has also been shown to directly participate in atheromatous lesion formation and insulin resistance and is recognized as a potent predictor of future cardiovascular disease (CVD) and diabetes mellitus (DM). An increase in CRP among children with OSA and a significant decrease after T&A treatment have been reported, but not in obese children. Analysis of measurements obtained before T&A revealed a correlation between CRP and body mass index (BMI) but not apnea hypopnea index. No BMI changes occurred pre- or postoperatively. No significant changes in CRP levels were observed before or after 6 months of T&A regardless of whether obese children had resolved or persistent OSA. The authors conclude that T&A can improve clinical signs and symptoms in obese children with OSA. However, OSA is not completely cured in all patients. Because changes in CRP levels are affected most strongly by obesity-related factors, which are similar before and after T&A, the risks for CVD and DM remain unchanged even when T&A therapy leads to dramatic improvements in OSA in obese children. More long-term data and studies looking at alternatives to T&A are needed in obese children with OSA.

R. B. Mitchell, MD

Postoperative Hemorrhage Following Adenoidectomy

Tomkinson A, Harrison W, Owens D, et al (Univ Hosp Wales, Cardiff, UK; Temple of Peace and Health, Cardiff, UK)

Laryngoscope 122:1246-1253, 2012

Objectives/Hypothesis.—To examine postoperative hemorrhage following adenoidectomy.

Study Design.—Prospective multicenter observational study.

Methods.—The Surgical Instrument Surveillance Programme (SISP) was established in 2003 to monitor tonsil and adenoid surgery in all hospitals in Wales. Data were examined between April 1, 2003 and June 30, 2008, for risk factors that may contribute to primary (R1) or secondary (R2) postoperative hemorrhage from the adenoid bed, of a severity sufficient to require a return to the operating room.

Results.—There were 5,588 procedures included, of which 4,225 included simultaneous tonsillectomy. The study included 2,903 (52%) males with a median age of 5.8 years (interquartile range [IQR], 4.5–7.7 years) and 2,685 (48%) females with a median age of 6.5 years (IQR, 5.0–9.1 years). There were 22 patients (0.4%; confidence interval [CI], 0.2–0.6) who returned to the operating room with a postoperative hemorrhage arising from the adenoid bed. These were exclusively R1 hemorrhage; there were no instances of R2 hemorrhage (0.0%; CI, 0.0-0.1). No specific risk factors for R1 hemorrhage could be identified. There were 38 patients in the adenotonsillectomy group who returned to operating room with a postoperative hemorrhage arising from the tonsil bed (0.5%; CI, 0.3-0.8). R1 was seen in 22 patients (0.5%; CI, 0.3-0.8) and R2 in 16 patients (0.4%; CI, 0.2-0.6).

Conclusions.—Adenoidectomy appears to be primarily a procedure performed in childhood. The rate of R1 hemorrhage following adenoidectomy is one in 200 (0.5%) and is similar to the R1 hemorrhage rate for tonsillectomy. R2 hemorrhage following an adenoidectomy appears to be extremely rare. In children, the risk of a serious primary hemorrhage following an adenotonsillectomy is double that of either procedure when performed alone.

▶ This is a unique study that looked specifically at postadenoidectomy as opposed to postadenotonsillectomy bleeding. In 2003, all hospitals in Wales commenced the use of specified single-use instruments for tonsil and adenoid surgery. The Surgical Instrument Surveillance Programme (SISP) collected data on complications rates for these procedures. The primary aim of this system was to determine whether surgery could be as safe with single-use instruments as it was with the equivalent reusable instruments. The data from the SISP (1363 [23%] patients underwent adenoidectomy alone) were used to report these findings. Nine categories of operative technique for adenoidectomy were available on the data sheet: curette, suction diathermy, bipolar diathermy, ultrasonic, potassium-titanyl-phosphate laser, CO_2 laser, microdebrider, or other. Unfortunately, cold curette was the most common method (96%), with other methods being very uncommon. As such, the ability to compare techniques is limited. Anecdotal experience suggests that postadenoidectomy bleeding has decreased significantly with new instrumentation. This study fails to address this issue. The conclusion is that cold curette was most commonly used to perform adenoidectomy in this cohort at a peak of 5 years of age. Serious primary hemorrhage requiring a return to the operating room was similar to tonsillectomy at approximately 1 in 200 (0.5%). The likelihood of a serious secondary hemorrhage was extremely rare, unlike a tonsillectomy. I expect the bleeding rates for suction cautery or coblation adenoidectomy are lower; this would make a good outcomes study.

R. B. Mitchell, MD

Pharyngeal flap versus sphincter pharyngoplasty for the treatment of velopharyngeal insufficiency: A meta-analysis

Collins J, Cheung K, Farrokhyar F, et al (McMaster Univ, Hamilton, Ontario, Canada)

J Plast Reconstr Aesthet Surg 65:864-868, 2012

Background.—Velopharyngeal insufficiency (VPI) has been reported in 5–20% of patients following cleft palate repair. Since VPI can limit communication, determining which operative procedure leads to the greatest improvement is of utmost importance. Since there is no consensus, this meta-analysis aims to determine which procedure results in the most significant resolution of VPI.

Methods.—Two independent assessors undertook a literature review for articles that compare procedures aimed at treating VPI. Study quality was determined using validated scales. Level of agreement was assessed using intra-class coalition coefficient analysis. The heterogeneity between studies was evaluated using I^2 and Cochran's Q-statistic. Random effect model analysis and forest plots were used to report a pooled odds ratio (OR) and 95% confidence intervals (CI) for treatment effect. A *p*-value of 0.05 was considered for statistical significance.

Results.—Two randomised controlled trials (RCTs) comparing pharyngeal flap to sphincter pharyngoplasty were obtained. A total of 133 patients were included, with follow-ups at 3–4 months. The pooled OR was determined to be 2.95 (95% CI: 0.66–13.23) in favour of the pharyngeal flap.

Conclusions.—Based on these RCTs, which currently compose the highest quality data that compares pharyngeal flap versus pharyngoplasty, the pooled treatment effect suggests a possible trend favouring pharyngeal flap.

▶ Surgery is the definitive treatment of velopharyngeal insufficiency (VPI) with the goal of creating a functional seal between the nasopharynx and the oropharynx during speech while avoiding nasal airway obstruction. The 2 most common surgical techniques include pharyngeal flap and sphincter pharyngoplasty. The purpose of this study is to determine the optimal surgical procedure for the treatment of VPI after cleft palate repair, though this is made difficult by the fact that these techniques are highly dependent on surgeon experience and may require individual tailoring to the size and nature of the velopharyngeal defect. The methodology of the study is sound and well described, although the available literature is limited to 2 randomized controlled trials (RCTs) with 133 patients—a relatively small number. The RCTs demonstrate a possible trend favoring the pharyngeal flap over sphincter pharyngoplasty for velopharyngeal insufficiency resolution. With regard to complications, the incidence of sleep apnea was noted to be similar in both groups, or slightly higher in the pharyngeal flap group. Complications and reoperations were low in both groups, with no statistically significant differences. Moreover, lengths of stay were similar in both groups. It is difficult to reach definitive conclusions other than to say that both procedures are good options and further data is needed.

R. B. Mitchell, MD

Predictors of Tonsillectomy after Previous Adenoidectomy for Upper Airway Obstruction

Gov-Ari E, Mills JC, Basler KJ (Univ of Missouri Dept of Otolaryngology—Head and Neck Surgery, Columbia)
Otolaryngol Head Neck Surg 146:647-652, 2012

Objective.—(1) Characterize risk factors for subsequent tonsillectomy in pediatric patients undergoing primary adenoidectomy for upper airway obstruction. (2) Compare rates of subsequent tonsillectomy between adenoidectomy patients with and without upper airway obstruction.

Study Design.—Historical cohort study with a nested case-control study. Cohort data were analyzed using Kaplan-Meier plots and a multiple regression model. Case-control data were analyzed using logistic regression.

Subjects and Methods.—Patients undergoing adenoidectomy without tonsillectomy at the University of Missouri between 1995 and 2010 were identified using billing records and selected chart review. A nested case-control study with detailed chart review was conducted to determine predictors of subsequent tonsillectomy in patients with upper airway obstruction.

Results.—Of 1291 patients identified in the historical cohort, 7.8% later underwent tonsillectomy. Age younger than 3 years ($P = .027$), female sex ($P < .0001$), and upper airway obstruction ($P = .001$) were found to be significant predictors of subsequent tonsillectomy. In the nested case-control study, potential predictors investigated included adenoidectomy indications, symptoms, smoke exposure, weight, comorbidities, and tonsil size at the time of adenoidectomy. Of these, only tonsil size was significant, with an increased odds of future tonsillectomy of 2.5 ($P = .01$) for each unit increase in tonsil size.

Conclusion.—Patients undergoing adenoidectomy for upper airway obstruction are likely to be at an increased risk of subsequent tonsillectomy when compared with those with other indications. Within this subgroup of patients with upper airway obstruction, young age, female sex, and large tonsil size may further increase the risk of subsequent tonsillectomy.

▶ This study addresses a practical problem that faces otolaryngologists that take care of children. The role of adenoidectomy alone for upper airway obstruction remains unclear. Situations arise in which patients with symptoms of obstructive sleep apnea syndrome (OSAS) are found to have large adenoids but small tonsils. Conversely, patients may present with nasal obstruction and mouth breathing alone, without other symptoms of OSAS (or a negative sleep study), but have incidentally large tonsils. It is expected that a certain percentage of patients undergoing adenoidectomy alone will eventually require tonsillectomy. The objective of this study was to characterize potential risk factors for subsequent tonsillectomy, particularly when adenoidectomy is performed for upper airway obstruction. A total of 101 (7.8%) patients later underwent tonsillectomy. Time to tonsillectomy ranged from 0.2 to 10.5 years, with a median of 1.8 years and with 92% of tonsillectomies occurring within 5 years. Based on a fitted multiple logistic regression model, significant independent predictors of subsequent tonsillectomy within the adenoidectomy cohort as a whole included age younger than 3 years, female sex, and an indication of upper airway obstruction at adenoidectomy. This study demonstrates that patients undergoing adenoidectomy for upper airway obstruction have an increased rate of subsequent tonsillectomy when compared with those with other indications. In addition, certain patients undergoing adenoidectomy for upper airway obstruction may be at especially increased risk of requiring subsequent tonsillectomy. The highest risk patients based on our data are those younger than 3 years, girls, and those with large tonsils. When considering whether to perform tonsillectomy at the time of adenoidectomy, the otolaryngologist needs to consider the added risk and morbidity of tonsillectomy versus the potential morbidity of undertreated airway obstruction and risk and morbidity of a second surgical procedure, particularly postoperative bleeding. This study does agree with previous publications on the subject. Unfortunately, the final decision about performing an adenoidectomy versus adenotonsillectomy is down to parent and surgeon preferences.

R. B. Mitchell, MD

Long-term Surgical Outcomes of Adenotonsillectomy for PFAPA Syndrome

Licameli G, Lawton M, Kenna M, et al (Children's Hosp, Boston, MA; Harvard Med School, Boston, MA)

Arch Otolaryngol Head Neck Surg 138:902-906, 2012

Objective.—To evaluate the long-term efficacy of adenotonsillectomy in the treatment of pediatric patients with PFAPA (periodic fever, aphthous stomatitis, pharyngitis, and cervical adenitis) syndrome.

Design.—Prospective case series.

Setting.—Tertiary care pediatric hospital.

Patients.—Pediatric patients meeting the criteria for PFAPA syndrome.

Interventions.—Tonsillectomy with adenoidectomy.

Main Outcome Measures.—Resolution of PFAPA symptoms.

Results.—A total of 124 patients (75 boys and 49 girls) underwent adenotonsillectomy from 2004 to 2011 for relief of cyclical fevers due to PFAPA syndrome. Of the 124 patients, 22 did not meet criteria for inclusion in this study because (1) they had less than 6 months of follow-up after surgery or (2) they were unavailable for follow-up; therefore, 102 patients were included in the study. The mean age at the time of surgery was 58 months (range, 18-179 months). The average duration of follow-up after adenotonsillectomy was 43 months (range, 6-98 months). Of 102 patients, 99 had complete resolution of their symptoms immediately after surgery.

Conclusions.—Our findings showed complete resolution of symptoms in 99 of 102 patients with PFAPA syndrome who were treated surgically.

Patients who meet the clinical criteria for PFAPA syndrome should be offered tonsillectomy and adenoidectomy as part of their treatment options.

► Periodic fever, aphthous stomatitis, pharyngitis, and cervical adenitis (PFAPA) syndrome is challenging to identify and treat because the physical findings are not specifically diagnostic. The hallmark of PFAPA is its periodic recurrence, with regular intervals of abrupt-onset high fever in early childhood. This is a follow-up study that demonstrates the long-term efficacy of adenotonsillectomy for the treatment of PFAPA syndrome along with a helpful review of the literature. Children who underwent adenotonsillectomy were followed for a minimum of 6 months. The primary outcome measure was time to cessation of fevers after surgery. Of 102 patients, 99 had complete resolution of their symptoms immediately after surgery. This large prospective series of surgically treated patients followed long term shows that adenotonsillectomy provides sustained relief of PFAPA syndrome symptoms in the great majority of cases. The authors mention that, not surprisingly, all parents of children treated with adenotonsillectomy were immensely grateful for the cessation of symptoms and improvement in their children's quality of life. Clearly, in carefully selected and properly diagnosed children, adenotonsillectomy can have an important curative role.

R. B. Mitchell, MD

Management of recurrent acute otitis media in children: systematic review of the effect of different interventions on otitis media recurrence, recurrence frequency and total recurrence time

Cheong KH, Hussain SSM (Ninewells Hosp and Univ of Dundee Med School, Scotland, UK)

J Laryngol Otol 126:874-885, 2012

Objective.—To conduct a systematic review comparing the effect of three interventions (prophylactic antibiotics, tympanostomy tube insertion and adenoidectomy) on otitis media recurrence, recurrence frequency and total recurrence time.

Methods.—Literature on recurrent otitis media was identified using the PubMed and Scopus search engines for the period January 1990 to March 2011. A hand search of the reference lists of relevant articles and textbooks was conducted to identify additional studies. Randomised, controlled trials with a minimum of 40 children and follow up of at least 12 months were included.

Results.—Eighteen publications were identified. Each was assessed using preset inclusion criteria; seven publications met these criteria.

Conclusion.—Prophylactic antibiotics are effective in reducing otitis media recurrence, recurrence frequency and total recurrence time. Tympanostomy tube insertion failed to reduce the prevalence of otitis media recurrence, but reduced the recurrence frequency and total recurrence time.

Adenoidectomy reduced otitis media recurrence; results on otitis media recurrence frequency differed but on average there was a reduction; however, the two studies with relevant data on total recurrence time had contradictory results.

▶ There are 3 main treatment modalities for recurrent otitis media: prophylactic antibiotics, adenoidectomy, and tympanostomy tube insertion. This article systematically reviews recent trials of recurrent otitis media treatment and prevention over the past 20 years, with the aim of assessing the efficacy of the 3 main treatment methods. The trend has been toward tympanostomy tube insertion, with adenoidectomy less frequently performed as the primary treatment and prophylactic antibiotics less commonly used because of concerns about resistance. Although the methodology of this review was good and all the articles included were randomized controlled studies of otitis media in children and assessed similar outcomes, there were multiple variables that made performing a meta-analysis difficult. The following conclusions can be reasonably made: First, prophylactic antibiotics are effective in improving all 3 otitis media outcomes assessed in this review. Treatment with prophylactic antibiotics reduces the prevalence of otitis media recurrence, the frequency of otitis media episodes, and the total time each child spends with otitis media. The effectiveness of prophylactic antibiotics was greater than that of tympanostomy tube insertion and adenoidectomy, in terms of reduction in otitis media recurrence and otitis media episode frequency. Second, tympanostomy tube treatment fails to prevent recurrence of otitis media but is effective in reducing the frequency of otitis media episodes and the total time spent with otitis media. Third, adenoidectomy is effective in reducing otitis media recurrence. Data on otitis media frequency differed among studies, but the mean result from the 3 relevant studies indicated that adenoidectomy reduces the frequency of otitis media episodes but has no benefit in the treatment of otitis media in children younger than age 2 years. Overall, this review supports current practice but would also support a reassessment of the risk-benefit equation of using prophylactic antibiotics in selected patients.

R. B. Mitchell, MD

Changes in Central Apnea Index Following Pediatric Adenotonsillectomy

Baldassari CM, Kepchar J, Bryant L, et al (Eastern Virginia Med School, Norfolk; Walter Reed Army Med Ctr, Washington, DC; et al)

Otolaryngol Head Neck Surg 146:487-490, 2012

Objectives.—To determine if there are changes in the central apnea index (CAI) when pediatric patients undergo adenotonsillectomy for obstructive sleep apnea (OSA).

Study Design.—Case series with chart review.

Setting.—Two tertiary children's hospitals.

Subjects and Methods.—Children between 1 and 16 years of age who underwent adenotonsillectomy for OSA and had both preoperative and postoperative full-night polysomnography (PSG) with CAI greater than 1 on preoperative PSG were eligible for inclusion. Central apnea was defined as the absence of both inspiratory effort and chest wall movement lasting longer than 20 seconds. Criteria for diagnosis of central sleep apnea (CSA) was CAI greater than 1.

Results.—A total of 101 children with OSA had preoperative and postoperative PSG. Fifteen of these patients had a preoperative CAI greater than 1. The mean age was 67.7 months (SD, 62.7 months). The CAI ranged from 1.1 to 11.1. The mean preoperative CAI was 3.9 (SD, 2.9), while the mean postoperative CAI was 1.9 (SD, 4.8). There was significant improvement ($P = .008$) of the CAI following adenotonsillectomy. Ninety percent of subjects with mild CSA (CAI between 1 and 5) had postoperative resolution of their disease. There was also significant improvement ($P = .004$) in the obstructive apnea hypopnea index (AHI), with the mean preoperative AHI of 22.8 (SD, 19.8) decreasing to an AHI of 5.5 (SD, 6.5) postoperatively.

Conclusions.—Children with OSA and mild CSA on preoperative PSG showed significant improvement in CAI following adenotonsillectomy. Future studies are needed to determine the clinical significance of CSA in children with OSA and to identify treatment strategies.

▶ Central sleep apnea (CSA) is characterized by episodes of apnea during sleep in the absence of airway obstruction. A central apnea index (CAI; number of central apneas per hour) greater than or equal to 1 is considered diagnostic for CSA in children. CSA can be primary in nature or can be associated with other medical conditions, including brainstem pathology such as Arnold-Chiari malformation, neurologic disorders such as Prader-Willi and Joubert syndrome, heart failure, and prematurity. Although the exact cause of CSA is unknown, this disorder likely involves a disruption or dysfunction of ventilatory control in the central nervous system.

The objectives of this study were (1) to determine the incidence of CSA in a population of children with obstructive sleep apnea (OSA) and (2) to assess whether there is improvement in the central apnea index in pediatric patients who undergo adenotonsillectomy for OSA. In this study, 15 of 101 (14.9%) subjects had CSA on preoperative polysomnography (PSG) and most children (73.3%) experienced resolution of CSA following adenotonsillectomy. Ninety percent of patients with mild CSA on preoperative PSG had no evidence of CSA following surgery. It is unclear why the CAI improves following adenotonsillectomy. CSA is believed to involve dysfunction of ventilatory control in the central nervous system, while OSA has been linked to anatomic obstruction and increased upper airway resistance. It may be that OSA leads to CSA in certain patients, and relief of obstruction leads to improvement in CSA. The authors conclude that children with OSA frequently have a CAI greater than 1 and that most pediatric patients with CSA, especially those with a CAI between 1 and 5, experience resolution of their disease after adenotonsillectomy. This is an important finding that helps in deciding if children with OSA and CSA should undergo adenotonsillectomy.

R. B. Mitchell, MD

A Systematic Review of Adenotonsillectomy as a Risk Factor for Childhood Obesity

Jeyakumar A, Fettman N, Armbrecht ES, et al (Saint Louis Univ, MO)

Otolaryngol Head Neck Surg 144:154-158, 2011

Objective.—Tonsillectomy is the most common major surgical procedure performed in children. There is evidence that tonsillectomy is associated with weight increase and may contribute to pediatric obesity. The study aimed to review the evidence that tonsillectomy with or without adenoidectomy is a risk factor for future obesity.

Data Sources.—Systematic literature search was performed using PubMed and Ovid.

Review Methods.—Systematic analysis of the literature from 1970 to 2009 on patients who underwent adenotonsillectomy (T&A) with preoperative and postoperative weight-based measurements.

Results.—Nine studies satisfied inclusion criteria. A total of 795 children were included. Preoperative weight ranged from normal to morbid obesity. In total, 656 children had demographic information recorded, and 53.35% of the children were male. Indication for surgery was not recorded in 336 patients. In 47.7% patients, the indication recorded was sleep-disordered breathing. The first group included 3 studies involving 127 children, and body mass index (BMI) increased by 5.5% to 8.2%. The second group included 3 studies involving 419 patients; the standardized weight scores increased in 46% to 100% of patients. The third group included 3 studies with 249 patients; the corrected weight increased postoperatively in 50% to 75% of patients. Morbidly obese patients (weight 130%-260% vs peers) remained unchanged postoperatively.

Limitations.—Each study was designed with different definitions of overweight and a range of follow-up periods. Demographic information was limited.

Conclusions.—A large population of normal and overweight children undergoing T&A gained a greater than expected amount of weight postoperatively, which suggests an association between T&A and weight gain. A significant need exists for a large study with consistent outcomes measured.

▶ This review is important reading for otolaryngologists who perform adenotonsillectomy (T&A) for sleep-disordered breathing (SDB) in children. There is increasing concern that T&A may be responsible for weight gain following surgery in normal and overweight children. Because SDB is more common in overweight or obese children, this can make the underlying sleep problem worse after T&A and may reverse any benefit of surgery. The article demonstrates an association between T&A and a greater than expected weight gain in normal and overweight children. However, there was lack of standardization in recording and obtaining data for weight, height, and body mass index and a variety of surgical techniques and study methodologies. Although it is important to treat pediatric obstructive sleep apnea and chronic tonsillitis appropriately with T&A,

the decision for surgery in normal and overweight children must be tempered with the possibility that T&A could cause further weight gain and obesity. A large population of normal and overweight children undergoing T&A gained a greater than expected amount of weight postoperatively, which suggests an association between T&A and weight gain. Studies are needed to determine which children may be at greatest risk for developing obesity and whether nonsurgical intervention is more appropriate in some children who are or may become overweight or obese.

R. B. Mitchell, MD

6 Rhinology and Skull Base Surgery

Basic and Clinical Research

The Effects of Systemic, Topical, and Intralesional Steroid Treatments on Apoptosis Level of Nasal Polyps

Kapucu B, Cekin E, Erkul BE, et al (GATA Haydarpasa Training Hosp, Istanbul, Turkey)

Otolaryngol Head Neck Surg 147:563-567, 2012

Objective.—The purpose of this study was to compare the apoptotic responses to systemic, topical, and intrapolyp injection of glucocorticoid with no treatment in nasal polyps.

Study Design.—Prospective, randomized controlled study.

Setting.—Tertiary training hospital.

Subjects and Methods.—The study was performed on 48 patients with nasal polyposis in the Department of Otorhinolaryngology between 2008 and 2009. Patients were assigned to 1 of 4 groups of 12 patients. Group A was treated with oral methylprednisolone 1 mg/kg/d, and the dose was tapered gradually. Group B received 0.3 mL triamcinolone acetonide (40 mg/mL), which was injected into polyp tissue. Group C was treated with topical 55 μg triamcinolone acetonide 2 times daily for 1 month. Group D received no medication. Samples were collected endoscopically after the seventh day for groups A and B, the first month for group C, and the first visit for group D. Apoptotic indexes were determined using the terminal deoxynucleotidyl transferase-mediated dUTP nick end labeling method.

Results.—Statistically significant differences in apoptotic index were found between each steroid-medicated group and the control group ($P_{D\text{-}A} = .0001$; $P_{D\text{-}B} = .003$; $P_{D\text{-}C} = .026$) and between groups A and C ($P_{A\text{-}C} = .012$). Group B did not differ significantly from either group A or C ($P_{A\text{-}B} = .11$; $P_{B\text{-}C} = .75$).

Conclusions.—The apoptotic index in nasal polyps treated with systemic, topical, and intrapolyp injection forms of glucocorticoids was

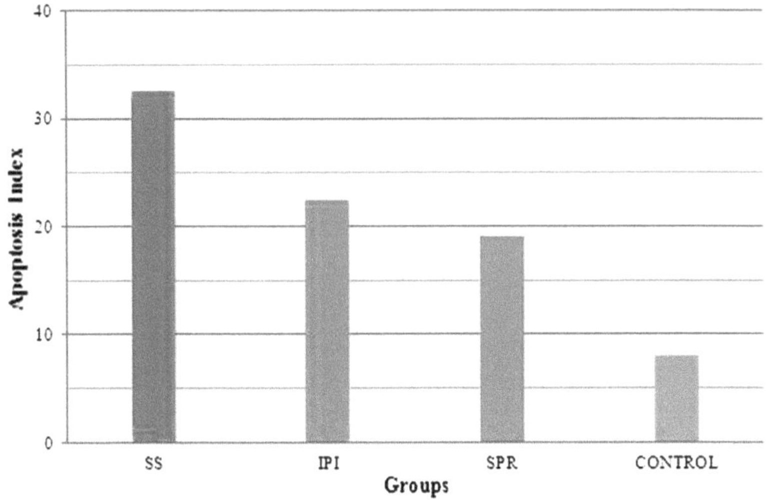

FIGURE 2.—Comparison of the distribution of apoptosis indexes among groups. The x-axis shows the groups and the y-axis shows the apoptosis index values of the groups. IPI, intrapolyp injection; SPR, spray; SS, systemic steroid. (Reprinted from Otolaryngology-Head and Neck Surgery. Kapucu B, Cekin E, Erkul BE, et al. The effects of systemic, topical, and intralesional steroid treatments on apoptosis level of nasal polyps. *Otolaryngol Head Neck Surg.* 2012;147:563-567, Copyright 2012, with permission from the American Academy of Otolaryngology-Head and Neck Surgery Foundation.)

higher than that in the control group. Systemic steroid treatment induced the most apoptosis (Fig 2).

▶ Apoptosis is physiologic cell death caused by developmental and environmental stimuli. The ability of various routes of steroid therapy to impact apoptosis in nasal polyps has not been previously studied in detail. Initiating apoptosis may be one mechanism by which steroids may reduce inflammation and polyposis. This study compared the apoptotic responses of nasal polyps to a variety of steroid treatment strategies. This prospective, controlled study randomly assigned 48 patients with nasal polyposis to 1 of 4 groups of 12 patients: Group A was treated with oral methylprednisolone 1 mg/kg/d gradually tapered, group B received 0.3 mL triamcinolone acetonide (40 mg/mL) intralesional injection, group C was treated with topical 55 μg triamcinolone acetonide 2 times daily for 1 month, and group D received no medication. Their primary outcome measure was degree of apoptosis seen in samples harvested after treatment. Samples were collected endoscopically, and apoptotic indexes were determined using the terminal deoxynucleotidyl transferase-mediated dUTP nick end labeling method. The results showed that apoptotic index in nasal polyps treated with systemic, topical, and intrapolyp injection forms of glucocorticoids was higher than that in the control group, and systemic steroid treatment induced the most apoptosis in those treated with steroids (Fig 2). Clearly, more basic science investigations like this one are needed to further elucidate how and why our current treatment strategies work.

R. Sindwani, MD

Anti-proliferative effect of glucocorticoids on mesenchymal cells in juvenile angiofibromas

Wendler O, Dlugaiczyk J, Birk S, et al (Univ Hosp Erlangen, Germany; Saarland Univ Med Ctr, Homburg/Saar, Germany)

Head Neck 34:1615-1621, 2012

Background.—Glucocorticoids (GCs) not only regulate metabolic and inflammatory mechanisms, but also are known to suppress tumor growth. Despite previous detection of glucocorticoid receptors (GRs) in juvenile angiofibromas, their distribution and function have not further been studied.

Methods.—Juvenile angiofibroma tissue ($n = 30$), nasal mucosa specimens ($n = 10$), subepithelial stroma of nasal mucosa ($n = 20$), and primary fibroblasts from juvenile angiofibroma ($n = 6$) and nasal mucosa samples ($n = 6$) were analyzed by quantitative reverse transcriptase-polymerase chain reaction (RT-PCR) and immunofluorescence staining. The antiproliferative effect of GCs (dexamethasone, prednisolone, and hydrocortisone) in vitro was assessed using a bromdeoxyuridine (BrdU) assay.

Results.—An upregulation of GR transcripts and protein was shown in juvenile angiofibroma tissue and primary mesenchymal cells compared to nasal mucosa. Application of GCs resulted in a significantly higher antiproliferative effect on juvenile angiofibroma versus nasal mucosa fibroblasts in vitro.

Conclusion.—Expression of GRs and antiproliferative effects of GCs on juvenile angiofibroma fibroblasts offer novel options for the treatment of this unique fibrovascular tumor (Fig 2).

▶ Glucocorticoid (GC) steroid receptors have been detected in juvenile angiofibromas and have been implicated in tumor suppression in other clinical settings. Despite this, little attention has been given to their potential role in juvenile nasopharyngeal angiofibromas (JNAs). This basic science study examines the presence and putative therapeutic role the GCs may have in these rare tumors. Juvenile angiofibroma tissue (n = 30), nasal mucosa specimens (n = 10), subepithelial stroma of nasal mucosa (n = 20), and primary fibroblasts from juvenile angiofibroma (n = 6) and nasal mucosa samples (n = 6) were analyzed by quantitative reverse transcriptase-polymerase chain reaction (RT-PCR) and immunofluorescence staining (Fig 2). The antiproliferative effect of GCs (dexamethasone, prednisolone, and hydrocortisone) in vitro was assessed using a bromodeoxyuridine assay. The study found upregulation of glucocorticoid receptor transcripts and protein in JNA tissue and primary mesenchymal cells compared with nasal mucosa. Application of GCs resulted in a significantly higher antiproliferative effect on juvenile angiofibroma vs nasal mucosa fibroblasts in vitro as well. The observation of GC-related growth inhibition in juvenile angiofibroma fibroblasts offers the future prospect of a preoperative treatment with GCs to reduce juvenile angiofibroma tumor size. The concept of a neoadjuvant hormone therapy in this rare fibrovascular tumor has been addressed previously using sex steroid hormones, albeit with controversial results, and these have been associated

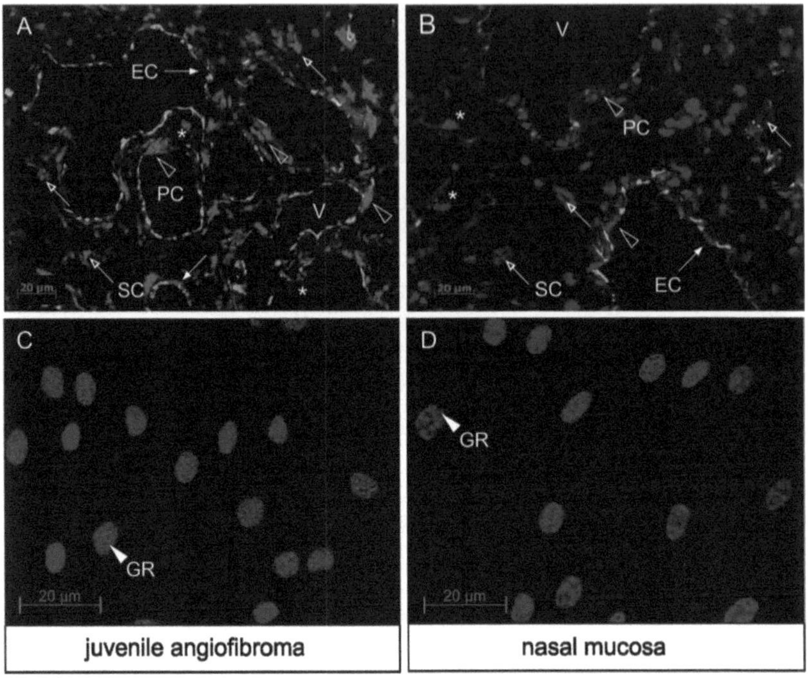

FIGURE 2.—Immunofluorescence staining of glucocorticoid receptor alpha (GRα) protein (red) in juvenile angiofibroma and nasal mucosa cryosections (A, B) as well as cultured fibroblasts (C, D). Cell nuclei were counterstained with diamidino-phenylindole (DAPI) (blue). Scale bar: 20 μm. (A) A strong signal for GRα protein (red) was detected in stromal cells (SC; open arrow) and perivascular cells (PC; open arrowhead) of juvenile angiofibromas, whereas a weak GRα protein expression was determined for endothelial cells (EC; filled arrow). Endothelial cells surrounding juvenile angiofibroma vessels (V) were stained by CD 31 (green). Most GRα signals were observed in the cytoplasm, but some nuclear staining was also found (*). (B) Weak immunofluorescence signals for GRα protein were obtained in stromal cells (SC, open arrow), perivascular cells (PC, open arrowhead), and endothelial cells (EC, filled arrow) of nasal mucosa cryosections. Vascular (V) endothelial cells were identified by staining CD31 (green). (C) Cultured juvenile angiofibroma fibroblasts displayed a prominent nuclear staining for GRα protein (red, filled arrowhead). (D) Weak nuclear GRα signals (red, filled arrowhead) were obtained for nasal mucosa fibroblasts. For Interpretation of the references to color in this figure legend, the reader is referred to web version of this article. (Reprinted from Wendler O, Dlugaiczyk J, Birk S, et al. Anti-proliferative effect of glucocorticoids on mesenchymal cells in juvenile angiofibromas. *Head Neck*. 2012;34:1615-1621, with permission from Head & Neck and John Wiley and Sons, www.interscience.wiley.com.)

with significant unwanted feminizing side effects. Preoperative administration of GCs might constitute an attractive treatment alternative. We look forward to further work to follow up on the exciting and novel findings of this study.

R. Sindwani, MD

General

Should Intranasal Splints Be Used After Nasal Septal Surgery?
Tang S, Kacker A (New York-Presbyterian/Weill Cornell Med College)
Laryngoscope 122:1647-1648, 2012

Background.—The use of intranasal splints after nasal septal surgery is designed to prevent intranasal adhesions and support septal position. Patients report significant discomfort is associated with the use of splints, so the benefits of their use were considered in relation to their associated disadvantages.

Methods.—A literature search over the previous 20 years identified six randomized controlled trials that compared the outcomes of septal surgery performed with and without the use of intranasal splints. Septal position, airway position, pain, and the development of complications such as intranasal adhesions were evaluated for the two approaches.

Results.—Intranasal adhesions occurred at similar rates in the two treatment groups for the majority of studies. Pain scores, however, tended to be higher in the splinted groups than in the nonsplinted groups. Splints showed no association with diminished rates of most other complications, including compromised postoperative Eustachian tube function and septal perforation.

Conclusions.—Conventional septal splints cause significantly greater postoperative pain that is not offset by significant reductions in complications. A recent randomized controlled trial has shown that a thinner splint may improve mucosal status and decrease postoperative discomfort; this may offer an attractive option.

► The simple answer to this relevant question is NO. This best practice article is a short and concise review of the literature on the use of nasal splints after septal surgery. Intranasal splints are widely used after nasal septal surgery for prevention of intranasal adhesions and support of septal position. However, they have been found to cause significant discomfort to patients, so their routine use has more recently been questioned. Conventional septal splints have been found in multiple large, randomized controlled trials (RCTs) to cause significantly increased postoperative pain without sufficient evidence of decreasing rates of intranasal adhesions or other clinically significant complications. As the report discusses, there have been 6 RCTs in the last 20 years comparing outcomes of septal surgery with and without the use of intranasal splints. Overwhelmingly, the negatives associated with them seem to outweigh the limited benefits that they provide, which, according to the literature, are quite minimal to nonexistent. So the short of it is that, in most cases, the routine use of splints does not confer any advantage to outcomes from septal surgery but are, however, associated with drawbacks, including patient discomfort and other complications (such as septal perforation). I do not use splints after septal surgery as a routine. Having said this, I may consider using a splint in the rare scenario in which dissection has led to multiple flap tears and I am concerned about an increased chance of possible septal perforation.

R. Sindwani, MD

Medical therapy vs surgery for chronic rhinosinusitis: a prospective, multi-institutional study with 1-year follow-up

Smith TL, Kern R, Palmer JN, et al (Oregon Health and Science Univ, Portland; Northwestern Univ, Chicago, IL; Hosp of the Univ of Pennsylvania, Philadelphia; et al)

Int Forum Allergy Rhinol 3:4-9, 2013

Background.—This study evaluated 1-year outcomes in patients with chronic rhinosinusitis (CRS) who were considered surgical candidates by study criteria and elected either medical management or endoscopic sinus surgery (ESS). In addition, some patients initially enrolled in the medical treatment arm crossed over to the surgery arm during the study period and their respective outcomes are evaluated.

Methods.—Adult subjects with CRS who failed initial medical therapy were prospectively enrolled into a nonrandomized, multi-institutional cohort. Subjects were included in 1 of 3 cohorts: medically managed, surgically managed, or crossover (from medical to surgical). The primary outcome measure was disease-specific quality-of-life (QOL). Bivariate and multivariate analyses compared QOL improvement between cohort groups.

Results.—Baseline comorbidity, QOL, and other disease severity measures were not different between the 3 cohorts. With 1-year follow up, surgical patients ($n = 65$) reported significantly more improvement than medically managed patients ($n = 33$; Rhinosinusitis Disability Index (RSDI), $p = 0.039$; Chronic Sinusitis Survey (CSS), $p = 0.018$). Seventeen subjects who had initially elected medical management crossed over to surgery during the follow-up period. QOL in the crossover cohort was initially stagnant or worsening followed by improvement after ESS (RSDI, $p = 0.035$; CSS, $p = 0.070$). At 1-year follow-up, higher frequency of improvement was found in the surgical cohort vs medical cohort for several outcomes (total CSS: 70.8% vs 45.5%; odds ratio [OR], 3.37; 95% confidence interval [CI], 1.27-8.90; $p = 0.014$).

Conclusion.—With 1 year of follow-up, patients electing ESS experienced significantly higher levels of improvement in outcomes compared to patients managed by medication alone. In addition, a crossover cohort who initially elected medical management experienced improvement in several outcomes after crossing over to ESS.

▶ The relative benefits of medical therapy vs. surgery for chronic rhinosinusitis (CRS) has been a hotly debated topic for many years. This article, which is a 1-year follow-up of the results from a group of patients presented earlier by this group,[1] looks at getting to the heart of this controversy. In a very realistic way, this multicentered study looks at outcomes in patients with CRS who were considered surgical candidates and elected either medical management or endoscopic sinus surgery. So although not randomized, the decision to enroll in either arm of the study was left to the patient, which, as mentioned, is the "real-world" way decisions for treatment actually occur. So patients were organized and compared in 3 cohorts: medically managed, surgically managed, or crossover (from medical to surgical). The study found that patients electing endoscopic sinus surgery (ESS) had significantly greater quality-of-life (QOL) improvements in addition to less exposure to oral antibiotics and oral steroids as well as fewer missed school and work days. A very interesting finding of the study was the experience of the so-called "crossover" group of patients (albeit only 17 in number). These patients initially had a poor response to medical therapy (which they opted for at the outset), but their QOL improved significantly once they had ESS. After 1-year follow-up, all 3 cohorts experienced significant and durable improvement in symptoms, with the surgical cohort demonstrating nearly twice as much improvement in most QOL domains. The crossover cohort's significant improvement in QOL after ESS suggests that lack of improvement/worsening in QOL may be a factor for patient decision-making regarding treatment. This is a very significant study that helps cement the beneficial role of ESS in the management of CRS.

R. Sindwani, MD

Reference

1. Smith TL, Kern RC, Palmer JN, et al. Medical therapy vs surgery for chronic rhinosinusitis: a prospective, multi-institutional study. *Int Forum Allergy Rhinol.* 2011;1:235-241.

Impact of Topical Nasal Steroid Therapy on Symptoms of Nasal Polyposis: A Meta-Analysis

Rudmik L, Schlosser RJ, Smith TL, et al (Univ of Calgary, Alberta, Canada; Med Univ of South Carolina, Charleston; Oregon Health and Science Univ, Portland)
Laryngoscope 122:1431-1437, 2012

Objectives/Hypothesis.—Topical steroid therapy is an important strategy in the management of chronic rhinosinusitis (CRS) with nasal polyposis. The objective of this study was to determine the impact of topical steroid therapy on nasal symptoms in patients with nasal polyposis.

Study Design.—Systematic review with meta-analysis using standardized methodology.

Methods.—Study inclusion criteria included: randomized, placebo controlled trials, nasal polyposis, and topical steroid therapy. Exclusion criteria included: failure to report at least one symptom-based outcome measure, concurrent use of systemic steroids, or mixed CRS cohorts (polyp and nonpolyp patients). Quantitative analysis was performed using a random effect model. The PRISMA guidelines for meta-analysis reporting were followed.

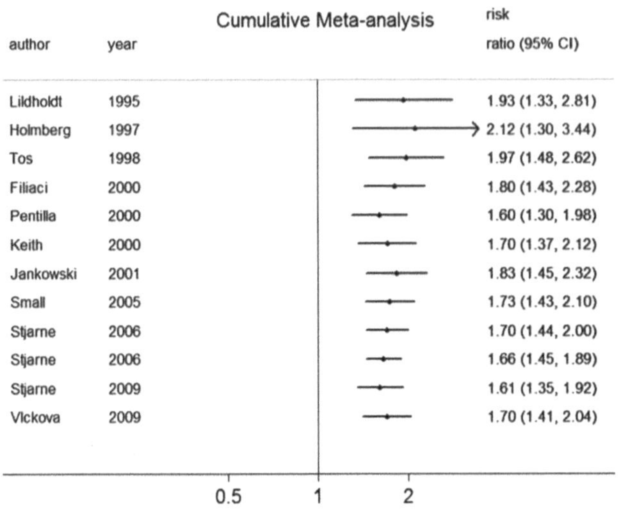

FIGURE 4.—Pooled relative risk adding one study at a time by year of publication. CI = confidence interval. (Reprinted from Rudmik L, Schlosser RJ, Smith TL, et al. Impact of topical nasal steroid therapy on symptoms of nasal polyposis: a meta-analysis. *Laryngoscope*. 2012;122:1431-1437, with permission from Laryngoscope and John Wiley and Sons, www.interscience.wiley.com.)

Results.—A total of 19 studies fulfilled eligibility. Seven studies were excluded from the meta-analysis due to significant heterogeneity in outcome reporting. A total of 12 studies were combined for quantitative analysis and demonstrated a pooled risk ratio of 1.72 (95% confidence interval, 1.41–2.09), indicating a significant improvement in nasal symptoms. All three topical steroid preparations (fluticasone, mometasone, and budesonide) resulted in symptom improvement. All seven studies excluded from the meta-analysis qualitatively confirmed the overall findings.

Conclusions.—Topical nasal steroid therapy improves nasal symptoms in CRS patients with nasal polyposis. Future studies will need to evaluate the impact on quality of life, preferably using validated disease-specific instruments (Fig 4).

▶ This systematic review and meta-analysis looks at the impact of nasal steroid sprays on patient-subjective nasal symptoms in chronic rhinosinusitis (CRS) and nasal polyps. As the authors discuss, many trials previously published have demonstrated an improvement in objective findings with the use of steroid sprays in this particular patient group (most notably in reducing polyp size, for example) but none has focused on actual symptom improvement, which, of course, is key. This is a well-conducted meta-analysis that pooled results from 12 randomized, placebo-controlled trials. The pooled data demonstrated a risk ratio of 1.72 (95% confidence interval, 1.41–2.09), indicating a significant improvement in nasal symptoms (Fig 4) and, of note, all 3 topical steroid preparations (fluticasone, mometasone, and budesonide) resulted in symptom improvement. The review concluded that there indeed is convincing, high-level evidence that topical nasal steroids improve patient symptomatology in CRS with polyposis, and it strongly recommended the use of topical steroids in the comprehensive management strategy of polyp patients. Most would agree that topical steroid delivery (in some form) to the sinonasal cavities in patients suffering with nasal polyps is a true cornerstone of maintenance therapy. This may not always take the form of a steroid spray, however, because steroids delivered in a variety of methods (eg, nebulization, high-volume irrigations) have also gained favor. This article nicely highlights that in addition to objective data, information on disease-specific symptoms and quality-of-life outcomes (preferably using validated, health-related quality-of-life instruments) are also very important.

R. Sindwani, MD

Management of intractable spontaneous epistaxis

Rudmik L, Smith TL (Univ of Calgary, Alberta, Canada; Oregon Health and Science Univ, Portland)

Am J Rhinol Allergy 26:55-60, 2012

Background.—Epistaxis is a common otolaryngology emergency and is often controlled with first-line interventions such as cautery, hemostatic agents, or anterior nasal packing. A subset of patients will continue to bleed and require more aggressive therapy.

Methods.—Intractable spontaneous epistaxis was traditionally managed with posterior nasal packing and prolonged hospital admission. In an effort to reduce patient morbidity and shorten hospital stay, surgical and endovascular techniques have gained popularity. A literature review was conducted.

Results.—Transnasal endoscopic sphenopalatine artery ligation and arterial embolization provide excellent control rates but the decision to choose one over the other can be challenging. The role of transnasal endoscopic anterior ethmoid artery ligation is unclear but may be considered in certain cases when bleeding localizes to the ethmoid region.

Conclusion.—This article will focus on the management of intractable spontaneous epistaxis and discuss the role of endoscopic arterial ligation and embolization as it pertains to this challenging clinical scenario (Tables 4 and 5).

► All otolaryngologists have a true distaste for managing epistaxis, yet nosebleeds continue to be a common reason for consultations, especially from the emergency department. Fortunately, most cases of epistaxis can be managed with conservative measures, although a subset of patients will continue to bleed and require an escalation of management. This article serves as an excellent review of the management decisions and options for the control of intractable nosebleeds. A nice description of the techniques of transnasal endoscopic sphenopalatine artery ligation (TESPAL) and control of the anterior ethmoid artery (AEA) is presented in a step-by-step manner (Tables 4 and 5). The review highlights that for posterior epistaxis, TESPAL and arterial embolization provide excellent control rates, but the decision to choose one over the other is multifactorial

TABLE 4.—Surgical Steps for TESPAL

Medialize middle turbinate
Lateral nasal wall incision posterior to the maxillary sinus (see Fig. 1 in the original article)
Elevate nasal mucosa
Identify ethmoid crest (marks the anterior limit of possible SPA location)
Tent up the SPA as it exits the SPF
Cauterize the SPA
Redrape the elevated nasal mucosa

SPA = sphenopalatine artery; TESPAL = transnasal endoscopic sphenopalatine artery ligation.

TABLE 5.—Surgical Steps for TEAEAL

Maxillary antrostomy and anterior ethmoidectomy
Define the lamina papyracea and ethmoid roof
Identify AEA canal (helpful to use image-guidance navigation)
Small opening made in lamina papyracea below the AEA canal (using small curette)
Unshell the bony fragments off the AEA adjacement to the lamina papyracea
Elevate posterior and anterior to the AEA (allow for clip placement)
Place small clip across the AEA next to the orbital periosteum

AEA = anterior ethmoid artery; TEAEAL = transnasal endoscopic anterior ethmoid artery ligation.

and not obvious. Decision making is influenced by numerous factors, including patient comorbidity, presence of anticoagulation, institution surgical and endovascular expertise, patient preference, and even health care costs. Advantages of TESPAL over embolization are: a lower risk for major complications (stroke, blindness, and soft-tissue ischemia), improved bleeding site localization, improved ability to diagnose less common etiologies of epistaxis, the option to perform immediate AEA ligation, and significantly lower health care costs. Advantages of embolization include avoiding general anesthesia (especially important in patients with significant comorbidities) and improved diagnosis of vascular abnormalities (including malformations or pseudoaneurysm). The article presents a cost analysis of the 2 interventions showing that TESPAL is significantly less expensive (approximately half as costly as embolization: $6000 versus $12 000, respectively) and outlines a management pathway placing surgical intervention as the preferred first choice of intervention for intractable epistaxis patients without any other major health issues (Fig 4 in the original article). Overall, a worthwhile review and excellent summary of everyone's least favorite topic.

R. Sindwani, MD

Antimicrobials and chronic rhinosinusitis with or without polyposis in adults: an evidenced-based review with recommendations

Soler ZM, Oyer SL, Kern RC, et al (Med Univ of South Carolina, Charleston; Northwestern Univ, Chicago, IL; et al)

Int Forum Allergy Rhinol 3:31-47, 2013

Background.—Chronic rhinosinusitis (CRS) is characterized by inflammation of the mucosa of the nose and paranasal sinuses. The role of bacterial or fungal infection in CRS is unclear, yet antimicrobials are commonly prescribed for this condition. Published guidelines offer little direction regarding antibiotic strategies for CRS. The purpose of this article is to provide an evidence-based approach to the use of antibacterial and antifungal antibiotics in the management of CRS.

Methods.—A systematic review of the literature was performed following recommendations of the Clinical Practice Guideline Manual, Conference on Guideline Standardization (COGS), and the Appraisal of Guidelines and Research Evaluation (AGREE). Inclusion criteria were: age ≥ 18 years old, chronic rhinosinusitis with or without polyps, antibiotic treatment as the experimental group, and clearly defined primary clinical endpoint. Studies involving patients with cystic fibrosis or acute invasive fungal sinusitis were excluded.

Results.—The review identified and evaluated the literature on 8 classes of antimicrobials for CRS: oral antibacterial antibiotics ≤ 3 weeks, oral antibacterial antibiotics > 3 weeks, macrolide antibiotics, intravenous antibacterial antibiotics, topical antibacterial antibiotics, oral antifungals, intravenous antifungals, and topical antifungals.

Conclusion.—Based on the available evidence, oral antibacterial antibiotics and prolonged macrolide antibiotics are considered therapeutic options in the treatment of CRS while the use of topical antibacterial antibiotics, intravenous antibacterial antibiotics and oral, topical, or intravenous antifungals would be *recommended against.* These evidence-based recommendations should not necessarily be applied to all patients with

TABLE 1.—Antibiotic Approaches for CRS Evaluated in Review

Antibacterial
Oral antibiotics (non-macrolide; shorter than 3 weeks treatment duration)
Oral antibiotics (non-macrolide; longer than 3 weeks treatment duration)
Macrolide class of antibiotics
Intravenous antibiotics
Topical antibiotics
Antifungal
Oral antibiotics
Intravenous antibiotics
Topical antibiotics

CRS = chronic rhinosinusitis.

CRS and are not intended to supersede clinical judgment based on individual patient circumstances (Table 1).

▶ This is an excellent review of the literature with recommendations on the role of antimicrobials in adult patients with chronic rhinosinusitis (CRS; with and without polyps). The authors looked at antibiotics, antifungals, and various routes of administration. The efficacy of 8 relevant antimicrobial therapeutic options was analyzed: oral antibacterial, antibiotics ≤3 weeks, oral antibacterial antibiotics >3 weeks, macrolide antibiotics, intravenous antibacterial antibiotics, topical antibacterial antibiotics, oral antifungals, intravenous antifungals, and topical antifungals (Table 1). All of these various therapeutic options have been used by most of us to some degree or another over the years, so the topic is very relevant and worthy of study. The article is well written and clearly laid out with pros and cons, risks of the medications, and recommendations where applicable. Based on the currently available evidence, oral antibacterial antibiotics and prolonged macrolide antibiotics are considered effective therapeutic options in the treatment of CRS, whereas the use of topical antibacterial antibiotics, intravenous antibacterial antibiotics, and oral, topical, or intravenous antifungals were recommended against. The authors did couch their findings by saying that "the evidence-based recommendations should not necessarily be applied to all patients with CRS and are not intended to supersede clinical judgment based on individual patient circumstances," leaving the door open for potential use of these other therapeutic options in selected patients. Overall, a thoughtful and meaningful review, but clearly more study on these other routes of delivery and therapies is required.

R. Sindwani, MD

Evolution and Future of Skull Base Surgery: The Paradigm of Skull Base Meningiomas

Di Maio S, Ramanathan D, Garcia-Lopez R, et al (Univ of Washington, Seattle)

World Neurosurg 78:260-275, 2012

Background.—Skull base meningiomas represent the paradigm for the evolution of skull base surgery within the past 50 years into a distinct neurosurgical subspecialty.

Methods.—From 2005 to 2011, 117 patients with cranial base meningiomas underwent surgical resection. Extent of resection, histologic grade, complications, functional status, and recurrence-free and overall survival data are presented.

Results.—The summary rate of gross total resection was 53.0%. The surgical complication and mortality rates were 17.9% and 0.9%, respectively. Five-year recurrence-free survival was 88.0% for grade I meningiomas. A total of 90.3% of patients had a Karnofsky performance score ≥ 80 at last follow-up.

Conclusions.—A large contemporary series of skull base meningiomas is presented. In addition, the evolution of surgical approaches to skull base meningiomas is reviewed, together with the current issues regarding radiation therapy, management of cavernous sinus tumor, oncologic management of atypical and malignant subtypes, molecular genetics, and future therapeutic options.

▶ This article is a very thorough account of meningioma surgery. Part historical perspective, part update, and part series presentation, the authors present their outcomes for 117 patients with cranial base meningiomas who underwent surgical resection. Extent of resection, histologic grade, complications, functional status, and recurrence-free and overall survival data are presented. The summary rate of gross total resection was 53.0%. The surgical complication and mortality rates were 17.9% and 0.9%, respectively. The authors highlighted that regardless of meningioma location, treatment objectives for cranial base meningiomas can be summarized in the following manner: (1) complete tumor resection, (2) preservation of patient's function and quality of life, (3) when the previous is not possible, a reasonable goal would be at least independence for daily living, (4) adjuvant or alternative treatment, such as fractionated radiotherapy or stereotactic radiosurgery, should be implemented when complete tumor resection is not possible. I enjoyed this article as much for its historical perspective and discussion of controversies as for its data presentation.

R. Sindwani, MD

Acute Bacterial Sinusitis in Children

DeMuri GP, Wald ER (Univ of Wisconsin School of Medicine and Public Health, Madison)

N Engl J Med 367:1128-1134, 2012

A 4-year-old girl who attends day care presents with rhinorrhea and a daytime cough that have been present for 12 days. She has not had fever, but her appetite is poor and her interest in activities is diminished. On physical examination, there is clear rhinorrhea present in the nasal passages. The remainder of the examination is unremarkable. Should she be treated with an antibiotic (Fig 1, Table 1)?

▶ It is not often that we get to include an article from the *New England Journal of Medicine* in these reviews. Although much of this article on acute bacterial (vs viral) sinusitis should be a review for otolaryngologists, it is included because it is well written, pertinent, and an excellent review of the available evidence. Topics explored include time course of disease, risk factors, recommended first-line antibiotics, dosing, adverse events, and the data for adjunctive medical therapy. The article also highlights that imaging is, of course, not necessary in the acute setting (unless, of course, an impending complication is suspected) and that imaging cannot distinguish between viral and bacterial etiologies. Again, well written and a good synopsis of the literature on the topic. With respect to the vignette

KEY CLINICAL POINTS

Acute Bacterial Sinusitis in Children

- In most instances, acute bacterial sinusitis in children follows a viral upper respiratory infection.
- Sinusitis in children has three predictable patterns of presentation: persistent, severe, and worsening symptoms.
- The diagnosis of acute bacterial sinusitis should be made on the basis of the history, generally without the use of imaging studies.
- *Haemophilus influenzae* appears to have become more common and *Streptococcus pneumoniae* less common as causes of acute bacterial sinusitis in children.
- Rates of beta-lactamase production in *H. influenzae* have increased in many geographic areas.
- Studies of the use of antimicrobial agents have had conflicting results, but findings generally support treatment.
- Amoxicillin–clavulanate should be considered as the first-line treatment for sinusitis in children.

FIGURE 1.—Key Clinical points. (Reprinted from DeMuri GP, Wald ER. Acute bacterial sinusitis in children. *N Engl J Med.* 2012;367:1128-1134, © 2012, Massachusetts Medical Society.)

TABLE 1.—Clinical Criteria for the Diagnosis of Acute Bacterial Sinusitis

Persistent symptoms
Nasal congestion, rhinorrhea, or cough
≥10 Days' duration without improvement
Severe symptoms
Temperature ≥38.5°C for 3–4 days
Purulent rhinorrhea for 3–4 days
Worsening symptoms
Return of symptoms after initial resolution
New or recurrent fever, increase in rhinorrhea, or increase in cough

presented—no weird and wonderful pathology here: The presumptive diagnosis is acute bacterial sinusitis, and they recommended a course of amoxicillin-clavulanate.

R. Sindwani, MD

Cost effectiveness of magnetic resonance imaging in the workup of the dysosmia patient

Decker JR, Meen EK, Kern RC, et al (Northwestern Univ, Chicago, IL)
Int Forum Allergy Rhinol 3:56-61, 2013

Background.—Intracranial causes of dysosmia are uncommon. Nonetheless, a missed intracranial disorder or neoplasm is worrisome. Magnetic resonance imaging (MRI) may be used in diagnosis; however, the cost effectiveness of this practice is unclear. We hypothesize that MRI scans for idiopathic dysosmia will demonstrate sufficient significant findings to be a cost-effective screening tool.

Methods.—Tertiary-care otolaryngology clinic records were queried for smell and taste disturbance. The patients underwent anosmia-protocol MRI of the brain for idiopathic dysosmia in 122 cases. Each MRI report was reviewed for dysosmia findings, intracranial neoplasms, and incidental findings.

Results.—MRI was normal in 44.3%, there were dysosmia-related findings in 25.4%, and incidental findings in 40.2%. The most common related diagnosis was occult frontoethmoid sinusitis (18.8%). The most common incidental diagnosis was small vessel disease (21.1%). Intracranial neoplasms were observed in 6 patients (4.9%). Nine patients had intracranial causes of dysosmia including olfactory meningiomas, infarct, trauma, and atrophy. MRI cost per dysosmia etiology diagnosis was $9445. Costs increased to $32,355 and $48,880 per intracranial cause or neoplasm, respectively. Cost to diagnose 1 causal intracranial neoplasm was $146,400. From 1997 to 2003, median medical malpractice settlements ranged from $625,616 for misdiagnosis to $682,500 for delay in treatment to $1,750,000 for brain injury. The median jury award was $975,000 for misdiagnosis, $1,550,000 for delayed treatment, and $6,000,000 for brain injury.

Conclusion.—MRI in idiopathic dysosmia yielded information regarding the diagnosis in one-quarter of cases. The implications of missing an intracranial neoplasm alone justify the cost of screening MRI for idiopathic dysosmia.

▶ As otolaryngologists, we are frequently asked to see patients with disturbances of smell and taste. After ruling out a sinonasal origin for the anosmia, some would advocate for an evaluation to exclude an intracranial etiology through imaging such as magnetic resonance imaging (MRI). The analysis of whether this is a sound practice, from a cost-effectiveness standpoint, is unresolved, and is the topic of this interesting article. Set in a tertiary-care setting, this study examined outcomes of 122 cases of idiopathic anosmia which were evaluated with MRI. Each MRI report was reviewed for dysosmia findings, intracranial neoplasms, and incidental findings. The study found that although the imaging was normal in 44%, there were dysosmia-related findings in a surprisingly high 25% of cases. The most common related diagnosis was occult frontoethmoid sinusitis (18.8%). Also noteworthy, intracranial neoplasms were observed in 5% of cases. The analysis showed that the cost to diagnose 1 causal intracranial neoplasm was $146 400. The authors present an interesting and thoughtful discussion arguing that the costs associated with missing an intracranial neoplasm justified ordering an MRI scan for cases of anosmia. For example, the median jury award was $975 000 for misdiagnosis and $1 550 000 for delayed treatment. Sobering numbers to say the least... The group concluded that a 5% incidence of intracranial lesion was too high to not evaluate for lesions routinely with MRI in the setting of idiopathic anosmia and recommended routine imaging in the workup of these patients. Based on their findings, I think these recommendations are sound, although I do think that a 5% risk seems high based on my own clinical practice. Having said this, I do routinely get MRIs for patients with idiopathic anosmia and think it is a justifiable expense, and in the rare setting in which a lesion is found, you and your patient will be happy that you did it. Further studies looking at the incidence of intracranial neoplasia in this population (eg, from other centers, different types of practices) would be beneficial.

R. Sindwani, MD

Exploring the Clinical Value and Implications of Routine Pathological Examination of Septoplasty Specimens

Haffey T, Pabon S, Hawley K, et al (Cleveland Clinic Foundation, OH; Case Western Reserve Univ School of Medicine, Cleveland, OH)
Laryngoscope 122:2373-2377, 2012

Objectives/Hypothesis.—During septoplasty, otherwise normal cartilage and bone are removed and routinely submitted for pathologic examination. According to the College of American Pathologists, however, the examination of bone and cartilage from septoplasty and rhinoplasty may be left to the pathologist's discretion. We explored the processing of tissues removed during septoplasty, examining the clinical value and implications of current practices.

Study Design.—Retrospective chart review.

Methods.—Our database was searched for septoplasty (CPT code 30520) procedures performed specifically for the indication of nasal obstruction.

Results.—Five hundred sixteen consecutive cases from 15 surgeons spanning a 2-year period were identified. In the majority of cases, septal tissues removed during surgery were submitted to pathology. The majority of cases (>90%) involved septoplasty performed in conjunction with another procedure, most commonly addressing the inferior turbinates. All septal specimens received gross examination by a pathologist, and a smaller fraction were also examined histologically. Gross findings included the qualitative appearance of the specimen and dimensional measurements of bone and cartilage fragments. No abnormalities were identified (by gross or histologic examination) in any of the specimens. Associated costs included specimen handling, storage, and pathology fees.

Conclusions.—In our health care system, it is common practice to submit tissues removed during septoplasty for pathologic examination. This study demonstrates that routine evaluation of septal tissues following surgery for obstruction has no clinical value whatsoever, and is associated with direct and indirect costs. Given the current health care climate, this practice should be further scrutinized and reconsidered.

▶ We live and practice in a very cost-conscious era in which quality and efficiency of health care delivery are at the forefront. This study examines the clinical value and implications of routine pathologic examination of septoplasty specimens removed during surgery for nasal obstruction. The probing question here is simple: Is there any clinical utility in examining the misshapen but otherwise normal cartilage and bone removed during septoplasty? According to the College of American Pathologists, the examination of bone and cartilage from septoplasty and rhinoplasty may be left to the pathologist's discretion. More than 500 consecutive cases from 15 surgeons spanning a 2-year period were analyzed. In most cases, septal tissues removed during surgery were submitted to pathology. Most cases (> 90%) involved septoplasty performed in conjunction with another procedure. All septal specimens received gross examination by a pathologist, and a smaller fraction were also examined histologically. No abnormalities were identified (by gross or histologic examination) in any of the specimens. A financial analysis found that associated costs included specimen handling, storage, and pathology fees, and, depending on the carriers, not sending septoplasty specimens was determined to have a minimal impact on reimbursement (likely financially net positive). This study nicely establishes that routine evaluation of septal tissues after surgery for obstruction has no clinical utility whatsoever, does not improve patient care, and is associated with direct and indirect costs. They recommend that this practice be reconsidered but advised surgeons to engage their pathology departments and hospital administration to seek clarification and consensus before altering current practices.

R. Sindwani, MD

EPOS 2012: European position paper on rhinosinusitis and nasal polyps 2012. A summary for otorhinolaryngologists

Fokkens WJ, Lund VJ, Mullol J, et al (Academic Med Ctr, Amsterdam, the Netherlands; Nose and Ear Hosp, London, UK; Hosp Clinic – IDIBAPS, Barcelona, Catalonia, Spain; et al)

Rhinology 50:1-12, 2012

The European Position Paper on Rhinosinusitis and Nasal Polyps 2012 is the update of similar evidence based position papers published in 2005 and 2007.

The document contains chapters on definitions and classification, we now also propose definitions for 'difficult to treat' rhinosinusitis, control of disease and better definitions for rhinosinusitis in children. More emphasis is placed on the diagnosis and treatment of acute rhinosinusitis. Throughout the document the terms chronic rhinosinusitis without nasal polyps (CRSsNP) and chronic rhinosinusitis with nasal polyps (CRSwNP) are used to further point out differences in pathophysiology and treatment of these two entities.

There are extensive chapters on epidemiology and predisposing factors, inflammatory mechanisms, (differential) diagnosis of facial pain, genetics, cystic fibrosis, aspirin exacerbated respiratory disease, immunodeficiencies, allergic fungal rhinosinusitis and the relationship between the upper and lower airways. The chapters on paediatric acute and chronic rhinosinusitis are totally rewritten.

Last but not least all available evidence for management of acute rhinosinusitis and chronic rhinosinusitis with or without nasal polyps in adults and children is analyzed and presented and management schemes based on the evidence are proposed. This executive summary for otorhinolaryngologists focuses on the most important changes and issues for otorhinolaryngologists.

The full document can be downloaded for free on the website of this journal: http://www.rhinologyjournal.com.

▶ An excellent summary of the available evidence on the diagnosis and management of rhinosinusitis and nasal polyps is the recently published European Position Paper on Rhinosinusitis and Nasal Polyps. This is a 2012 update of a similar document published last in 2007. The article does a good job of distilling diagnostic criteria, care pathways, and management options based on evidence available. (The summary for otolaryngologists is a shorter, to-the-point version.) In addition to routine classification and diagnostic schemes, this group also worked to define difficult to treat patients. Management algorithms for chronic rhinosinusitis without nasal polyps (CRSsNP), chronic rhinosinusitis with nasal polyps, and pediatric chronic rhinosinusitis (CRS) are discussed in the article (see Figs 1 and 2 in the original article). This executive summary for otorhinolaryngologists focuses on the most important changes and issues for otorhinolaryngologists in the management of CRS patients. A significant change from the prior 2007 guidelines is the categorization of patients with CRSsNP. In 2007, patients were categorized solely on symptoms, but now it is recommended that the endoscopic examination findings contribute to categorization as well. In moderate/severe disease, signs of mucosal disease at endoscopy are also required. The most important change in the management of adults with CRS without nasal polyps is the changed place of long-term antibiotics. This is based on some recent conflicting data on the impact of long-term macrolide use. The level of evidence for macrolides in all patients with CRSsNP is Ib, and strength of recommendation is now only a C based on 2 double-blind, placebo-controlled studies (of approximately the same size) that were contradictory: One showed a benefit and the other did not. It appears that there may be better efficacy in using long-term macrolides in CRSsNP in patients with normal immunoglobulin E (IgE) specifically, but perhaps not for those with elevated IgE. This executive summary is a focused and quick read that is useful in reviewing the current key issues and recommendations for the management of CRS.

R. Sindwani, MD

'Conchae bullosis': a rare case with bilateral triple turbinate pneumatisations

Ozturan O, Yenigun A, Degirmenci N, et al (Bezmiâlem Vakif Univ, Istanbul, Turkey)

J Laryngol Otol 127:73-75, 2013

Background.—Concha bullosa is the pneumatisation of intranasal conchae (usually the middle turbinate, and rarely the inferior or superior turbinate); however, the term is generally used to describe aeration of the

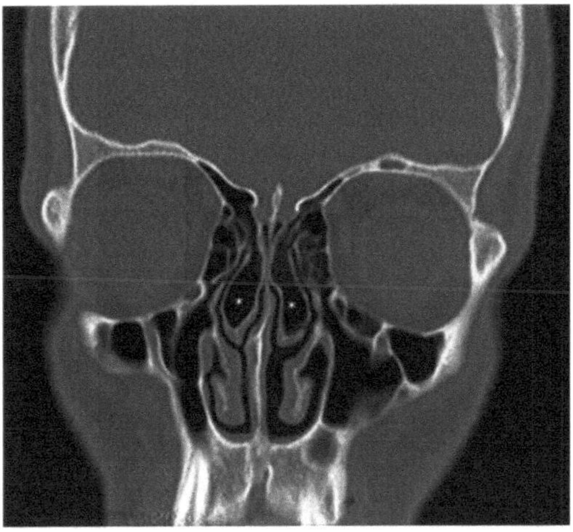

FIGURE 1.—Coronal computed tomography section showing bilateral, expansive middle turbinate pneumatisation. (Reprinted from Ozturan O, Yenigun A, Degirmenci N, et al. 'Conchae bullosis': a rare case with bilateral triple turbinate pneumatisations. *J Laryngol Otol.* 2013;127:73-75, with permission of Cambridge University Press.)

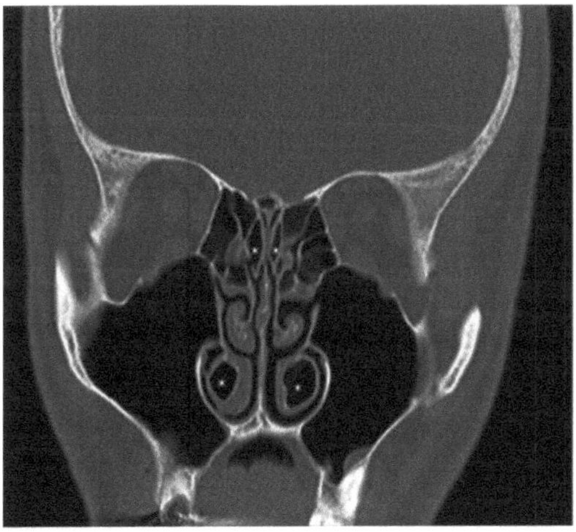

FIGURE 2.—Coronal computed tomography section showing bilateral superior and inferior turbinate pneumatisation. (Reprinted from Ozturan O, Yenigun A, Degirmenci N, et al. 'Conchae bullosis': a rare case with bilateral triple turbinate pneumatisations. *J Laryngol Otol.* 2013;127:73-75, with permission of Cambridge University Press.)

middle concha. Superior concha bullosa is a rare finding, and only a few cases of inferior concha bullosa have been reported in the medical literature. When symptomatic, concha bullosa may cause various problems including nasal congestion, headache, postnasal drip, anosmia and, sometimes, epiphora.

Methodology.—Computed tomography, following history-taking and physical examination, is a valuable tool in diagnosing turbinate pneumatisation. This article presents a very rare case with bilateral triple conchae pneumatisations.

Results.—The symptomatology, diagnosis and treatment options for cases of multiple concha bullosa are discussed. The surgical interventions performed in the presented case are briefly described.

Conclusion.—The presented patient had pneumatisation of all six turbinates. In such cases, we propose that this condition be termed 'conchae bullosis' rather than 'conchae bullosa', in a similar fashion to the use of nasal polyposis as the plural form of nasal polyp (Figs 1 and 2).

▶ This is a rare case report of conchae bullosis or pneumatization of all 6 of the patients' turbinates (conchae). The authors present the case of a 23-year-old man with continuous nasal congestion, nasal drip, and intermittent facial pain of 10 years' duration. The images of the computed tomography (CT) scan show significant pneumatization in all 6 turbinates (inferior, middle, and superior). It is also relevant that there is little (if any) associated mucosal disease present in any of the images and the conchae are also noted to be fully aerated (without air fluid levels, mucosal thickening, or opacification). The patient was taken to surgery and the lateral aspects of the middle and inferior conchae were resected (nothing was done to the superior conchae). According to the report, there were no complications and the patient's symptoms resolved, with the duration of follow-up not provided. I found the CT findings and the considerations discussed for surgical resection of pneumatized turbinates (in a general context) in this article meritorious, but I do have some reservations about the indications for surgery in the patient presented. The authors do make the statement that "when symptomatic, concha bullosa may cause various problems..." but provide no references for this and do not elaborate on how one determines that the concha(e) is/are responsible for a patient's symptoms. Can pneumatizations in and of themselves (in the absence of mucosal disease) cause the symptoms cited? Further, I take issue with the reference to any concha bullosa (or multiples thereof) as a condition, as is done throughout the article. So, although I do agree with the nomenclature proposed of conchae bullosis for this observation, I would like to remind readers that there are a plethora of different pneumatization patterns possible in the sinonasal tract—this case of conchae bullosis being merely one such example—and that in the absence of associated mucosal or sinus disease they represent variations of normal anatomy and do not require any management whatsoever. Perhaps the only exception to this may be the symptom of nasal obstruction, I suppose. I encourage readers to look at this interesting CT scan and see if you agree with the procedures performed.

R. Sindwani, MD

Etiology of Nasal Polyps in Cystic Fibrosis: Not a Unimodal Disease

Steinke JW, Payne SC, Chen PG, et al (Univ of Virginia Health Systems, Charlottesville)

Ann Otol Rhinol Laryngol 121:579-586, 2012

Objectives.—The objective was to determine whether the polyp subtypes observed in cystic fibrosis (CF)—related sinusitis were similar to those observed in non—CF-related sinusitis.

Methods.—Polyp and mucus samples were collected from CF patients who presented for sinus surgery. The polyps underwent histologic and cytochemical evaluation for the presence of lymphocyte cell populations and their respective cytokine markers. The mucus samples were evaluated for DNA content.

Results.—Of the polyps, 42% had an eosinophilic infiltrate, of which 80% had an additional mixed neutrophilic infiltrate. Of the remaining polyp samples, 42% did not have a granulocytic infiltrate, consistent with non-eosinophilic polyps. All samples had CD138-positive plasma cells. The mucus samples from the patients with CF showed higher extracellular DNA concentrations than did the mucus samples from patients with non-CF sinus disease.

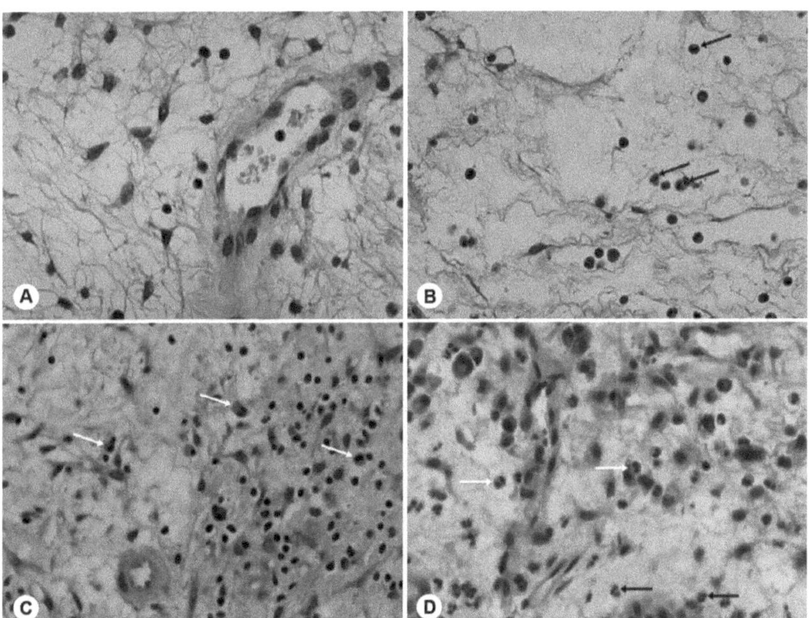

FIGURE 1.—Hematoxylin-eosin (H&E) staining of cystic fibrosis (CF) polyps. Arrows indicate relevant cell types. **A**) Paucigranulocytic nasal polyp (NP; original ×200). **B**) Polymorphonuclear cell (PMN) infiltration without eosinophils (original ×200). **C**) Eosinophilic infiltration without PMNs (original ×200). **D**) Both eosinophils PMNs within same field (original ×400). (Reprinted from Steinke JW, Payne SC, Chen PG, et al. Etiology of nasal polyps in cystic fibrosis: not a unimodal disease. *Ann Otol Rhinol Laryngol.* 2012;121:579-586, © 2012, Annals Publishing Company.)

Conclusions.—Cystic fibrosis–related polyps demonstrated an eosinophil-based dichotomy similar to that of idiopathic non–CF-related polyps. Many also demonstrated neutrophilic infiltrate, indicating that chronic mucus stasis and infection complicate the disease. Agents capable of reducing extracellular DNA may help manage sinusitis in CF patients (Fig 1).

► There are different types of nasal polyp subtypes based on histopathologic assessment. This article evaluated whether the polyp subtypes observed in cystic fibrosis (CF)-related sinusitis were similar to those observed in non-CF-related sinusitis. Polyp and mucus samples were examined. Of the polyps, 42% had an eosinophilic infiltrate, of which 80% had an additional mixed neutrophilic infiltrate. Of the remaining polyp samples, 42% did not have a granulocytic infiltrate, consistent with noneosinophilic polyps. The CF mucus samples showed higher extracellular DNA concentrations than did the mucus samples from patients with non-CF sinus disease. The authors demonstrated that CF-related polyps were similar to idiopathic polyps in that they showed an eosinophil-based dichotomy. Many also demonstrated neutrophilic infiltrate, however, which was different and unique to CF (Fig 1). It was suggested that this may support that chronic mucus stasis and infection complicate CF, and that targeting this issue should be part of the overall treatment strategy in these patients. This study shows some very interesting findings of polyps in CF when compared with those in patients without this condition.

R. Sindwani, MD

Multi-Institutional Evaluation of a Sinus Surgery Checklist

Soler ZM, Poetker DA, Rudmik L, et al (Med Univ of South Carolina, Charleston; Med College of Wisconsin, Milwaukee; Univ of Calgary, Alberta, Canada; et al)

Laryngoscope 122:2132-2136, 2012

Objectives/Hypothesis.—To examine the frequency of safe surgical practices specific to endoscopic sinus surgery (ESS) before and after implementation of a checklist at four institutions across North America.

Study Design.—Prospective, multi-institutional, observational study.

Methods.—Consecutive surgeries were observed at four institutions before (n = 100) and after (n = 100) implementation of the ESS Checklist. A passive observer documented whether 10 specific tasks were performed by the surgical team during the course of each case. The frequency with which each item was performed was tabulated, and differences across institutions were evaluated using the Pearson χ^2 test. Improvement in the frequency of each single item between pre- and postintervention time periods was assessed by the McNemar χ^2 test.

Results.—Successful performance of all 10 tasks in the prechecklist period was not observed for any ESS case at any of the four study sites.

Step 1: Preparation [Surgeon(s) Only] Timing: Prior to Intubation

* Lead Surgeon Reviews (Assisting Surgeon(s) Confirm)

- ☐ Correct CT/MRI displayed in room (patient, date, sidedness)
- ☐ Image guidance in room, proper scan uploaded, correct views available (if necessary for case)
- ☐ Important anatomic variations identified and discussed among surgical team (skull base erosion, dehiscent lamina papyracea, Onodi cell, etc)

Step 2: Pause/Time-Out [Full Operative Team] Timing: Prior to Instrumentation

Review/Confirm Roles Vary by Institution

- ☐ Complete standardized surgical checklist
  -WHO-equivalent (site, procedure, antibiotics, etc)
  -Exact organization expected to vary by institution

* Surgeon Reviews (Anesthesia, Nursing, and Tech Teams Confirm)

- ☐ Topical epinephrine/cocaine/oxymetazoline stained and labeled appropriately
- ☐ Injectable anesthetic labeled and left unstained
- ☐ Suction cautery/bipolar immediately available in room
- ☐ Hemostatic materials immediately available in room
- ☐ Method of specimen collection (sidedness, microdebrider trap, fresh/formalin)

Step 3: Completion [Surgeon, Nursing, Tech] Timing: Prior to Extubation

* Surgeon Reviews (Nursing and Tech Teams Confirm)

- ☐ Pledget count correct
- ☐ Documentation of materials left in situ (stents, spacers, packing)
- ☐ Specimen properly collected, labeled, and sent to pathology

FIGURE 1.—The Endoscopic Sinus Surgery Checklist. ESS, endoscopic sinus surgery; CT = computed tomography; MRI = magnetic resonance imaging; WHO = World Health Organization. Image reproduced from: Soler ZM, Smith TL. Endoscopic sinus surgery checklist. *Laryngoscope* 2012;122:137–139. (Reprinted from Soler ZM, Poetker DA, Rudmik L, et al. Multi-institutional evaluation of a sinus surgery checklist. *Laryngoscope*. 2012;122:2132-2136, with permission from Laryngoscope and John Wiley and Sons, www.interscience.wiley.com.)

As might be expected, performance of any individual task was highly variable, ranging from 14% to 95%. After implementation of the ESS Checklist, successful performance of all 10 tasks during an individual surgery increased from 0% to 87% across all institutions, a change that was highly significant ($P < .001$). Significant increases in the performance of individual tasks was observed for nine of 10 items across all institutions ($P \leq .031$ for all).

Conclusions.—Significant heterogeneity exists with regard to performance of specific tasks aimed at minimizing error during ESS. Utilization of the ESS Checklist standardized practice across four institutions and significantly increased the likelihood that individual safety tasks were performed during the course of sinus surgery (Fig 1).

▶ It is well established that complications from sinus surgery, although rare, can be devastating. It is also true that otolaryngology lawsuits happen most commonly for cases involving endoscopic sinus surgery (ESS). There is great attention to doing whatever possible to reduce the number of errors during surgical procedures. There has been significant emphasis in the quality and safety arena to using checklists to standardize protocols and minimize errors. This also would be expected to result in an improvement in quality and outcomes, as it would minimize variations in practice. This study evaluated the frequency of safe surgical practices specific to ESS before and after implementation of a checklist (Fig 1) at several institutions. A passive observer audited whether 10 specific tasks were performed by the surgical team during the course of each case. The study found that successful performance of all 10 tasks in the prechecklist period was not observed for any ESS case at any of the 4 study sites, but after implementation of the ESS Checklist, successful performance of all 10 tasks during an individual surgery increased significantly. The group concluded that significant heterogeneity exists with regard to performance of specific safety-related tasks and that utilization of the ESS Checklist could standardize practice across institutions and significantly increased the likelihood that individual safety tasks are performed by the surgery team. The authors discuss how several specific practices have been advocated to help minimize errors that might occur during ESS, including correct display of radiographic imaging, identification of anatomic abnormalities, and proper labeling and staining of topical vasoconstrictors. These specific surgical practices are typically adopted by surgeons as means of minimizing error based on their prior training and personal experience. The adoption and use of an ESS Checklist served to standardize practice across institutions and led to significant increases in the performance of nearly every task. There has been an explosion in the use of medical checklists in all aspects of patient care (borrowed from the airline industry), a trend that establishes that the use of checklists does standardize procedures and minimize errors. The ESS Checklist appears to accomplish these 2 very important goals for sinus surgery. I am certain that we will hear a great deal more about checklists, safety, and quality metrics in the future.

R. Sindwani, MD

Efficacy and safety of the "mother's kiss" technique: A systematic review of case reports and case series

Cook S, Burton M, Glasziou P (Buxted Med Centre, UK; Oxford Univ Hosps Natl Health Service Trust, UK; Bond Univ, Gold Coast, Queensland, Australia)
CMAJ 184:E904-E912, 2012

Background.—Foreign bodies lodged in the nasal cavity are a common problem in children, and their removal can be challenging. The published studies relating to the "mother's kiss" all take the form of case reports and case series. We sought to assess the efficacy and safety of this technique.

Methods.—We performed a comprehensive search of the Cochrane library, MEDLINE, CINAHL, Embase, AMED Complementary and Allied Medicine and the British Nursing Index for relevant articles. We restricted the results to only those studies involving humans. In addition, we checked the references of relevant studies to identify further possibly relevant studies. We also checked current controlled trials registers and the World Health Organization search portal. Our primary outcome measures were the successful extraction of the foreign object from the nasal cavity and any reported adverse effects. We assessed the included studies for factors that might predict the chance of success of the technique. We assessed the validity of each study using the Newcastle–Ottawa scale.

TABLE 3.—Overall Rates of Success for the Mother's Kiss Technique in the 8 Included Studies

Study	Success Rate, % (*n*/*N*)	Type of Object: Smooth, Regular	Type of Object: Irregular
Case series			
Botma et al.[1]	79 (15/19)	5/7 (beads, buttons, pebbles)	10/12 (vegetable matter, sponge, tissue paper, magnet)
Purohit et al.[12*]	65 (20/31)	13/17	7/13
Backlin[13]	100 (8/8)	2/2 (beads)	6/6 (sunflower seed, plastic doll's shoe, Styrofoam chip, plastic toy piece, popcorn kernel, crayon piece)
Wagner[14]	100 (2/2)		2/2 (piece of wiener sausage, small stone)
Taylor et al. [15]	49 (41/84)	Not specified	Not specified
Alleemudder et al. [16]	63 (5/8)	0/2 (plastic beads)	5/6 (toy part, sponge, eraser, pea, rubber tire, raisin)
Case reports			
Hore[17]	100 (1/1)	1/1(small polystyrene bead)	
Manca[18]	100 (1/1)	1/1 (white scented bead)	

Editor's Note: Please refer to original journal article for full references.
*Discrepancy between number of patients and number of objects removed appears in original study by Purohit et al. Attempts to contact the authors of the original study for clarification were unsuccessful.

Results.—Eight relevant published articles met our inclusion criteria. The overall success rate for all of the case series was 59.9% (91/152). No adverse effects were reported.

Interpretation.—Evidence from case reports and case series suggests that the mother's kiss technique is a useful and safe first-line option for the removal of foreign bodies from the nasal cavities of children (Table 3).

▶ Admittedly, I had no idea what the "mother's kiss" technique was or what it was used for before I read this article from a Canadian journal (and I'm even Canadian). To be honest, the catchy title of the technique is what drew my attention to the article. So as it turns out, the "mother's kiss" was first described in 1965 and is used to remove a foreign body from a child's nose. The mother, or other trusted adult, places her mouth over the child's open mouth, forming a firm seal as if about to perform mouth-to-mouth resuscitation. While occluding the unaffected nostril with a finger, the adult then blows until they feel the resistance caused by closure of the child's glottis, at which point the adult gives a sharp exhalation to deliver a short puff of air into the child's mouth. This puff of air passes through the nasopharynx, out through the unoccluded nostril, and, if successful, results in the expulsion of the foreign body. Pretty clever, given how challenging and distress-causing removing foreign bodies can be. Of course, the adult is coached on what to do at the start of the procedure and the child is told the adult is going to give them a "big kiss" to keep them as calm as possible. The procedure can be repeated a number of times if not initially successful. This article reviewed the literature on the efficacy and safety of this technique. Eight relevant published articles were included, yielding an overall success rate of 60% (91/152). No adverse effects were reported. Although a review of only case reports and series', the study found that the mother's kiss appears to be a safe and effective technique for first-line treatment in the removal of a variety of nasal foreign bodies (Table 3). In addition, the authors noted that it may prevent the need for general anesthesia in some cases. Further studies are needed to compare different positive-pressure techniques and to test their efficacy in specific situations. A very interesting technique.

R. Sindwani, MD

Aerodynamic Investigation of the Correlation Between Nasal Septal Deviation and Chronic Rhinosinusitis

Li L, Han D, Zhang L, et al (Capital Med Univ, Beijing; et al)
Laryngoscope 122:1915-1919, 2012

Objectives/Hypothesis.—To compare the aerodynamic differences around ostiomeatal complex between the convex side and concave side in patients with concurrent nasal septal deviation and chronic rhinosinusitis, and to explore the potential correlation between nasal septal deviation and chronic rhinosinusitis occurrence from the perspective aerodynamics.

Study Design.—Retrospective case series.

Methods.—Fifty-six patients with concurrent nasal septal deviation and chronic rhinosinusitis were recruited. Nasal septal deviation was divided into mild, moderate, and severe deviations according to deviation angle. Using computational fluid dynamics, indices such as maximal velocity, maximal turbulence kinetic energy, maximal wall shear stress, and minimal temperature around the ostiomeatal complex were calculated and compared between the convex side and concave side, and among patients with varying severities of deflection.

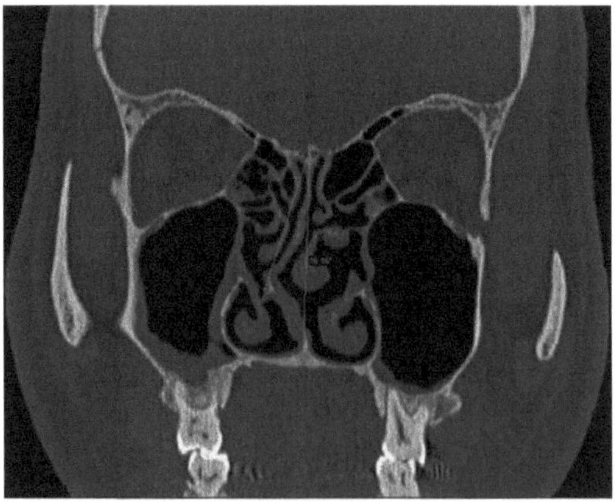

FIGURE 1.—Measurement of deviation angle. [Color figure can be viewed in the online issue, which is available at wileyonlinelibrary.com.] (Reprinted from Li L, Han D, Zhang L, et al. Aerodynamic investigation of the correlation between nasal septal deviation and Chronic rhinosinusitis. *Laryngoscope*. 2012;122:1915-1919, with permission from Laryngoscope and John Wiley and Sons, www.interscience.wiley.com.)

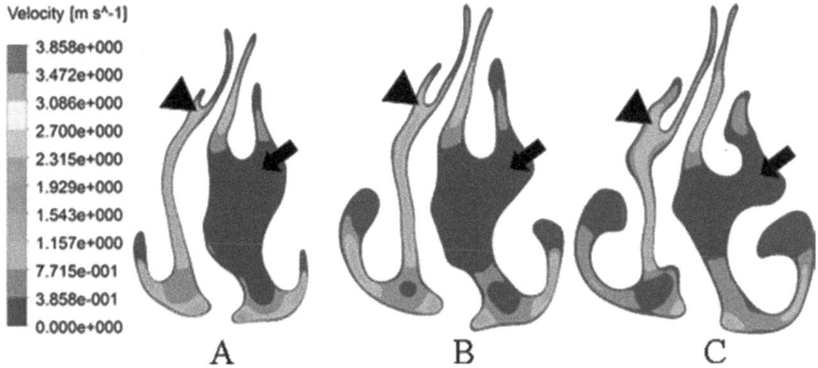

FIGURE 2.—Velocity contour of three consecutive coronal planes around the ostiomeatal complex (OMC). The arrows point to the lower velocity around the OMC in the concave side. The triangles point to the higher velocity around the OMC in the convex side. [Color figure can be viewed in the online issue, which is available at wileyonlinelibrary.com.] (Reprinted from Li L, Han D, Zhang L, et al. Aerodynamic investigation of the correlation between nasal septal deviation and Chronic rhinosinusitis. *Laryngoscope.* 2012;122:1915-1919, with permission from Laryngoscope and John Wiley and Sons, www.interscience.wiley.com.)

Results.—The proportion for mild, moderate, and severe deviations was 12.5%, 32.1%, and 55.4%, respectively. Significant differences for maximal velocity, maximal wall shear stress, maximal turbulence kinetic energy, and minimal temperature around the ostiomeatal complex between the convex side and concave side could be detected. No significant difference of aerodynamic characteristics around the osteomeatal complex could be detected with the increasing of deviation angles. The incidence for chronic rhinosinusitis in convex, concave, and bilateral sides was 16.1%, 25%, and 58.9%, respectively.

Conclusions.—From the aerodynamics perspective, both sides of nasal cavity have the potential to predispose the occurrence of chronic rhinosinusitis in patients with nasal septal deviation. The increased deviation angle did not aggravate aerodynamic disturbance around the osteomeatal complex. The contributing role of nasal septal deviation in the pathogenesis of chronic rhinosinusitis should not be emphasized in excess (Figs 1 and 2).

▶ The role of the nasal septal deviation (NSD) in chronic rhinosinusitis (CRS) has been questioned for some time. Although it is thought to have only a small contributing role on CRS occurrence according to some recent literature, the mechanism related to the impact of NSD on the pathogenesis of CRS has not yet been validated by objective avenues. Aerodynamics were hypothesized to constitute one of the mechanisms relating to the occurrence of CRS in NSD patients. This article, although a bit technical at times, is a very fascinating read. The purpose of the study was to compare the aerodynamic differences around the ostiomeatal complex (OMC) between the convex side and concave side in patients with concurrent NSD and CRS, to investigate the impact of septum deviation with varying deflection severities on aerodynamic characteristics around OMC, and ultimately to explore the potential correlation between

NSD and CRS occurrence from the aerodynamics perspective. It looks at 56 patients with concurrent NSD and CRS and analyses the degree of septal deviation (according to deviation angle, Fig 1) and also uses computational fluid dynamics (indices such as maximal velocity, maximal turbulence kinetic energy, maximal wall shear stress, and minimal temperature) to compare the impact of the deviation on both sides of the nose. Most patients had severe deviations (55%). No significant difference of aerodynamic characteristics around the ostiomeatal complex could be detected with the increase of deviation angles (Fig 2). The study concluded that at least from an aerodynamics perspective, both sides of the nasal cavity have the potential to predispose the occurrence of CRS in patients with NSD. The increased deviation angle did not aggravate aerodynamic disturbance around the ostiomeatal complex, as has been hypothesized in the past, and it appears that a NSD is not a major contributing factor to the occurrence of CRS.

R. Sindwani, MD

Low-Frequency Ultrasound for Biofilm Disruption in Chronic Rhinosinusitis With Nasal Polyposis: In Vitro Pilot Study

Karosi T, Sziklai I, Csomor P (Univ of Debrecen, Hungary)

Laryngoscope 123:17-23, 2013

Objectives/Hypothesis.—Microbial biofilms have been implicated in the pathogenesis of chronic rhinosinusitis with nasal polyposis (CRSwNP). Although biofilms are characterized by an extremely high resistance against chemical and physical agents, low-frequency ultrasound (LFU) treatment has been suspected to be an efficient and safe method for biofilm disruption.

Study Design.—Basic science experimental study.

Methods.—A total of 10 patients with CRSwNP undergoing endoscopic sinus surgery were analyzed. Two series of identical nasal polyps (n = 20) were processed to hematoxylin-eosin (HE) and Gram staining and to continuous-wave LFU treatment (5 minutes, 0.4 MHz, 37°C), respectively.

Results.—Presence of microbial biofilms was confirmed in all patients with CRSwNP. HE staining showed a strong correlation with the results of Gram protocol in biofilm detection. In the LFU-treated group (n = 10), a significantly decreased inflammatory cell count was found in the subepithelial layer of nasal polyps ($P < .001$). In addition, bacterial biofilms were completely removed from the surface of the epithelial layer. Microscopic tissue injuries or significant temperature changes were not detected due to LFU treatment.

Conclusions.—Between in vitro conditions, LFU treatment appeared to be a reliable and microscopically safe method for the disruption of microbial biofilms in CRSwNP. These results may provide a basis for a prospective human study investigating the efficacy and safety of this therapeutic

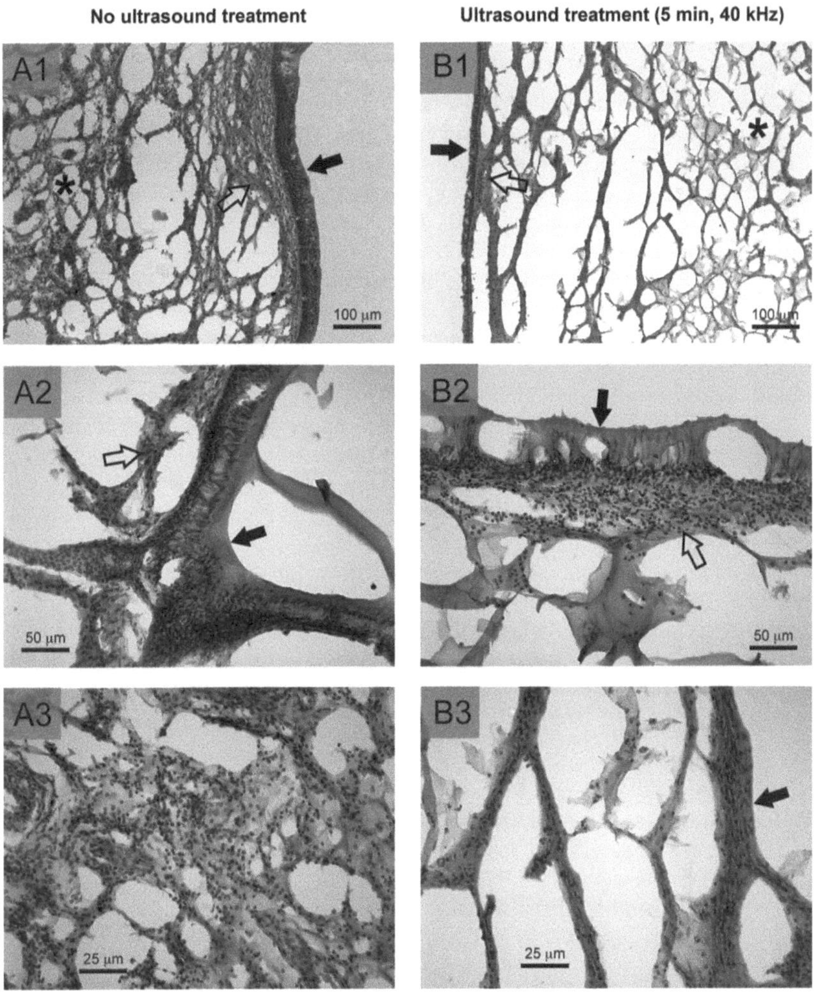

FIGURE 1.—Microphotographs of nasal polyps stained by hematoxylin-eosin before and after low-frequency ultrasound treatment. (A1) At low magnification, a columnar epithelium with eosinophilic polysaccharide layer can be detected (black arrow). The submucosal layer is marked by a white arrow, whereas the black asterisk indicates the stromal layer with massive infiltration of inflammatory cells. (A2) Microbial biofilm is displayed as a dense, eosinophilic structure on the surface of epithelial layer (black arrow). The white arrow shows the submucosa. (A3) Stromal substance of the nasal polyp is heavily infiltrated by eosinophil and neutrophil granulocytes and also by plasmocytes. (B1) At low magnification, a columnar epithelium without biofilm-like structures can be detected (black arrow). The submucosal layer is marked by a white arrow, whereas black asterisk indicates the hypocellular stromal layer. (B2) The respiratory epithelium shows intact architecture without any signs for superficial biofilm presence (black arrow). The white arrow shows the intact submucosal layer. (B3) The stromal layer represents as a hypocellular structure with sporadic inflammatory cells and intact connective tissue web. (Reprinted from Karosi T, Sziklai I, Csomor P. Low-frequency ultrasound for biofilm disruption in chronic rhinosinusitis with nasal polyposis: in vitro pilot study. *Laryngoscope*. 2013;123:17-23, with permission from Laryngoscope and John Wiley and Sons, www.interscience.wiley.com.)

modality alone or in combination with antibiotics or topical steroids in biofilm-positive cases of CRSwNP (Fig 1).

▶ The concerns over the role of biofilms in chronic rhinosinusitis (CRS) continue to abound. As another option to target biofilms in CRS, some novel work has suggested that continuous or pulsed-wave low-frequency ultrasound (LFU) treatment is a reliable and safe method for biofilm removal. This preliminary study investigates the effectiveness and microscopic findings of low-frequency, continuous-wave ultrasound treatment in biofilm disruption in CRS with nasal polyposis (CRSwNP) in vitro. The study examined specimens from 10 patients (20 specimens) with CRSwNP undergoing endoscopic sinus surgery and subjected them to LFU in vitro. Specimens were processed and treated with continuous-wave LFU treatment (5 minutes, 0.4 MHz, 37°C). In the LFU-treated group ($n = 10$), a significantly decreased inflammatory cell count was found in the subepithelial layer of nasal polyps. In addition, bacterial biofilms were completely removed from the surface of the epithelial layer (Fig 1). In this in vitro experiment, LFU treatment appeared to disrupt microbial biofilms in CRSwNP. The authors postulated that ultrasound-induced movement, intravascular microstreaming, and the escape effect of leukocytes at the surgical resection surface of nasal polyps might be responsible for the histological findings observed. The experiments demonstrated the presence of biofilms in all patients; unfortunately, there was no control group and only a small number of subjects were included. Nevertheless, this is a very promising study and the use of this technology to combat biofilms deserves further inquiry.

R. Sindwani, MD

Topical therapies in the management of chronic rhinosinusitis: an evidence-based review with recommendations

Rudmik L, Hoy M, Schlosser RJ, et al (Univ of Calgary, Alberta, Canada; Med Univ of South Carolina, Charleston; et al)

Int Forum Allergy Rhinol 2012 [Epub ahead of print]

Background.—Topical therapies have become an integral component in the management plan for chronic rhinosinusitis (CRS). Several topical therapy strategies have been evaluated, but a formal comprehensive evaluation of the evidence has never been performed. The purpose of this article is to provide an evidence-based approach for the utilization of topical therapies in the management of CRS.

Methods.—A systematic review of the literature was performed and the guidelines for development of an evidence-based review with recommendations were followed. Study inclusion criteria were: adult population > 18 - years old; chronic rhinosinusitis (CRS) based on published diagnostic criteria; and clearly defined primary clinical end-point. We focused on reporting higher-quality studies (level 2b or higher), but reported on lower-level studies if the topic contained insufficient evidence. We excluded drug-eluting spacer and stent therapy from this review.

TABLE 5.—Estimated Topical Sinonasal Medication Costs

Medication	Unit	Estimated Market Cost Per Unit ($)	Estimated Per Day Cost ($)
Neilmed saline sinus rinse bottle	1 box with 50 salt packages	11.99	0.24
Mometasone furoate (Nasonex)	17-g bottle	134.40	4.48
Fluticasone propionate (generic)	16-g bottle	18.31	0.61
Fluticasone propionate (Flonase)	16-g bottle	92.31	3.08
Fluticasone furoate (Veramyst)	10-g bottle	114.82	3.83
Budesonide (Rhinocort)	9-g bottle	121.58	4.05
Ciclesonide (Omnaris)	12.5-g bottle	42.00	1.40
Beclomethasone dipropionate monohydrate	25-g bottle	144.00	4.80
Flunisolide (Nasalide)	25-mL bottle	65.22	2.17
Triamcinolone acetonide (Generic)	17-g bottle	81.91	2.73
Triamcinolone acetonide (Nasocort)	17-g bottle	124.51	4.15
Budesonide respule (0.5 mg/2 mL)	1 respule	4.19	4.19
Budesonide respule (1 mg/2 mL)	1 respule	4.97	4.97
Prednisolone 1% drop	15-mL bottle	42.14	2.81
Ciprofloxacin-dexamethasone (0.3/0.1%) drop	8-mL bottle	157.93	10.51
Dexamethasone 0.1% drop	15-mL bottle	78.07	5.20
Mupirocin 2% ointment	22-g tube	18.62	2.66
Nebulized tobramycin	5 mL	7.64	7.64

Results.—This review identified and evaluated the literature on 5 topical therapy strategies for CRS: saline irrigation, topical steroid, topical antibiotic, topical antifungal, and topical alternatives (surfactant, manuka honey, and xylitol irrigations).

Conclusion.—Based on the available evidence, sinonasal saline irrigation and standard topical nasal steroid therapy are *recommended* in the topical treatment of CRS. Nonstandard (off-label) topical sinonasal steroid therapies can be an option for managing CRS. The evidence *recommends against* the use of topical antifungal therapy and topical antibiotic therapy delivered using nebulized and spray techniques in routine cases of CRS. There is insufficient clinical research to provide recommendations for alternative therapies or topical antibiotic therapy delivered using other delivery methods (eg, irrigations) (Table 5).

▶ As we are all well aware, neither surgery nor medical therapy can cure chronic rhinosinusitis (CRS). Even after surgical intervention, delivering drugs effectively to the site of infection/inflammation remains a worthwhile goal. A major advantage of endoscopic sinus surgery (ESS) is creating an open and accessible cavity, which has been demonstrated to optimize sinonasal penetration of topical drug therapy. Because the majority of patients will require ongoing medical therapy to control infection and/or inflammation after ESS, the creation of an open sinus cavity has become a critical component to improve topical drug delivery and provide sustained symptom control. Over the past few years, there has been a proliferation of medications and means (eg, nebulization, irrigations, gelatinous vehicles) used to deliver these medications directly into the nose and sinuses. This review, with practice recommendations, aims to identify topical medical therapy strategies and promote an evidence-based approach to their use. This is a very well-organized analysis of 5 topical strategies: saline irrigation, topical steroid, topical antibiotic, topical antifungal, and some emerging topical alternatives. It summarizes available knowledge on these therapies according to the headings: aggregate evidence, benefit, harm, cost benefit-harm assessment, value judgment, and recommendation level, which I found easy to read and informative. Another very interesting perspective provided by the article is the cost per day of using these therapies, summarized in Table 5. Based on the best available evidence, the management of CRS would include sinonasal saline irrigation and standard topical nasal steroid therapy. Also, the authors suggested that there is an option for the use of nonstandard (off-label), high-concentration topical sinonasal steroid therapy as well. The evidence suggests that topical sinonasal antibiotic therapy delivered using either a nebulized or spray technique fails to provide clinical benefit, and when combined with a preponderance for harm, the group recommended against its use in routine cases of CRS. There also was strong evidence to recommend against the use of topical antifungal therapy in the management of CRS. No recommendations for or against topical surfactant (baby shampoo), Manuka honey, or xylitol irrigations were possible because of a lack of research on these agents. We are definitely going to see more about topical drug delivery for CRS—stay tuned.

R. Sindwani, MD

Mapping the Frontal Sinus Ostia Using Virtual Endoscopy

Dearking AC, Pallanch JF (Mayo Clinic, Rochester, MN)

Laryngoscope 122:2143-2147, 2012

Objectives/Hypothesis.—To determine the relative location of the frontal sinus opening to other frontal cells using virtual endoscopy; and to assess whether the relative location of the frontal sinus ostium can be predicted.

Study Design.—Retrospective analysis of high-resolution computed tomography scans from 50 adult patients without frontal sinus disease or previous sinus surgery.

Methods.—Using virtual endoscopy software, 100 frontal recesses were mapped for the presence and relative position of the frontal sinus ostium to the following cells: agger nasi (ANC); frontal bullar; frontal types 1, 2, and 3; supraorbital ethmoid; suprabullar; and intersinus septal cells.

Results.—ANC and frontal type 3 cells were present in 92% and 45% of frontal recesses, respectively. All other cell types had a prevalence of ≤ 25%. Fifty percent of recesses had two rows of ostia anterior to posterior (AP), and the frontal opening was anterior in 52%. When there were three rows of cells AP (39%), the frontal opening was in the center in 64% of cases. Thirty-five percent of recesses had two rows of ostia medial to lateral (ML), and the frontal opening was medial 80% of the time. When there

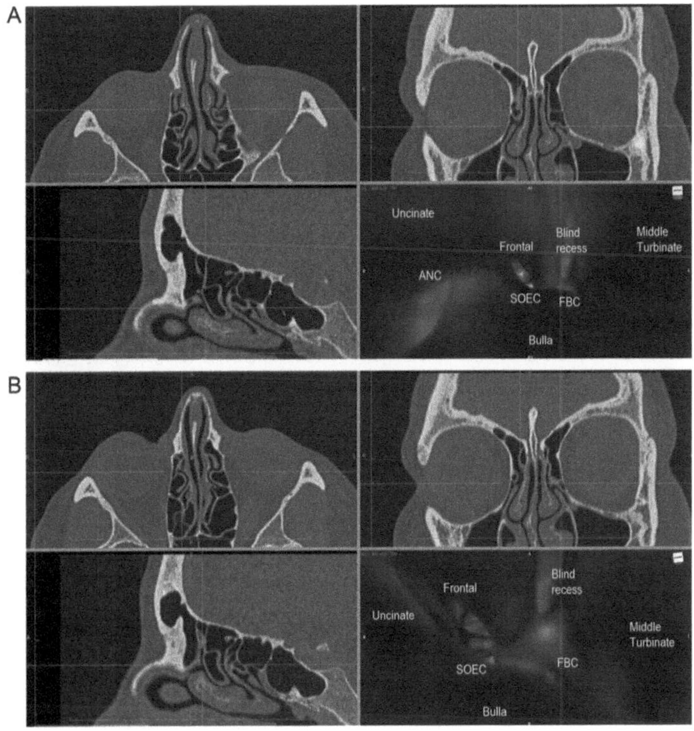

FIGURE.—Example of a right side frontal recess map with triplanar computed tomography (CT) views and the corresponding virtual endoscopy view. (A) This was the standard starting location used for creating each frontal recess map. The starting position was the trifurcation where the uncinate, the ethmoid bulla, and the middle turbinate are all visualized on both triplanar CT and virtual endoscopy. Upper left: axial CT image; upper right: coronal CT image; lower left: sagittal CT image; lower right: virtual endoscopy image. The uncinate, ethmoid bulla, and middle turbinate are labeled on the virtual endoscopy image, as well as the five openings in this frontal recess. (B) Magnified view of the same right side frontal recess map as in A. The opening to the frontal sinus is anterior to the supraorbital ethmoidal cell (SOEC), anterior and lateral to the frontal bullar cell (FBC), and lateral to the blind recess. ANC = agger nasi cell. (Reprinted from Dearking AC, Pallanch JF. Mapping the frontal sinus ostia using virtual endoscopy. *Laryngoscope*. 2012;122:2143-2147, with permission from Laryngoscope and John Wiley and Sons, www.interscience.wiley.com.)

were three rows of openings ML (45%), the frontal opening was in the center 56% of the time.

Conclusions.—The frontal sinus recess is variable and complex. Virtual endoscopy can be used to analyze the frontal recess and assist in presurgical planning. Although there is variability in the ostial configuration present in the frontal recess, the probable position of the frontal sinus ostium can be predicted (Fig).

► This study looks at the varied anatomy of the frontal sinus drainage pathway using virtual endoscopy and assessed whether the relative location of the frontal sinus ostium can be predicted. Fifty adult computed tomography scans were evaluated with virtual endoscopy software, and 100 frontal recesses were mapped for the presence and relative position of the frontal sinus ostium to a variety of cells. Agger nasi and frontal type 3 cells were present in 92% and 45% of frontal recesses, respectively, whereas all of the other cells were significantly less common (≤25%). Because of the immense variability, a simple methodology of finding the frontal sinus outflow tract could not be consistently identified. The authors concluded that the frontal sinus recess is variable and complex and suggest virtual endoscopy can be used to analyze the frontal recess and assist in presurgical planning. These types of analyses are useful in establishing incidence of various anatomic cells and improving understanding of surgical anatomy of trainees and surgeons and may indeed augment surgical planning. The challenge, however, remains reliably translating this information to real-time decision making that a surgeon has to perform in the operating room.

R. Sindwani, MD

Evaluation of Adult Pott's Puffy Tumor: Our Five Cases and 27 Literature Cases

Akiyama K, Karaki M, Mori N (Kagawa Univ, Japan)
Laryngoscope 122:2382-2388, 2012

Objectives/Hypothesis.—Pott's puffy tumor (PPT) is defined as one or more subperiosteal abscesses of the frontal bone based on osteomyelitis. PPT is observed predominantly in the adolescent age group and rarely in adults. Some parameters affecting prognosis and an appropriate surgical approach for antecedent frontal sinusitis have not been elucidated due to the rarity of patients with adult PPT.

Study Design.—Retrospective patient record and literature study.

Methods.—Five patients from our cohort and 27 patients identified in a literature search formed the study group.

Results.—The incidence rate of intracranial complications was lower than in previous reports at 29.0%. There was no correlation between the incidence rate of intracranial complications and each patient's parameters. It was indicated that the department first consulted by the patients was possibly related to the initial diagnosis and the incidence rate of intracranial complications.

Conclusions.—Although the incidence rate of major complications is lower than in children and later than in earlier published adult cases, patients are still at high risk of serious intracranial complications. Early diagnosis and adequate treatment may contribute to reducing the incidence rate (Fig 2).

▶ Pott's puffy tumor (PPT) is defined as 1 or more subperiosteal abscesses of the frontal bone based on osteomyelitis, which is usually seen as a complication of frontal sinusitis or after head trauma in adolescents. It is a very rare complication resulting from the advent of antibiotic therapy, but it does still occur. This retrospective study analyzed 32 cases (5 patients and 27 cases identified in a literature search) and demonstrated an intracranial complication rate of 29%, which is

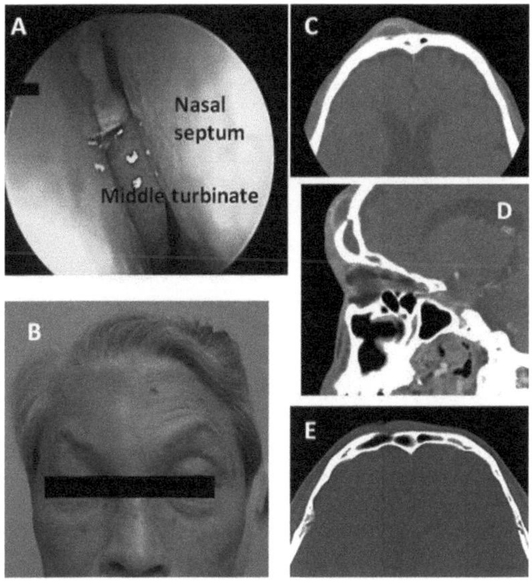

FIGURE 2.—(A) Right nasal cavity image of patient 30 showing pus arising from the middle meatus. (B) Preoperative photograph of patient 30 showing right forehead swelling and redness. (C, D) Preoperative axial and sagittal enhanced computed tomography (CT) of patient 30, revealing destruction of the anterior wall of the right frontal sinus and right forehead subperiosteal abscess. (E) Postoperative axial CT showing pneumatization of the bilateral frontal sinus and disappearance of puffy tumor. [Color figure can be viewed in the online issue, which is available at wileyonlinelibrary.com.] (Reprinted from Akiyama K, Karaki M, Mori N. Evaluation of adult pott's puffy tumor: our five cases and 27 literature cases. *Laryngoscope.* 2012;122:2382-2388, with permission from Laryngoscope and John Wiley and Sons, www.interscience.wiley.com.)

lower than previously noted. There were no identifiable risk factors for patients developing these major complications seen in the study. This study shows that the rate of intracranial complications is still significant with PPT, and early diagnosis and adequate treatment may contribute to reducing poor outcomes.

R. Sindwani, MD

Postraumatic frontal sinus obliteration with calvarial bone dust and demineralized bone matrix: a long term prospective study and literature review

Rodríguez IZ, Uceda MIF, Lobato RD, et al (12 de Octubre University Hospital, Madrid, Spain)

Int J Oral Maxillofac Surg 42:71-76, 2013

Defining the ideal material for frontal sinus obliteration remains controversial. Autogenous cancellous bone is effective because of its biological properties: it undergoes fast revascularization acting as an active scaffold for bone healing, but is linked to additional donor site morbidity. Bone dust harvesting from the skull surface produces no sequelae but availability

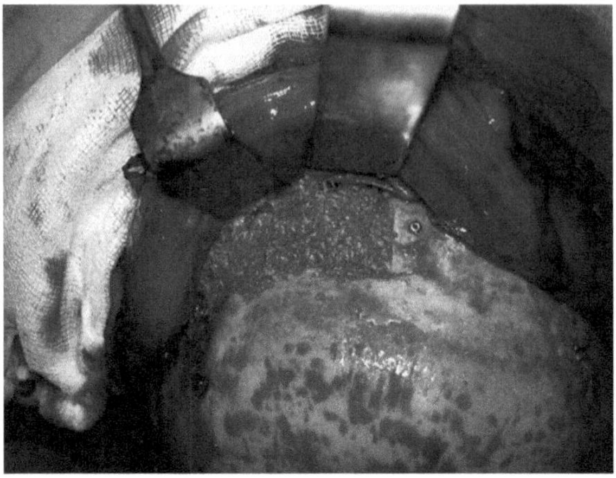

FIGURE 1.—Frontal sinus obliteration. (Reprinted from International Journal of Oral and Maxillofacial Surgery. Rodríguez IZ, Uceda MIF, Lobato RD, et al. Postraumatic frontal sinus obliteration with calvarial bone dust and demineralized bone matrix: a long term prospective study and literature review. *Int J Oral Maxillofac Surg*. 2013;42:71-76, Copyright 2013, with permission from the International Association of Oral and Maxillofacial Surgeons.)

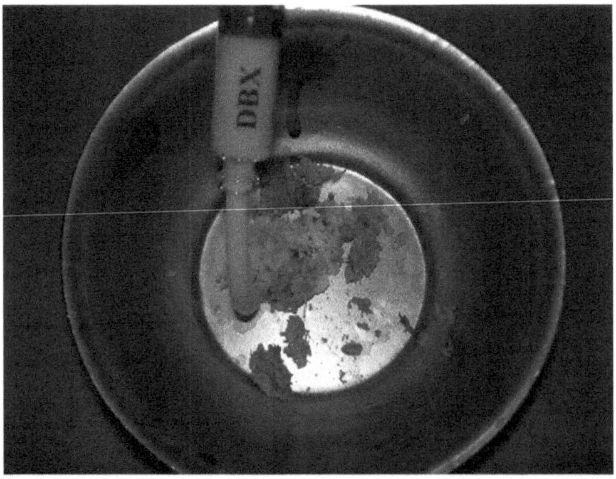

FIGURE 3.—Calvarial bone dust associated with DBX. (Reprinted from International Journal of Oral and Maxillofacial Surgery. Rodríguez IZ, Uceda MIF, Lobato RD, et al. Postraumatic frontal sinus obliteration with calvarial bone dust and demineralized bone matrix: a long term prospective study and literature review. *Int J Oral Maxillofac Surg*. 2013;42:71-76, Copyright 2013, with permission from the International Association of Oral and Maxillofacial Surgeons.)

is limited. Many efforts have been made to overcome these drawbacks, and an ideal bone substitute sought. Demineralized Bone Matrix (DBX; Musculoskeletal Transplant Foundation, Edison, NJ, USA) is a commercially available product composed of demineralized bone particles reduced after proper processing of human bone in combination with sodium hyaluronate. It generates an osteoconductive surface and it is also a source of

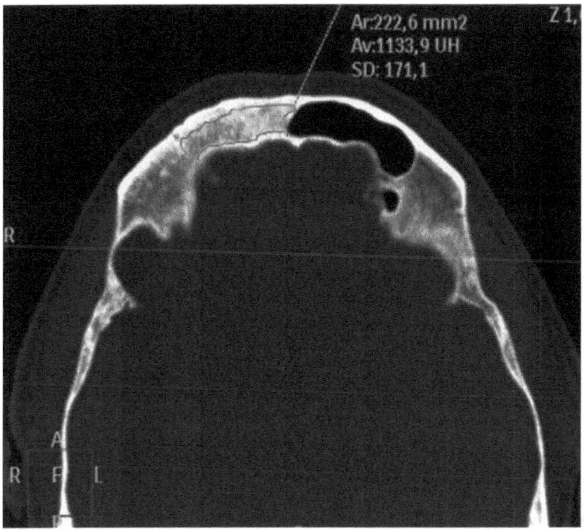

FIGURE 5.—Postobliteration frontal sinus with high bone density 24 months after surgery. (Reprinted from International Journal of Oral and Maxillofacial Surgery. Rodríguez IZ, Uceda MIF, Lobato RD, et al. Postraumatic frontal sinus obliteration with calvarial bone dust and demineralized bone matrix: a long term prospective study and literature review. *Int J Oral Maxillofac Surg*. 2013;42:71-76, Copyright 2013, with permission from the International Association of Oral and Maxillofacial Surgeons.)

osteoinductive factors. Radiological follow-up using computed tomography is a very reliable method of following-up ossification and detecting the early signs of possible complications. The authors present their clinical series of postraumatic frontal sinus obliteration using a mixture of calvarial bone dust and DBX shell, with long-term radiological monitoring. The technique was demonstrated to be effective, reliable, stable in the long term and associated with minimal morbidity (Figs 1, 3, and 5).

▶ During frontal sinus obliteration, the mucosa of the frontal sinus is meticulously removed, the outflow to the sinonasal tract below is abolished, and the cavity is obliterated. Over the years, several materials have been employed to obliterate the frontal sinus cavity, including different alloplastic materials, pedicled flaps, and, most commonly, fat. Each of these options has its drawbacks, and the ideal material for obliteration remains obscure. The authors suggest that obliterating with bone (or bone substitute) is ideal and report their experience with a demineralized bone matrix (DBX), a commercially available product made of demineralized cadaveric bone. They present their results with this technique in 18 patients with surgically treated frontal sinus fractures and a total of 30 sinus cavities obliterated with bone chips plus DBX (Figs 1 and 3) between 2005 and 2008. An average follow-up of 36 months was achieved. Computed tomography scans at 6 and 24 months postoperatively showed the presence of cortical bone in these patients (Fig 5), and the complication rate was low with no issues related to the material being used. Complete obliteration with sinus volume maintenance and new bone formation was seen in all cases. This is a good-sized series exhibiting an interesting technique (product) for obliteration. I do see the advantages of having the cavity filled with bone most importantly in the follow-up of these patients, which is much more easily interpreted radiographically than it would be for obliterations performed with soft-tissue materials (ie, fat). However, I would point out that complications such as mucocele takes years to develop, so a follow-up of 36 months (only 24 months radiographically) is not really "long term," as is suggested in the article. Having said this, short-term complications such as infection of the material used would be likely captured in this time frame, and I do think the authors have made a good case for the use of this material in frontal obliteration. It should be noted that there were no conflicts of interest disclosed by the authors for this commercially available product.

R. Sindwani, MD

Intranasal Hydrocodone-Acetaminophen Abuse Induced Necrosis of the Nasal Cavity And Pharynx

Alexander D, Alexander K, Valentino J (Univ of Kentucky College of Medicine, Lexington)

Laryngoscope 122:2378-2381, 2012

Objectives.—Two million new users will abuse prescription narcotics this year, most commonly hydrocodone. The most commonly prescribed form is hydrocodone-acetaminophen (HA). Many individuals crush the tablets and snort the product to take advantage of the rapid transmucosal delivery of narcotics. The resultant pathology of intranasal hydrocodone acetaminophen abuse (INHAA) has been described only in a few case studies.

Study Design.—Retrospective chart review.

Methods.—Two private and one academic otolaryngology practices in Kentucky searched their patient charts for patients with morbidity from

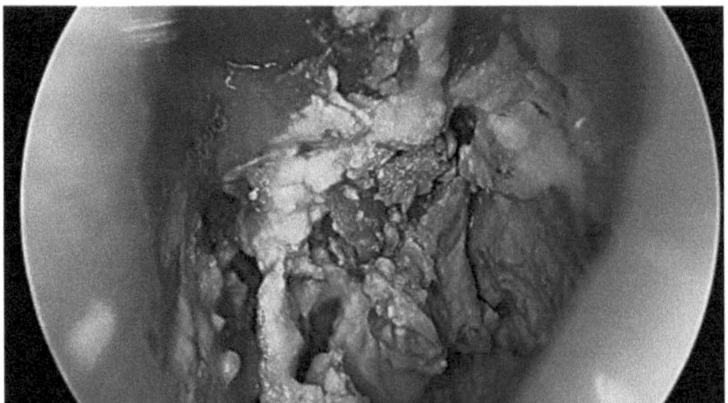

FIGURE 1.—Acute INHAA nasal manifestations of injury. The characteristic crusty, white exudate is noted overlying the necrotic and ulcerated mucosal surfaces. (Reprinted from Alexander D, Alexander K, Valentino J. Intranasal hydrocodone-acetaminophen abuse induced necrosis of the nasal cavity and pharynx. *Laryngoscope*. 2012;122:2378-2381, with permission from Laryngoscope and John Wiley and Sons, www.interscience.wiley.com.)

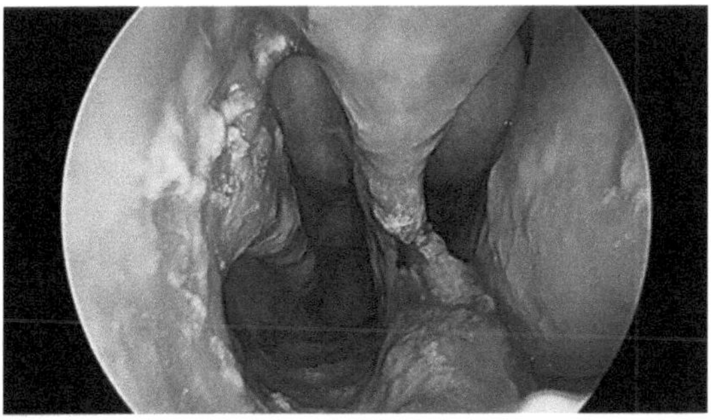

FIGURE 2.—Near total perforation of the nasal septum, post-debridement. This endoscopic photograph taken within a week of initial debridement and cessation of INHAA demonstrates healing of mucosa and clear cessation of the soft tissue destruction. (Reprinted from Alexander D, Alexander K, Valentino J. Intranasal hydrocodone-acetaminophen abuse induced necrosis of the nasal cavity and pharynx. *Laryngoscope*. 2012;122:2378-2381, with permission from Laryngoscope and John Wiley and Sons, www.interscience.wiley.com.)

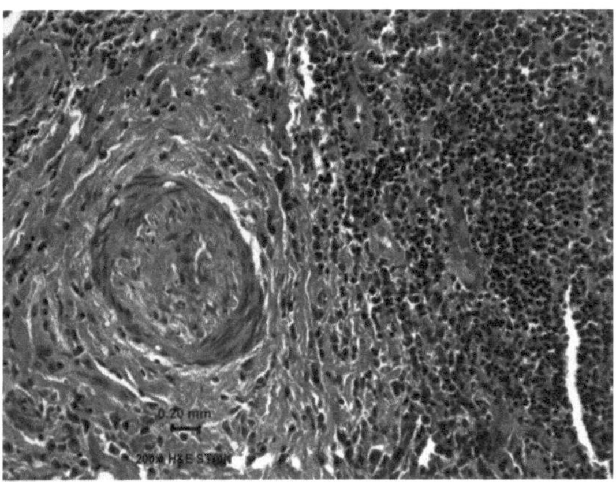

FIGURE 3.—Biopsy of involved nasal tissue. This high power magnified photomicrograph demonstrates extensive superficial exudates with underlying granulation tissue. The deep tissue on the septum shows extensive fibrous proliferation with a mixed chronic inflammatory cell infiltrate. There is no vasculitis present. There is intimal proliferation of some obliterative vasculopathy. There are scattered fragments of necrotic cartilage and focal osteonecrosis. (Reprinted from Alexander D, Alexander K, Valentino J. Intranasal hydrocodone-acetaminophen abuse induced necrosis of the nasal cavity and pharynx. *Laryngoscope*. 2012;122:2378-2381, with permission from Laryngoscope and John Wiley and Sons, www.interscience.wiley.com.)

intranasal abuse of hydrocodone acetaminophen tablets. We identified thirty-five patients who presented for treatment between 2004 and 2011.

Results.—The majority of patients will initially deny the behavior, frequently delaying diagnosis. Physical exam findings of white powder covering an underlying nasal mucosal necrosis are characteristic of this condition during active INHAA. Follow up was limited as only 26% returned for follow-up care. Patients commonly presented with orofacial-nasal pain (43%) andsino-nasal congestion and discharge (43%). Active necrosis or prior tissue loss was noted in 77% of patients. Fifty-one percent of patients presented with septal perforations, and 26% with palatal perforations. Two cases of invasive fungal sinusitis were clearly documented, with one resulting in death.

Conclusions.—The vast majority of cases presented with characteristic physical findings that included acute necrosis of soft tissue, which can progress to destroy oronasal structures. In the absence of invasive fungal disease, the condition is self-limited after cessation of INHAA and performance of local nasal debridement and nasal hygiene (Figs 1-3).

▶ Hydrocodone-acetaminophen (HA; Percocet) is one of the most commonly prescribed and widely abused medications. Many individuals crush the tablets and snort the product intranasally. This large series describes the dangers of this practice and presentation and management options. The first time one encounters this entity, it can be quite striking, invoking considerations of midline destructive processes and even invasive fungal sinusitis. This study analyzes 35 cases and reminds readers that the majority of patients will initially deny abusing the drug. Physical exam findings of white powder covering an underlying nasal mucosal necrosis are characteristic (Figs 1-3). Patients commonly presented with orofacial-nasal pain, congestion, and discharge. Necrosis and tissue loss is present in the majority, with many patients presenting with septal and even palatal perforations. Of great concern, 2 cases in this series of invasive fungal sinusitis were also identified. Management includes cessation of the abuse, ruling out the presence of invasive fungal disease (especially in the immunocompromised patient), nasal debridement, and nasal hygiene. In most cases, the effects were locally destructive but self-limiting. The article presents a nice discussion of possible mechanisms of how the damage occurs. Unlike the destructive properties of cocaine abuse, which are thought to be a result of its vasoconstrictive properties and causes local ischemic injury and inflammation, hydrocodone and acetaminophen lack these vasoconstrictive properties. The authors theorize that high concentrations and local hyperosmotic conditions could be responsible for the tissue necrosis seen. The clinician should consider this entity in a patient presenting with severe oronasal pain with crusty, white exudate overlying necrotic mucosa in the oronasal cavities.

R. Sindwani, MD

A 10-Year Review of Frontal Sinus Fractures: Clinical Outcomes of Conservative Management of Posterior Table Fractures

Choi M, Li Y, Shapiro SA, et al (McMaster Univ, Hamilton, Ontario, Canada; Indiana Univ, Indianapolis; Wishard Memorial Hosp, Indianapolis, IN)

Plast Reconstr Surg 130:399-406, 2012

Background.—Frontal sinus cranialization is commonly indicated for posterior table fractures with significant comminution, displacement, or cerebrospinal fluid leaks. This study assessed the clinical outcomes of conservative management.

TABLE 2.—Frontal Sinus Posterior Table Fracture Patterns and Features

Feature	Categorization	*n* (Incidence %)
Open/closed	Open	8 (14)
	Closed	51 (86)
Pattern	Noncomminuted, nondisplaced	32 (54)
	Comminuted and/or displaced	27 (46)
CSF leak	Present	11 (19)
	Absent	48 (81)
Management	ORIF and sinus preservation	7 (12)
	Obliteration	5 (8)
	Cranialization	1 (2)
	Nonoperative	46 (78)
Intracranial infections		1 (2)

CSF, cerebrospinal fluid; ORIF, open reduction and internal fixation.

Methods.—A 10-year retrospective review of all frontal sinus fractures treated at a level 1 trauma center was performed using medical records and radiographic images.

Results.—A total of 875 patients with frontal sinus fractures were identified, and 68 had posterior table involvement. Nine died within the first 48 hours from other injuries. The remaining 59 patients constituted the study population. Average follow-up approached 1 year (342 days). The more common mechanisms of injury were blunt interpersonal violence (29 percent) and motor vehicle accidents (27 percent). Concurrent central nervous system injury was common (73 percent), and the average Glasgow Coma Scale score was 12.7. Posterior wall fracture pattern was nondisplaced and noncomminuted in 33 patients (54 percent) and comminuted and/or displaced in 27 (46 percent). Cerebrospinal fluid leak was recorded in 11 patients (19 percent). Conservative management was the more common strategy (78 percent), followed by open reduction and internal fixation with sinus preservation (12 percent), obliteration (8 percent), and cranialization (2 percent). Of the 27 patients with comminuted and/or displaced fractures, 16 (59 percent) underwent conservative management, and 11 (41 percent) underwent surgical management, but only one patient (2 percent) underwent cranialization. There was no incidence of intracranial infection, except for one patient who died from encephalitis secondary to a gunshot wound to the head.

Conclusion.—The vast majority of frontal sinus fractures involving the posterior table, including those with comminution, displacement, or cerebrospinal fluid leaks, can be safely managed without cranialization.

Clinical Question/Level of Evidence.—Therapeutic, IV (Table 2).

▶ Frontal sinus cranialization is a fairly radical procedure in which the posterior table of the frontal sinus is resected and the frontal lobes are permitted to move anteriorly and occupy the dead space that once was the frontal sinus. It is performed through a craniotomy approach, and this has significant morbidity associated with it. The indications for this procedure include: significant posterior table comminution, displacement, or cerebrospinal fluid (CSF) leaks. This 10-year study retrospectively looked at clinical outcomes of conservative management in these situations at a level 1 trauma center. Although a total of 875 patients with frontal sinus fractures were identified, only 68 had posterior table involvement, with only 59 that had significant posterior table involvement. As expected, the leading causes of injury were blunt trauma and motor vehicle accidents. Posterior wall fracture pattern was nondisplaced and noncomminuted in 33 patients (54%) and comminuted and/or displaced in 27 (46%). CSF leak was recorded in 11 patients (19%) (Table 2). Conservative management was elected in the majority of these (almost 80%), followed by open reduction with internal fixation with sinus preservation (12%), obliteration (8%), and cranialization was selected in a very small number (2%). The authors demonstrated that the large majority of frontal sinus fractures involving the posterior table can be safely managed without cranialization. This was true even in significant comminution, displacement, and CSF leak. There indeed has been a trend in clinical practice to avoid cranialization over the past decade or so. Most of us have done far fewer cranializations of late and no longer use minimal displacement, minor comminution, or even CSF leak as a strict indication to cranialize. As the article supports, these patients tend to do well with conservative therapy or procedures other than cranialization. In addition to the associated morbidity of this procedure, long-term surveillance, an issue not addressed by this study (with only a year follow-up), can be very challenging in cranialized and even obliterated sinuses. Maintaining an aerated and functioning frontal sinus makes follow-up (endoscopically or radiographically) much easier.

R. Sindwani, MD

Outcomes

One Year after Endoscopic Sinus Surgery in Polyposis: Asthma, Olfaction, and Quality-of-Life Outcomes

Ehnhage A, for the NAFS Study Group (Karolinska Institutet, Stockholm, Sweden)

Otolaryngol Head Neck Surg 146:834-841, 2012

Objective.—Nasal polyposis is a disease known to be associated with asthma. The long-term effects of surgical treatment on lower airways have not been sufficiently studied.

Study Design.—One-year follow-up of a double-blind, randomized, placebo-controlled study.

Setting.—The study was conducted at the Karolinska University Hospital, Stockholm, Sweden.

Subjects and Methods.—Fifty-one patients, age 18 years or older, with nasal polyposis and asthma were evaluated 1 year after endoscopic sinus surgery (ESS). Outcomes included dyspnea/cough scores, mean daily peak expiratory flow rate, spirometry, butanol test, olfaction scores, peak nasal inspiratory flow, polyp scores, and health-related quality of life (SF-36).

Results.—The short-term postsurgery improvements in asthma symptom scores, daily peak expiratory flow rate, all nasal parameters including olfaction, and quality-of-life scores were generally maintained 1 year after ESS.

Conclusion.—Endoscopic sinus surgery had beneficial long-term effects on asthma, olfaction, and quality of life in patients with nasal polyposis. This is the first study to show long-term benefits of ESS on butanol tests in patients with nasal polyposis.

▶ Goals for the management of nasal polyposis include removing the polyps, opening the nasal airway, improving smell, minimizing risk of polyp recurrence, and improving a patient's overall quality of life (QOL). It is well known that polyps are associated with asthma, and there is a lack of understanding of the long-term outcomes of endoscopic sinus surgery (ESS). This article reports a 1-year follow-up of a double-blind, randomized, placebo-controlled study in 51 Swedish patients with nasal polyposis and asthma who underwent ESS. A variety of nasal, QOL, and lower airway (asthma) outcomes were analyzed. This prospective follow-up study of nasal polyposis and concomitant asthma patients establishes that ESS can have long-term benefits on lower airways, upper airways, and QOL. This offers direct support for the popular "one airway, one disease" hypothesis.

R. Sindwani, MD

Olfactory Function in Patients With Postinfectious and Posttraumatic Smell Disorders Before and After Treatment With Vitamin A: A Double-Blind, Placebo-Controlled, Randomized Clinical Trial

Reden J, Lill K, Zahnert T, et al (Univ of Dresden Med School, Germany)

Laryngoscope 122:1906-1909, 2012

Objectives/Hypothesis.—In this study we investigated the effectiveness of vitamin A in postinfectious and posttraumatic smell disorders. A possible effect of vitamin A is likely due to the stimulation of regeneration and repair of the peripheral olfactory system.

Study Design.—Double-blind, randomized, placebo-controlled clinical trial.

Methods.—A total of 52 patients (age range, 20–70 years; mean age, 52 years) participated, 26 of whom received placebo (7 male, 19 female) and another 26 verum (8 male, 18 female). A standardized history was obtained in each patient. Olfactory function was measured by means of the Sniffin' Sticks test kit, a validated technique to investigate odor thresholds, odor discrimination, and odor identification. Vitamin A was prescribed at a dose of 10,000 IU per day for 3 months. Follow-up testing was performed on average 5 months after the first investigation.

Results.—Forty-four percent of all patients reported recovery of their sense of smell; 29% of the participants exhibited significant improvement in measured olfactory function. However, there was no significant difference between the outcome of patients receiving verum or placebo.

Conclusions.—The systemic application of vitamin A at a dose of 10,000 IU per day for 3 months does not appear to be useful in the treatment of postinfectious or posttraumatic olfactory loss.

▶ Loss of smell is a very disturbing symptom that has a major impact on quality of life and implications on a patient's ability to react in potentially dangerous situations. Common causes include viral infections or upper respiratory tract infections, chemical reference substances, and head injuries. Up until now, only a few controlled studies have been performed on possible treatment options for these patients. A growing body of literature has suggested that vitamin A improves peripheral olfactory fiber regeneration and may be of benefit. This very well performed double-blind, randomized, placebo-controlled trial looked at the effects of vitamin A in postinfectious and posttraumatic smell disorders. Fifty-two patients were enrolled. Olfactory function was measured by means of the Sniffin' Sticks test kit. Half of the patients received placebo while the other half received 10 000 IU per day for 3 months of vitamin A. Follow-up testing was performed for an average of 5 months. Results showed that 44% of all patients reported recovery of their sense of smell, and 29% of the participants exhibited significant improvement in smell testing. However, there was no significant difference in the vitamin A treatment group compared with those receiving placebo. The group concluded that at the dose and duration of treatment used in the study, the systemic application of vitamin A was not useful in the treatment of postinfectious or posttraumatic olfactory loss. Interestingly, they did suggest that perhaps high concentration of direct topical application of vitamin A to the olfactory clefts, or possibly even higher systemic dosing regimens, might show some benefit. It is uncommon to see such a well-designed and executed clinical study in smell research. More work is required.

R. Sindwani, MD

Risk of stroke among patients with rhinosinusitis: A population-based study in Taiwan

Wu C-W, Chao P-Z, Hao W-R, et al (Taipei Med Univ, Taiwan; et al)

Am J Rhinol Allergy 26:278-282, 2012

Background.—Research has found evidence that chronic inflammation may promote atherosclerotic disease. The purpose of this study was to test the hypothesis that rhinosinusitis is a risk factor for stroke.

Methods.—This prospective cohort study comprised patients recorded on the Taiwan Longitudinal Health Insurance Database 2005 (LHID2005) who had received a diagnosis of rhinosinusitis (n = 53,653) between January 1, 2004 and December 31, 2005. A control group (1:4) drawn from the same database was matched for age and gender (n = 214,624). Each patient was followed up using data entered until the end of 2006. Cox proportional hazard regressions were performed to evaluate the hazard ratios (HRs) after adjusting for potential confounding factors.

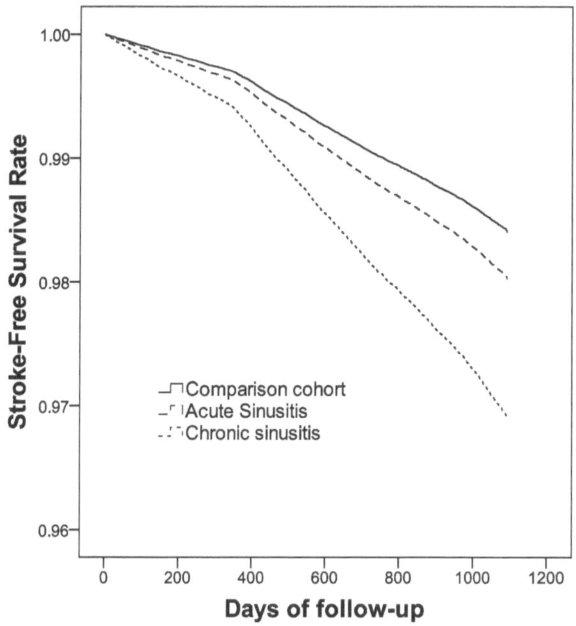

FIGURE 1.—A plot of stroke-free survival curves based on the Kaplan-Meier analysis for patients with acute and chronic sinusitis and the age- and gender-matched comparison cohort. (Courtesy of Wu C-W, Chao P-Z, Hao W-R, et al. Risk of stroke among patients with rhinosinusitis: a population-based study in Taiwan. *Am J Rhinol Allergy.* 2012;26:278-282, with permission from OceanSide Publications, Inc.)

Results.—We found that patients with rhinosinusitis were more likely to suffer strokes than the control population, after adjusting for potential confounders (adjusted HR, 1.39; 95% confidence interval [CI], 1.28–1.50). The HR of stroke was 1.39 (95% CI, 1.28–1.51) for acute sinusitis patients, and 1.34 (95% CI, 1.04–1.74) for chronic sinusitis patients.

Conclusion.—Both acute and chronic sinusitis are risk factors or markers for stroke that is independent of traditional stroke risk factors. Further research in this important area of epidemiology is warranted (Fig 1).

▶ This is a provocative study that looked at whether acute and chronic sinusitis are risk factors for stroke. In addition to the well-known risk factors of stroke, such as hypertension, diabetes, hyperlipidemia, smoking, obesity, and urbanization level, there is a theory that inflammation and chronic infection may also play an important role in strokes. A relationship between sinusitis and ischemic strokes has been suggested, and the anatomic proximity of the paranasal sinuses and internal carotid artery suggests that inflammation of the sinuses could easily extend to the intracranial vasculature. There is, of course, very little data on this. This population-based study examined the association between sinusitis and stroke in the Taiwanese using a government health care database. A prospective cohort of patients with the diagnosis of rhinosinusitis (n = 53 653) was matched with a control group drawn from the same database (n = 214 624). Their analysis showed that after adjusting for potential confounding factors, patients with rhinosinusitis were significantly more likely to suffer strokes than the control population. This was true for both acute and chronic sinusitis (Fig 1). This is the first large-scale study to show that acute and chronic sinusitis are risk factors for stroke. The exact relation between stroke and sinusitis is not fully understood. The article suggests that several possible mechanisms, including intracranial complications of sinusitis leading to ischemia and inflammation, contribute to atherosclerotic plaque formation. To be critical, there is not a lot of solid evidence for either of these putative mechanisms in the literature at the present time. And although there are significant shortcomings with this type of database-oriented, population-based study, the results are very interesting and warrant further study.

R. Sindwani, MD

Paranasal Sinus Exostoses: An Unusual Complication of Topical Drug Delivery Using Cold Nasal Irrigations

Haffey T, Woodard T, Sindwani R (Cleveland Clinic Foundation, OH)

Laryngoscope 122:1893-1897, 2012

Objectives/Hypothesis.—The use of topical drug delivery through nasal irrigations can minimize systemic side effects and deliver higher concentrations of drugs directly to diseased sinus mucosa. Complications related to this popular method of treatment are not well described. We present our experience with paranasal sinus exostosis (PSE), a new diagnostic entity that appears to be a complication of cold nasal irrigations.

Study Design.—Retrospective chart review.

Methods.—Retrospective chart reviews were performed on patients within the Cleveland Clinic Foundation from 2005 to 2011. Six patients were identified with sinus exostoses. A literature review for "sinonasal exostoses" and "paranasal sinus exostoses" was performed using PubMed.

Results.—Six patients with PSE were identified at the Cleveland Clinic Foundation between 2005 and 2011. All patients had undergone sinus surgery, and none had documented evidence of PSE prior to surgery. There was no evidence of worsening PSE once the cold irrigations were stopped. No patients showed any resolution of PSE over time. None of our patients has progressed to have disease burden significant enough to require intervention.

Conclusions.—PSE is a rare condition that mirrors a well-described otologic process; exostoses of the external auditory canal. PSE appears to be a complication of cold nasal irrigations. It does not resolve with the halting of cold irrigations, but does not appear to progress further after intervention. PSE only affects postoperative patients. With the evolving trend to treat postoperative sinus disease topically, the clinician should be aware of the

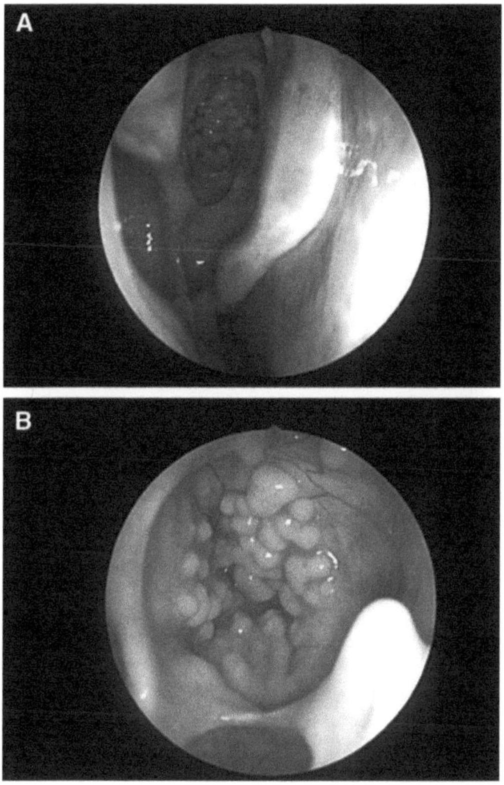

FIGURE 2.—(A) Endoscopic image showing paranasal sinus exostosis lesions along the right skull base. (B) Magnified image of right skull base lesions. (Reprinted from Haffey T, Woodard T, Sindwani R. Paranasal sinus exostoses: an unusual complication of topical drug delivery using cold nasal irrigations. *Laryngoscope*. 2012;122:1893-1897, with permission from Laryngoscope and John Wiley and Sons, www.interscience.wiley.com.)

dangers of cold irrigations, and patients should be counseled accordingly (Figs 2 and 3).

▶ There has been a growing trend toward the use of topical drug delivery directly to diseased sinus mucosa though techniques including nebulization, aerosolization, and nasal irrigation. The advantages of topical treatment are that systemic effects and complications of oral medications are avoided and a higher concentration of drug can be delivered directly to the site of infection or inflammation. Complications related to this popular method of treatment are not well described. This article characterizes a new clinical entity known as "paranasal sinus exostoses" (PSE), which appears to be a complication of cold nasal irrigations.

Six post-endoscopic sinus surgery patients admitted to using a variety of cold nasal irrigations, and the article describes relevant clinical, pathologic, and radiographic findings (Figs 2 and 3). There was no evidence of worsening PSE after the cold irrigations were stopped, and no patients showed any resolution of PSE

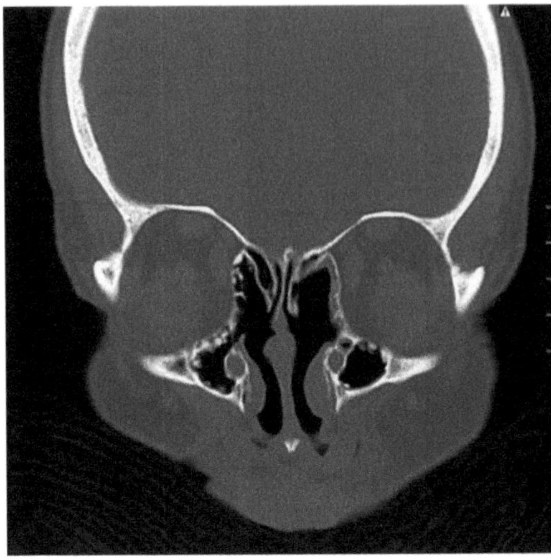

FIGURE 3.—Noncontrast coronal computed tomography in a postoperative patient showing exostoses along the lamina and luminal surfaces of the maxillary sinuses. (Reprinted from Haffey T, Woodard T, Sindwani R. Paranasal sinus exostoses: an unusual complication of topical drug delivery using cold nasal irrigations. *Laryngoscope*. 2012;122:1893-1897, with permission from Laryngoscope and John Wiley and Sons, www.interscience.wiley.com.)

over time. None of the lesions required surgery for management. The authors concluded that PSE is a rare condition that mirrors a well-described otologic process: exostoses of the external auditory canal. PSE appears to occur only in postoperative sinus cavities. With the evolving trend to treat postoperative sinonasal disease topically, clinicians should be educated about the need for refrigerated storage of many common topical medications so that they can educate their patients about the correct use and specific need to let the solutions warm to room temperature prior to use.

R. Sindwani, MD

Surgical Technique

Endoscopic Endonasal Resection of Anterior Skull Base Meningiomas

Padhye V, Naidoo Y, Alexander H, et al (The Queen Elizabeth Hosp, South Australia, Australia; Wellington Hosp, New Zealand; et al)

Otolaryngol Head Neck Surg 147:575-582, 2012

Objective.—Anterior cranial fossa (ACF) meningiomas are difficult to surgically manage. Endoscopic transnasal approaches have increasingly been used as a minimally invasive route and thus offer significant advantages. However, a paucity of literature describing the intraoperative challenges and postoperative outcomes of this technique still exists.

Study Design.—Case series with chart review.

Setting.—The Royal Adelaide Hospital, Flinders Medical Centre, Wellington Hospital.

Subjects and Methods.—Fifteen consecutive patients who underwent endoscopic resection of ACF meningiomas between 2004 and 2010 by the South Australian and Wellington Skull Base Units. Demographic and clinical information was compiled by reviewing patient charts and operation notes. Safety and efficacy of the procedure, role of a team approach, and areas for further improvement were analyzed.

Results.—Of the patients, 87% were women. Tumor locations: 8 olfactory groove, 2 tuberculum sellae, 1 clinoidal, 1 jugum sphenoidale, 1 planum sphenoidale, 1 subfrontal, and 1 midline ACF floor. Commonest presenting symptom was visual change. Mean volume of tumor was 25.69 cm^3, with a size area of 7.28 cm^2. Five were revision cases. None had previous endonasal surgery. Average operating times decreased over time. Gross total removal was achieved in 14, with no deaths. Four patients had postoperative cerebrospinal fluid (CSF) leak. Rate of CSF leak decreased over time. Sixty percent of patients reported visual improvement. Two patients had radiological evidence of recurrence.

Conclusion.—ACF meningiomas can be safely removed endonasally, offering significant advantages over the traditional transcranial approach for suitable tumors. Early audit of this approach shows results achieved by this unit are comparable with the published literature.

▶ The endoscopic techniques for skull base surgery have continued to evolve and proliferate. This study nicely describes the intraoperative challenges and postoperative outcomes of endoscopic resection of anterior cranial fossa (ACF) meningiomas. Compared with published series on extracranial approaches, the results of this study are comparable. This report also shows steady improvement in results (from 2004 to 2010) with increasing experience of the surgeons. There have been fewer complications, including cerebrospinal fluid (CSF) leaks, which improved from a rate of 25% in earlier years to less than 10% more recently. This is the second-largest series of ACF meningiomas resected endoscopically reported in the literature and nicely demonstrates that ACF meningiomas can be safely removed endonasally. It does, however, have some limitations. Longer operating times are required, and intraoperative bleeding may compromise the safety and completeness of the resection. Reconstruction also remains a challenge. Overall, this is a very well-written article that does an excellent job of highlighting the endoscopic approach used for meningioma resection. It also presents a very thoughtful discussion of some key issues in endoscopic skull base surgery, including techniques used to control the anterior ethmoidal artery and how the skull base may be best reconstructed to minimize CSF leak. The authors have been able to reduce their CSF leaks considerably by using multilayered reconstructions and the pedicled septal flap, which has become a true workhorse in endonasal skull base surgery. Criteria useful in patient selection for the endoscopic versus transcranial approach are also explored. This is definitely worth the read for those surgeons performing endoscopic skull base surgery.

R. Sindwani, MD

The Young's procedure for severe epistaxis from hereditary hemorrhagic telangiectasia

Richer SL, Geisthoff UW, Livada N, et al (St Vincent's Med Ctr, Bridgeport, CT; Hosps of the City of Cologne, Germany; et al)

Am J Rhinol Allergy 26:401-404, 2012

Background.—Surgical treatment of epistaxis in hereditary hemorrhagic telangiectasia (HHT) has historically been managed with the laser procedure or the septodermoplasty procedure. For transfusion-dependent patients with severe epistaxis we have been performing the Young's procedure or surgical closure of the nostrils. The objective of this study was to report treatment of severe epistaxis related to HHT with the Young's procedure and assess patient outcome.

Methods.—Patients with severe iron or blood transfusion–dependent epistaxis who underwent a Young's procedure in three otolaryngology HHT centers were reviewed. Patients were evaluated for postoperative epistaxis and subjective outcome.

Results.—Forty-three patients underwent a Young's procedure for severe epistaxis and were observed for a mean of 34 months. The procedure was well tolerated by all patients and 30 of 36 patients (83%) experienced complete cessation of bleeding after the Young's procedure. Patients had a mean increase in hemoglobin of 4.68 g/dL after the procedure. The average Glasgow Benefit Inventory score after surgery was 43.56. No patients requested a reversal of the procedure.

Conclusion.—The Young's procedure is a safe and efficacious procedure with complete cessation of epistaxis in most patients with severe epistaxis and HHT (Fig 1).

► Epistaxis is the most frequent symptom in hereditary hemorrhagic telangiectasia (HHT). Almost all surgical treatments of epistaxis in HHT are only temporizing measures and include laser coagulation or cautery or injection of Avastin or septodermoplasty. The Young's procedure, which is surgical closure of the nostril originally described in 1967, is another surgical alternative that offers the possibility of complete cessation of epistaxis. This is the largest report in the literature of Young's procedure in HHT: 43 patients from 3 HHT centers. This was done for very severe, transfusion-dependent epistaxis in patients with HHT. Most patients had experienced multiple procedures before electing surgical nostril closure that was generally performed bilaterally under general anesthesia (Fig 1). The procedure was well tolerated by all patients, and 83% experienced complete cessation of bleeding. Notably, no patients requested a reversal of the procedure. The study concluded that the Young's procedure is a safe and efficacious procedure that can offer complete cessation of bleeding in severe HHT epistaxis. This article is very intriguing as this procedure had somewhat fallen out of favor because of concerns over tolerability and impact on quality of life related to smell disturbance, hyponasal voice, and inability to breath through the nose. The article nicely presents the pros for this procedure, which are that it is reversible, not disfiguring, and appears to be generally well tolerated. The

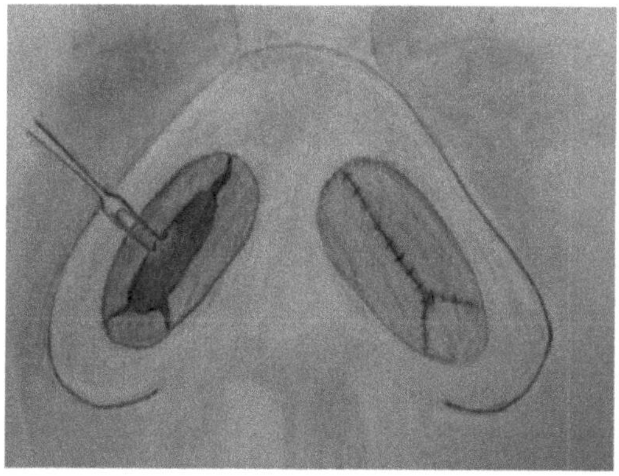

FIGURE 1.—In the Young's procedure, a circumferential incision is made at the mucocutaneous junction. Three radial flaps are raised to the alar rim and sutured with inverted mattress sutures to surgically close the nostril. (Reprinted from Richer SL, Geisthoff UW, Livada N, et al. The Young's procedure for severe epistaxis from hereditary hemorrhagic telangiectasia. *Am J Rhinol Allergy.* 2012;26:401-404, with permission from OceanSide Publications, Inc.)

study also shows quite dramatic results, and I agree that no other procedure or treatment (even though far less morbid) offers the chance for complete cessation of epistaxis or even lasting improvements for the most part. The Young's procedure appears to be a reemerging option for the most severe patients with HHT epistaxis. Results from other centers and surgeons with the Young's procedure would be beneficial.

R. Sindwani, MD

The Outside-In Approach to the Modified Endoscopic Lothrop Procedure

Chin D, Snidvongs K, Kalish L, et al (St Vincent's Hosp, Sydney, Australia; Macquarie Univ, Sydney, Australia; Univ of Sydney, Australia)

Laryngoscope 122:1661-1669, 2012

Objectives/Hypothesis.—Drilling in modified endoscopic Lothrop procedure (MELP) is traditionally described as commencing from the frontal recess (FR). This is challenging when the FR is involved by tumor, inflammatory disease, or scarring. The outside-in MELP, where the limits of the sinusotomy are first defined and the FR is addressed last, is described.

Study Design.—Case-control study.

Methods.—Patients undergoing MELP, using the standard or outside-in approach, for inflammatory disease or endoscopic skull base surgery were assessed. Data were collected on demographics, disease characteristics, and FR involvement. Operative time was calculated from intraoperative video recording. Time points recorded were times to frontal sinus and recess connected for outside-in MELP and completion of Lothrop cavity for both groups. Perioperative complications (infection, skin breach or contusion,

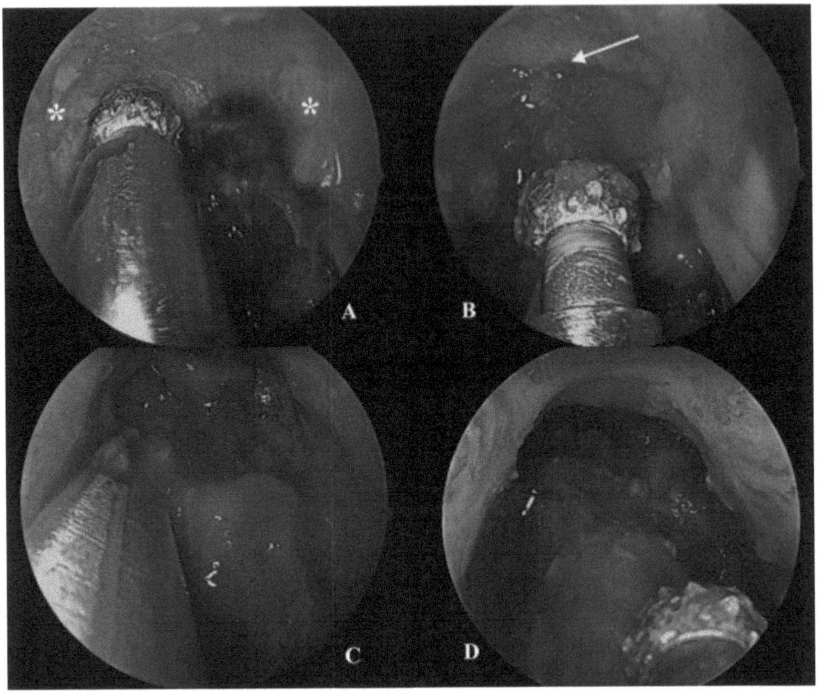

FIGURE 9.—Intraoperative pictures of a patient who had outside-in modified endoscopic Lothrop procedure for persistent nasal polyposis. (A) The frontal process of the maxilla has been drilled, and the periosteum (white asterisks) of the skin is identified on both sides. (B) The frontal sinus mucosa has just been visualized (white arrow), and subsequent drilling occurs between the periosteum bilaterally until the whole frontal sinus floor is removed before entering the mucosa. (C) The frontal recess is connected to the previously drilled Lothrop cavity with a 2-mm Kerrison rongeur. (D) The Lothrop cavity is completed. (Reprinted from Chin D, Snidvongs K, Kalish L, et al. The outside-in approach to the modified endoscopic lothrop procedure. *Laryngoscope*. 2012;122:1661-1669, with permission from Laryngoscope and John Wiley and Sons, www.interscience.wiley.com.)

surgical emphysema, orbital bleeding, cerebrospinal fluid leak, and intracranial complications) were recorded.

Results.—Thirty patients (67% female) with a mean age ± standard deviation of 56.0 ± 10.8 years underwent MELP (24 outside-in, six standard). Time for Lothrop completion was shorter for outside-in MELP (30.60 ± 14.10 minutes vs. 69.66 ± 64.52 minutes, $P = .002$). Among outside-in MELP, mean time to frontal sinus floor discovery was 8.41 ± 6.29 minutes, to recess connected 26.50 ± 12.45 minutes, and were similar regardless of pathology. The time for Lothrop cavity completion was shorter for tumor cases (24.63 ± 6.49 minutes) than for chronic rhinosinusitis without polyps (35.87 ± 20.18 minutes) and chronic rhinosinusitis with polyps (34.62 ± 11.56 minutes) ($P = .05$). One patient had skin edema. No other complications were recorded.

Conclusions.—The outside-in MELP is technically feasible and safe. Its advantage is a wide approach to the frontal sinus with development of the Lothrop cavity en route resulting in short predictable operative times.

TABLE 1.—Surgical Steps and Tips for the Outside-In Modified Endoscopic Lothrop Procedure

Step No.	Surgical Step	Figure No.	Tip
1	Remove mucosa over frontal process	1A,B	Use the medial orbital wall as the lateral limit
2	Create septal window	2	Stay in the upper half of the middle turbinate and use the first olfactory fascicle as the posterior limit
3	Remove mucosa of nasal cavity underlying the floor of the frontal sinus	3	Do not mistake the emissary veins for the olfactory fascicles
4	Drill down the remaining upper bony septum	4	Gives wide access
5	Find the periosteum on each side	5A,B	Develop the plane on a broad front gives wider access
6	Remove the bone between the lateral limits	6	Keep a broad front and the sinus floor is very quickly discovered
7	Continue to remove bone anterior to the frontal recess	7	Have confidence that the recess still lies between the surgeon and anterior cranial fossa
8	Remove the bone between the created cavity and the true frontal recess	8A,B	Complete the cavity, with mucosal care if required, using a 2-mm Kerrison ronguer

Defining the limits of the dissection early provides a robust and efficient approach (Fig 9, Table 1).

▶ Over the past 2 decades, the modified endoscopic Lothrop procedure (MELP; also known as the endoscopic modified Lothrop) has become established as a safe and effective option in managing a variety of frontal sinus issues,[1] and it has more recently been used in coordination with procedures involving the anterior skull base. Traditionally, bony removal of the floors and interfrontal septations proceeds after both frontal ostia are identified. Usually the less challenging side is pursued first because finding the frontal sinus can be difficult due to the disease processes that usually necessitate this procedure (eg, tumors, scarring, new bone formation). This article describes a variation on performing the MELP using an outside-in approach in which drilling is commenced away from the frontal without identifying the frontal ostium at all (Table 1). The outside-in MELP avoids initial dissection in the frontal recess completely and starts anterior to the frontal sinus where bone drilling begins and proceeds in a posterior direction until the sinus is eventually entered (Fig 9). The authors describe their technique and compared outcomes with the traditional technique in 30 patients (24 had the new outside-in procedure). Operative time and complications were noted. The time for the procedure was significantly shorter for outside-in MELP, and only 1 complication using this technique was encountered (skin edema). The authors concluded that outside-in MELP is technically feasible and safe and highlighted advantages, including speed (in their hands) and easier drilling. The pivotal concept in the outside-in MELP is that the dissection is not related to frontal recess anatomy, and the recess is always between surgeon and skull base until the end of the procedure. A major criticism of this technique is that instead of drilling away from the skull base as during a traditional MELP, this technique advocates drilling toward the skull base, which seems inherently more dangerous. The authors attempt to address this by arguing that this is not a major concern because the frontal floor and recess are always between the surgeon and the skull base during this approach. Although this is true, I still think drilling toward the skull base is not ideal. Another issue is that the start of the procedure is drilling from the anterior aspect of orbit to orbit, which is an unfamiliar region to be operating in for less experienced surgeons. I do agree that the outside-in approach would be ideal in circumstances when it may be impractical or ill-advised to commence drilling at the frontal recess, such as when it is occupied by tumor or in the setting of significant bleeding, for example. I commend the authors for a very innovative modification to the MELP. I do think that more experience with this technique is required to establish its advantages and disadvantages, and I would still suggest that most surgeons use navigation for this type of procedure—regardless of whether you perform it inside out or outside in.

R. Sindwani, MD

Reference

1. Anderson P, Sindwani R. Safety and efficacy of the endoscopic modified Lothrop procedure: a systematic review and meta-analysis. *Laryngoscope*. 2009;119: 1828-1833.

Endoscopic sinus surgery might reduce exacerbations and symptoms more than balloon sinuplasty

Koskinen A, Penttilä M, Myller J, et al (Helsinki Univ Central Hosp, Finland; Univ of Tampere, Finland; Päijat-Häme Central Hosp, Lahti, Finland)
Am J Rhinol Allergy 26:e150-e156, 2012

Background.—Endoscopic sinus surgery (ESS) is considered after medical therapy failure of chronic rhinosinusitis (CRS). The balloon sinuplasty dilates the natural ostium without moving mucosa or bone. It still lacks evidence from randomized controlled trials. The aim of this retrospective controlled study was to compare the symptom outcomes after maxillary sinus surgery with either the ESS or the balloon sinuplasty technique. No previous or additional sinonasal operations were accepted.

Methods.—Two hundred eight patients with CRS without nasal polyps underwent either balloon sinuplasty or ESS. The patients who met with the inclusion criteria (n = 45 in ESS group and n = 40 in balloon group) replied to a questionnaire of history factors, exacerbations, and a visual analog scale (VAS) scoring of the change in symptoms, on average 28 ± 6 (mean ± SD) months postoperatively.

Results.—The groups were identical in the response rate (64%), patient characteristics, and the improvement in all of the asked symptoms. Patients with CRS-related comorbidity and/or present occupational exposure had a statistically significantly better symptom reduction after ESS than after balloon sinusotomy. Moreover, the balloon sinusotomy group reported a statistically significant higher number of maxillary sinus punctures and antibiotic courses during the last 12 months.

Conclusion.—ESS might be superior to balloon sinuplasty, especially in patients with risk factors. There is a need to perform more controlled studies on the treatment choices of CRS.

▶ The use of balloon catheter technology (BCT) continues to gain popularity, although the effectiveness of this technique in comparison to traditional endoscopic sinus surgery remains unknown. In this retrospective, controlled study, adult chronic rhinosinusitis (CRS) patients underwent primary bilateral maxillary sinus procedures with either the balloon sinuplasty or the endoscopic sinus surgery (ESS) technique. This was only done on primary cases, and the ESS was limited to only an uncinectomy and middle meatal antrostomy (ie, an ethmoidectomy was not performed in either group). The aim of this study was to compare, using a questionnaire, the number of exacerbations and the change in symptoms between the procedures. The study included CRS patients without polyps (n = 45 in ESS group and n = 40 in balloon group) who replied to a questionnaire of history factors, exacerbations, and a visual analog scale (VAS) scoring of the change in symptoms 28 months postoperatively. Patients with CRS-related comorbidity and/or present occupational exposure had a statistically significantly better symptom reduction after ESS than after balloon sinusotomy. Moreover, the balloon sinusotomy group reported a statistically significant higher number of maxillary sinus punctures and antibiotic courses during the past 12 months. Both groups did improve postoperatively. The authors concluded that ESS might be superior to balloon sinuplasty, especially in patients with risk factors, and called for a more rigorous study design to examine the question of effectiveness of the 2 techniques. There indeed is a need to perform more controlled studies on the treatment choices of CRS. This study has some major flaws, which the authors discuss, including: a small sample size, a survey design that introduces issues including recall bias, use of a nonvalidated questionnaire and VAS scores, and studying disparate populations (the balloons were performed in a private sector whereas the ESS was on patients in the public sector), which the authors admitted may have different socioeconomic factors at play. The reason I included this study despite its poor design methodology is that it at least tried to compare apples to apples with respect to which sinuses were addressed. A major issue in most BCT studies has been having patients in the ESS arm subjected also to an ethmoidectomy, which is a major confounder. This study critically looked at only opening or dilating the maxillary sinus, which more aptly examines the fundamental question of whether dilatating an ostium with a balloon is inherently better. The authors also found the catheter technology disease in the BCT group to be milder than in those who underwent traditional surgery. Although we still have a lot to examine with respect to the functionality and role of BCT in CRS, we are starting to have some clarity, albeit only glimpses of it. It seems as though the role of the balloon may be slowly evolving to be, as this study suggests, useful for some surgeons to treat milder disease in patients without major CRS risk factors. Perhaps there is only limited ethmoid involvement, for example. This would leave the more involved and severely diseased patient on the spectrum of

CRS to be managed (eg, at the outset or after failure of the balloon technique with a more traditional ESS approach. Other indications for the balloon, such as revision procedures where the visible ostium is noted to be stenosing or isolated frontal disease, also continue to be refined and explored.

R. Sindwani, MD

Evaluation of inferior turbinate hypertrophy in patients with congenital and traumatic nasal septum deviation

Korkut AY, Islim F, Gulseven Ciftci S, et al (Vakif Gureba Training and Res Hosp, Istanbul, Turkey; Bakirkoy Dr Sadi Konuk Training and Res Hosp, Istanbul, Turkey)

J Laryngol Otol 126:784-788, 2012

Objective.—To compare mucosal and bony measurements in patients with congenital and traumatic nasal septum deviation and compensatory inferior turbinate hypertrophy.

Methods.—The study examined 50 patients with nasal septum deviation (25 congenital and 25 traumatic) and compensatory inferior turbinate hypertrophy in the contralateral nasal cavity, confirmed by computed tomography.

Results.—The study compared inferior turbinate measurements on the concave and convex sides of the septum, in the congenital and traumatic groups. Measurements comprised: the shortest distance from the median line to the medial border of the conchal bone; the distances from the most medial part of the conchal mucosa and the conchal bone to the lateral line; the projection angle of the inferior turbinate; and the widest parts of the whole inferior turbinate and the inferior turbinate conchal bone. The

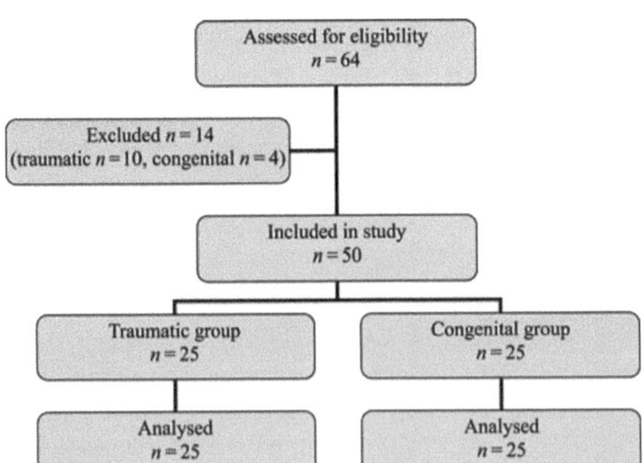

FIGURE 4.—Flowchart showing the patient selection process. (Reprinted from Korkut AY, Islim F, Gulseven Ciftci S, et al. Evaluation of inferior turbinate hypertrophy in patients with congenital and traumatic nasal septum deviation. *J Laryngol Otol.* 2012;126:784-788, with permission of Cambridge University Press.)

differences between the concave and convex side measurements were compared in the congenital group versus the traumatic group; for three measurements, the difference between these two groups was statistically significant ($p < 0.05$).

Conclusion.—The present study findings suggest that the conchal bone has a marked influence on nasal patency in patients with congenital septal deviation. These findings supported the decision to excise the inferior turbinate bone at the time of septoplasty, especially when treating congenital septal deviation (Fig 4).

▶ There are a variety of turbinate procedures we perform for inferior turbinate hypertrophy. Interestingly, some of these are done targeting the soft tissue of the turbinate, whereas others resect the bony concha. None of the studies on compensatory inferior turbinate hypertrophy has compared patients with traumatic and congenital septal deviations. This group hypothesized that the etiology of the septal deviation (congenital or traumatic) altered its duration and, thus, influenced the degree of turbinate mucosal hypertrophy and conchal bone development that occurred in reaction, which is an interesting premise. Based on this hypothesis, the study compared a variety of mucosal and bony measurements in patients with congenital and traumatic nasal septum deviation and compensatory inferior turbinate hypertrophy. The study examined 50 patients with nasal septum deviation (25 congenital and 25 traumatic) and compensatory inferior turbinate hypertrophy in the contralateral nasal cavity, confirmed by computed tomography. The differences between the concave and convex side measurements were compared in the congenital group vs the traumatic group for 3 measurements, and the difference between these 2 groups was statistically significant. The findings of the study suggest that the conchal bone has a marked influence on nasal patency in patients with congenital septal deviation, but in traumatic deviations it is more often the soft tissue of the inferior turbinate that hypertrophies. Key findings of this study include the nasal septum deviation commonly causes contralateral compensatory inferior turbinate hypertrophy, septal deviation may be traumatic or congenital in origin, and, in the latter, the conchal bone has more effect on nasal patency. The authors feel that turbinate bone resection at the time of septoplasty in congenital cases should be advocated, and they suggest that traumatic septal deviations occurring later in life cause compensatory changes involving only the turbinate mucosa—and that in this setting, perhaps managing only the mucosa is adequate. The results of this study are very intriguing, and I believe their hypothesis is meritorious. Central to their cause, however, is the ability to differentiate congenital from traumatic septal deviations that I think clinically is extremely difficult. The study labeled a patient with a congenital deviation if he or she had no history of significant nasal trauma before the age of 17; they argued that, as such, trauma could affect bone development. Patients often have a difficult time thinking of an "index" trauma that may have caused their deviated nasal septum and many people have some form of trauma in their younger years that could be implicated. In addition, it is worthwhile highlighting that most patients with the complaint of nasal obstruction do not get any imaging (which would help distinguish bony vs soft-tissue hypertrophy of the turbinated) and so the choice of turbinate procedure to be performed is essentially left to the experience (ie, habits) of the surgeon. A very thought-provoking article.

R. Sindwani, MD

Non-pedicled vs vascular pedicled nasal flap in repair of cerebrospinal fluid rhinorrhea

Aguilar Cantador J, Jurado-Ramos A, Gutiérrez Jodas J, et al (Univ of Cordoba, Spain)

Acta Otolaryngol 132:1192-1196, 2012

Conclusions.—In our study, pedicled nasal flap (NF) did not provide better results than free nasal graft (NG) for primary closure of cerebrospinal fluid (CSF) rhinorrhea. In the future, a multicenter randomized study would be needed to confirm this result. The choice of surgical technique will depend on the surgeon's experience, and the position and size of the defect.

Objectives.—To evaluate our results in repairing CSF leaks, comparing the two techniques we used: free NG and pedicled NF.

Methods.—A total of 33 patients diagnosed with CSF rhinorrhea were operated on between June 2000 and May 2010; 17 were women. The mean age was 44.7 years (± 13.0). Twenty-two (66.6%) NFs of the middle and lower turbinate and septum were performed, the rest being NGs of the middle and lower turbinate only. A descriptive statistical analysis and a Kaplan–Meier survival analysis were carried out and the log-rank statistic was used to compare both techniques.

Results.—In the present study, 78% of defects were closed in all cases; NF was used in 86% (19) and NG in 63.63% (7). The mean follow-up was 71.5 (95% confidence interval (CI), 56.9–86.1) months. There were no statistically significant differences ($p > 0.05$) (Fig 2).

▶ Endonasal repairs of cerebrospinal fluid (CSF) leaks and skull base defects have traditionally been made using a wide range of substances, including fatty tissue, fascia, muscle, cartilage, turbinal mucosa, and alloplastic materials. These techniques have been improved by the use of vascular pedicled nasal flaps (NF) of the inferior and middle turbinates and the septum. Endoscopic approaches have allowed these to be designed, manipulated, and inserted with high efficiency and a low incidence of morbidity. However, even with the use of these modern endoscopic reconstructive techniques, failures do occur. So which graft type offers the best results? This study aimed to answer this long-standing question. The authors compared their results with 2 techniques for CSF leak repair: the pedicled NF and the nonpedicled nasal graft (NG). Over a 10-year period, 33 CSF leaks were managed with 22 (66.6%) using NFs (pedicled turbinate and septal flaps) and the remainder with free nasal grafts. The authors admitted that the free grafts were performed routinely in the early years, and they switched to the pedicled flap technique in more recent years (an obvious shortcoming of the study). The study found that about 80% of defects were closed in all cases with no statistical difference between the 2 techniques. According to

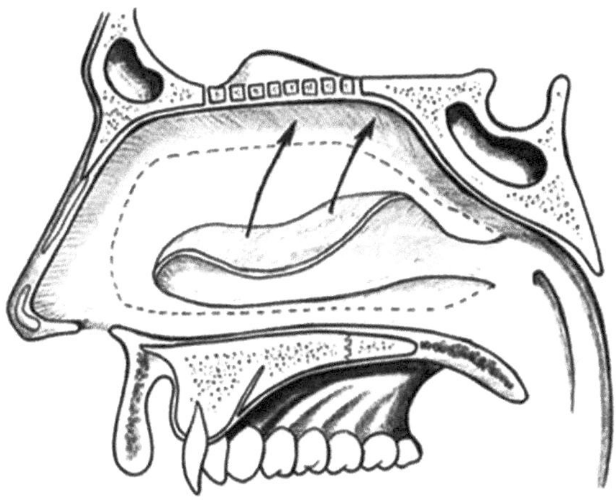

FIGURE 2.—Vascular pedicled nasoseptal flap. The arrows show that the rotation must continue to cover the defect. (Aguilar Cantador J, Jurado-Ramos A, Gutiérrez Jodas J, et al. Non-pedicled vs vascular pedicled nasal flap in repair of cerebrospinal fluid rhinorrhea. *Acta Otolaryngol.* 2012;132:1192-1196, reprinted by permission of Taylor & Francis Ltd, http://www.informaworld.com.)

this study, the pedicled NF did not provide better results than free NG for primary closure of CSF rhinorrhea, which is consistent with other reports in the literature for noncomplicated CSF leaks. I do think the report may have been inadequately powered to note a difference in these 2 techniques and, as mentioned, the retrospective design used is not ideal. Some of the downsides to using a pedicled graft compared with a free piece of mucosa in this context are that the pedicled graft takes a little longer to harvest, and it is not as easily manipulated and ideally placed at the site of the defect because of geometric constraints. In addition, reach of the pedicled graft could be an issue, and concerns have been raised that the farthest extent of the pedicled graft should have some redundancy of tissue placed over the defect to allow for adequate coverage after anticipated contracture during healing. The authors discuss that the choice of surgical technique depends on the surgeon's experience/preference and the position and size of the defect, with which I would agree. I would also add, however, that the complexity of the defect and the pathology being managed are also relevant. Although data for this may be somewhat lacking, many of us do consider using pedicled flaps for higher-risk CSF leaks, revision procedures, and more complicated skull base reconstructions. Recent literature suggests that the posterior pedicled nasoseptal flap (or the Hadad-Bassagasteguy flap, Fig 2) is becoming the workhorse in more complex skull base reconstructions. This flap has proven to be a reliable and versatile reconstructive technique for extensive defects of much of the ventral skull base. However, given the excellent success rate and the ease and simplicity of use of a free mucosal graft, I think the free graft really is the go-to choice for more routine CSF leaks.

R. Sindwani, MD

Role of Frontal Sinus Surgery in Nasal Polyp Recurrence

Bassiouni A, Wormald P-J (Univ of Adelaide, Australia)

Laryngoscope 123:36-41, 2013

Objectives/Hypothesis.—Patients with aggressive nasal polyp recurrence form an important subgroup of patients with refractory sinus disease. The objectives of this study were to establish patterns of polyp recurrence and evaluate the effect of frontal sinus surgery (Draf 2a vs. Draf 3) on polyp recurrence.

Study Design.—Retrospective cohort study reviewing 338 consecutive operations.

Methods.—Polyp recurrence was defined according to the Lund-Kennedy mucosal edema score. Survival analysis methods were used for statistics.

Results.—After complete sphenoethmoidectomies, Draf 2a frontal sinusotomies, and middle meatal antrostomies persistent polyp recurrence occurred in 19.8% of patients after 6 months and increased to 22.7% of patients after 12 months. Polyps first recurred in the area of the frontal sinus/ostium (55%) followed by the ethmoids (38%). Asthma and aspirin sensitivity were the most important variables affecting recurrence (hazard ratios, 1.71, 1.79, respectively; $P < .05$) The Draf 3 procedure was a significant factor in reducing recurrence, especially in asthma and aspirin intolerant patients. The overall revision rate was 18% (follow-up duration > 12 months, median = 29 months), with a 37% revision rate in the FESS group versus 7% in the Draf 3 group ($P < .001$). Survival analysis showed that the Draf 3 significantly reduced the risk of revision (hazard ratio = 0.258, $P = .0026$).

Conclusions.—Nasal polyposis is characterized by a high rate of recurrence. The presence of asthma or aspirin intolerance leads to more aggressive recurrence, and in these patients the Draf 3 drillout procedure becomes a good option for improved long-term outcomes and reducing the need for revision surgery (Table 2).

▶ A large majority of patients with polyps have recurrences, making the polyps challenging to manage. This is a large retrospective cohort study of 338 consecutive operations that examines patterns of polyp recurrence and also explores the

TABLE 2.—Analysis of 127 Known Sites of Recurrences

Site of Recurrence	Frequency (%)
Frontal sinus area (including around the frontal ostium, frontal recess, or inside the frontal sinus itself)	70 (55.1)
Ethmoid cavities, including the sphenoethmoidal recess	48 (37.8)
Maxillary sinus and ostium	4 (3.1)
Olfactory recess	3 (2.4)
Middle meatus	2 (1.6)
Total	127

effect of frontal sinus surgery (Draf 2a vs Draf 3) on polyp recurrence. The findings were quite informative and thought-provoking. First, polyp recurrence was noted initially in the area of the frontal sinus/ostium in more than 50% of patients, followed by the ethmoid sinus (Table 2). As expected, asthma and acetylsalicylic acid (ASA) sensitivity were the most important variables affecting recurrence. The most important finding of the article was that the Draf 3 procedure (endoscopic modified Lothrop procedure, or frontal drill out procedure) was a significant factor in reducing polyp recurrence, especially in asthma and ASA-sensitive patients. The authors also found that a larger frontal opening improved management of recurrences because having this procedure performed significantly reduced the need for revision surgery. The explanation for these findings is not clear. The authors explored theories, including that a greater reduction in the mucosal inflammatory load leads to better long-term outcomes, and they suggested that there may be advantages of removing the inferior part of the middle turbinate, which occurs with the Draf 3 procedure. Another very interesting hypothesis was that opening up the frontals widely using a Draf 3 allows for more complete removal of polyps; the authors expand on this, suggesting that removing polyps at their bases is key because the highest concentration of eosinophils is present in the pedicle.[1] This becomes critical in the asthma and ASA-intolerant subgroups, they argue, because these groups exhibit higher degrees of mucosal eosinophilia. The larger frontal sinus opening created during a Draf 3 procedure increases the ability of the surgeon to decrease the disease load by providing better access to the frontal sinuses, ventilate the sinuses better, and also provide access for postoperative topical drug therapy, which can contribute to better long-term disease management. A very stimulating article with very interesting findings and implications for more aggressive surgery in higher-risk polyp patients.

R. Sindwani, MD

Reference

1. Min YG, Kim YJ, Yun YS. Distribution of eosinophil granule proteins in nasal mucosa of atopic patients with nasal polyposis. *ORL J Otorhinolaryngol Relat Spec.* 1996;58:82-86.

7 Thyroid and Parathyroid

Basic and Clinical Research

Suspicious Cervical Lymph Nodes Detected after Thyroidectomy for Papillary Thyroid Cancer Usually Remain Stable Over Years in Properly Selected Patients

Robenshtok E, Fish S, Bach A, et al (Memorial Sloan-Kettering Cancer Ctr, NY; et al)

J Clin Endocrinol Metab 97:2706-2713, 2012

Context.—The risk of loco-regional recurrence in papillary thyroid cancer (PTC) patients ranges from 15–30%. However, the clinical significance of small-volume loco-regional recurrence detected by highly sensitive ultrasonography is unclear.

Objective.—Our objective was to describe the natural history of abnormal cervical lymph nodes (LN) diagnosed after initial treatment.

Design.—We conducted a retrospective cohort study.

Patients.—166 PTC with patients who had at least one abnormal LN outside the thyroid be on ultrasound and selected for active surveillance were included.

Main Outcome Measure.—LN growth during a period of active surveillance was the primary outcome.

Results.—Most patients had classical PTC (85%) and an intermediate risk of recurrence (77%). The median LN size at the start of the observation period was 1.3 cm (range, 0.5–2.7 cm) in largest diameter, with all nodes having at least one abnormal sonographic characteristic (70% of patients had LN with at least two abnormal features). In almost all patients, the LN were in the lateral neck, primarily in levels 3 (43%) and 4 (58%). After a median follow-up of 3.5 yr, only 20% (33 of 166) grew at least 3 mm, 9% (15 of 166) grew at least 5 mm, and 14% (23 of 166) resolved. None of the clinical or sonographic features were predictive of LN growth (positive predictive value range = 0.21–0.57). There were no local complications (nerve damage or local invasion) related to the abnormal nodes and no disease-related mortality.

Conclusions.—Suspicious cervical LN in the lateral neck usually remain stable for long periods of time in properly selected PTC patients and can be safely followed with serial ultrasounds.

▶ This selected article addresses the controversial issue of managing recurrent/persistent cervical nodal disease. It is generally accepted that in papillary thyroid carcinoma, cervical lymph node metastases do not affect overall survival. Based on this premise, several therapeutic options are available to manage such regional recurrences; they include repeated radioiodine (I-131) ablations, ultrasound-guided ethanol injections, minimally invasive excision of metastatic lymph nodes, and cervical lymphadenectomy. The authors of this retrospective study, based on their results, suggest that relatively small (1–2 cm) cervical lymph nodes, suspicious for recurrent/residual metastatic papillary carcinoma, may remain stable for prolonged periods and are safe to be observed with serial high-resolution ultrasound examinations performed at 6- to 12-month intervals. This, needless to say, applies only to patients who fall into good prognostic category and those in whom (as already stated above) presence or absence of cervical metastases will not affect their disease-specific survival. Based on this logic and supported by the data of this selected study, fine-needle aspiration followed by subsequent management of positive lymph nodes should be reserved only for those patients in whom there was a significant progression in the size of those nodes. This, of course, is a very attractive therapeutic option for a conservative surgeon, but it is often hard to follow through because of anxiety of the patient and, more often than not, the patient's endocrinologist.

M. Gapany, MD

Complications of Central Neck Dissection in Patients with Papillary Thyroid Carcinoma: Results of a Study on 1087 Patients and Review of the Literature

Giordano D, Valcavi R, Thompson GB, et al (Ctr for Clinical and Basic Res (IRCCS), Reggio Emilia, Italy; Mayo Clinic College of Medicine, Rochester, MN; et al)

Thyroid 22:911-917, 2012

Background.—Prophylactic central neck dissection (CND) has been proposed in the treatment of patients affected by papillary thyroid carcinoma (PTC) with clinically negative neck lymph nodes. The procedure allows pathologic staging of lymph nodes of the central compartment and treatment of the micrometastases. Nevertheless, the morbidity that its routine use adds to the total thyroidectomy must be taken into account. The aim of this study was to characterize the morbidity that CND adds to the total thyroidectomy.

Methods.—This was a retrospective study of 1087 patients with PTC and clinically negative neck lymph nodes. Patients were divided into three study groups: Group A, total thyroidectomy; Group B, total thyroidectomy and ipsilateral CND; Group C, total thyroidectomy and bilateral CND.

Primary endpoints of the study were evaluated by comparing the rates of transient and permanent recurrent laryngeal nerve (RLN) injury and hypoparathyroidism in the three study groups.

Results.—Analysis of data showed no significant differences in the rate of transient (Group A: 3.6%, Group B: 3.9%, and Group C: 5.5%; $p = 0.404$) and permanent (Group A: 1%, Group B: 0.5%, and Group C: 2.3%; $p = 0.099$) RLN injury between the three study groups. Both ipsilateral CND and bilateral CND were associated with a higher rate of transient hypoparathyroidism (Group: A 27.7%, Group B: 36.1%, and Group C: 51.9%; $p = 0.014$; odds ratio [OR]: 1.477; 95% confidence interval [CI]: 1.091–2.001; $p < 0.001$; OR: 2.827; 95% CI: 2.065–3.870, respectively). Bilateral CND had a higher rate of permanent hypoparathyroidism (Group A: 6.3%, Group B: 7%, and Group C: 16.2%; $p < 0.001$; OR: 2.860; 95% CI: 1.725–4.743).

Conclusions.—The increased rates of transient and permanent hypoparathyroidism in our series suggest a critical review of indications for the routine use of prophylactic CND for PTC. Prophylactic CND ipsilateral to the tumor associated with total thyroidectomy may represent an effective strategy for reducing the rate of permanent hypoparathyroidism. Concomitant completion contralateral paratracheal lymph node neck dissection should be performed in presence of lymph node metastasis on intraoperative frozen-section pathology. This approach limits the use of bilateral CND to patients with intraoperative pathological findings of lymph node metastases.

▶ It is generally accepted that in papillary thyroid carcinoma, cervical lymph node metastases do not affect overall survival. However, presence of cervical lymph node metastases is associated with increased incidence of loco-regional recurrence, justifying intraoperative removal of clinically or radiographically positive cervical lymph nodes in both lateral and central compartments. On the other hand, the issue of prophylactic cervical lymphadenectomy in clinically and radiographically negative cases remains subject to significant controversy. This holds particularly true for the prophylactic central compartment lymphadenectomy, which is associated with increased risk for recurrent laryngeal nerve injury and permanent hypoparathyroidism. The high incidence of central compartment micrometastases in clinically negative cases (50%–60%) is often used by proponents of prophylactic neck dissection to justify their approach, whereas the detractors cite increased incidence of complications without proven benefit of survival or even change in the course of the disease to justify their objection. To make things even more confusing, the American Thyroid Association recently came out with a recommendation to consider lymph node dissection (basically leaving the decision to individual surgeon) in all patients undergoing thyroidectomy for papillary thyroid carcinoma, regardless of whether the nodes are enlarged.

This selected article thoroughly addresses the issue of complications associated with central compartment neck dissection in papillary thyroid carcinoma. The authors caution against routine use of prophylactic neck dissection and call for critical review of indications for this operation.

Many experienced thyroid surgeons report that reoperation for central compartment lymphadenopathy is not associated with increased risk of complications or loco-regional recurrence compared with central compartment lymphadenectomy performed at the time of thyroidectomy. It appears, therefore, logical and prudent to recommend observation for clinically negative central compartment and surgery only for clinically or radiographically positive nodes. In my practice, in addition to outlined philosophy, I use risk stratification to guide my surgical approach: prophylactic central compartment lymphadenectomy in high-risk patients and no lymphadenectomy in patients with low-risk scores.

M. Gapany, MD

Diagnostics

BRAF V600E Mutation Independently Predicts Central Compartment Lymph Node Metastasis in Patients with Papillary Thyroid Cancer

Howell GM, Nikiforova MN, Carty SE, et al (Univ of Pittsburgh School of Medicine, PA; Univ of Pittsburgh, PA)

Ann Surg Oncol 20:47-52, 2013

Purpose.—This study was designed to examine whether available preoperative clinical parameters, including B-type Raf kinase (*BRAF*) V600E mutation status, can identify patients at risk for central compartment lymph node metastasis (CLNM).

Methods.—Under an institutional review board-approved protocol, we conducted a single-center, retrospective review of all patients who had initial thyroidectomy for histologic papillary thyroid carcinoma (PTC) during 2010. The presence of CLNM was examined for correlation with available preoperative clinical parameters, including tumor size, gender, age, and *BRAF* mutation status.

Results.—Cervical lymph node resection and molecular testing on FNAB or histopathologic specimen was performed on a consecutive series of 156 study patients with histologic PTC. Overall, CLNM was diagnosed in 37% and 46% were *BRAF*-mutation-positive. *BRAF* positivity was the only clinical parameter associated with CLNM (*BRAF*, $p = 0.002$; tumor size ≥ 2 cm, $p = 0.16$; male gender, $p = 0.1$; age ≥ 45 years, $p = 0.3$) and remained an independent predictor of CLNM on multiple logistic regression analysis (odds ratio (OR) 3.2, $p = 0.001$). The PPV and NPV of *BRAF* positivity for CLNM was 50 and 74%, respectively. When restricting the analysis to the subset of 38 patients who had molecular testing performed preoperatively on FNAB, the PPV and NPV of *BRAF* positivity for CLNM was 47 and 91%, respectively, and *BRAF* positivity was still a significant predictor of CLNM on both univariate (OR 8.4, $p = 0.01$) and multivariate (OR 9.7, $p = 0.02$) analyses.

Conclusions.—Of the commonly used clinical parameters available preoperatively, the *BRAF* V600E mutation is the only independent predictor of CLNM in PTC and can be utilized to guide the extent of initial surgery.

▶ B-type Raf kinase (BRAF) is an oncogene strongly linked to papillary thyroid cancer. A point mutation resulting in a valine to glutamate alteration at codon 600 (V600E) has been reported to occur in up to 80% of papillary thyroid cancers. There is also strong evidence that *BRAF* V600E mutation can be a predictor of aggressive tumor behavior, resulting in local recurrence and regional and distant metastases.

In this selected study, the authors have shown that *BRAF* V600E mutation can be a strong predictor of central compartment neck metastases in papillary thyroid carcinoma. Furthermore, their data suggest that preoperative *BRAF* testing of fine-needle aspirate (FNA) specimens could be a valuable preoperative screening method in determining whether patients are at risk for having central neck metastases. Although the positive predictive value of such preoperative screening does not exceed 50%, the negative predictive value can be as high as 90% and could successfully identify patients who would not be befit from prophylactic central neck dissection.

Preoperative screening of FNA specimens for *BRAF* mutation, thus, might be of great value in assigning risk for malignancy in suspicious specimens or even determining the extent of the planned operation.

M. Gapany, MD

A Prospective Evaluation of Quick Intraoperative Parathyroid Hormone Assay at the Time of Skin Closure in Predicting Clinically Relevant Hypocalcemia after Thyroidectomy

Lang BH-H, Yih PC-L, Ng KK (Univ of Hong Kong, Pokfulam, Hong Kong SAR, China)

World J Surg 36:1300-1306, 2012

Background.—Post-thyroidectomy hypocalcemia is a major contributing factor in delayed hospital discharge and dissuading surgeons from ambulatory thyroidectomy. We prospectively evaluated the accuracy and reliability of quick parathyroid hormone level measurement at skin closure (PTH-SC) in predicting clinically relevant hypocalcemia (i.e., patients requiring calcium ± calcitriol supplements on hospital discharge).

Methods.—Of the 117 patients who underwent a total or completion total thyroidectomy and PTH-SC, 17 (14.5 %) had hypocalcemic symptoms or adjusted calcium <1.90 mmol/L requiring calcium and/or calcitriol supplements on discharge. Serum calcium was checked regularly in the perioperative period until stabilization and an additional quick PTH was checked on the following morning (PTH-D1). Univariate and multivariate analyses were performed to evaluate potential preoperative clinicopathologic factors and postoperative day 0 biochemical indicators. Youden's index and the area under the ROC curve (AUC) were used to determine the best cutoff value and predictability of significant variables or criteria, respectively.

Results.—In the multivariate analysis, low preoperative adjusted calcium ($p = 0.041$) and low PTH-SC ($p = 0.001$) were the two independent variables associated with hypocalcemia. PTH-SC (≤1 or >1 pmol/L) had a higher specificity (95.0%) and AUC (0.887) than serial calcium monitoring or PTH-D1 alone. Although 3/98 of patients with PTH-SC >1 pmol/L required calcium supplements on discharge, they required only the minimum amount to maintain normocalcemia.

Conclusion.—PTH-SC is an accurate and reliable means of predicting clinically relevant hypocalcemia. It would be reasonable to discharge those with PTH-SC >1 pmol/L on the same operative day as the risk of life-threatening hypocalcemia would seem unlikely.

▶ This is the second article selected for this year's YEAR BOOK that focuses on prevention of serious hypocalcemia after thyroid surgery. The current trend in thyroid surgery is reducing it to ambulatory surgery or 23-hour observation level. To this end, algorithms have been developed to monitor and predict postoperative hypocalcemia through serial measurement of postoperative ionized calcium or parathyroid hormone (PTH) levels using rapid PTH assay. Others have been simply routinely prescribing calcium and vitamin D supplementation in all thyroidectomy patients without the need for any postoperative hospital observation. In this selected study, authors have evaluated the efficacy for predicting hypocalcemia using a rapid PTH assay performed on serum samples collected at the very end of the thyroidectomy operation (ie, at skin closure). They found this method to be very accurate, but not 100% accurate (because there are no 100% accurate predictive methods).

It appears thus that surgeons, who prefer to perform total thyroidectomies (or completion thyroidectomies) as ambulatory operations, have a choice between several fairly accurate methods to predict and prevent potentially dangerous hypocalcemia.

M. Gapany, MD

The Impact of Thyroid Nodule Size on the Risk of Malignancy and Accuracy of Fine-Needle Aspiration: A 10-Year Study from a Single Institution

Shrestha M, Crothers BA, Burch HB (Walter Reed Natl Military Med Ctr, Bethesda, MD)

Thyroid 22:1251-1256, 2012

Background.—False-negative rates for thyroid fine-needle aspiration (FNA) vary from 0.4% to 13%, but the effect of nodule size on the accuracy of thyroid FNA remains controversial. We hypothesized that large thyroid nodule size does not contribute to the risk of malignancy or the risk of a false-negative FNA.

Methods.—All thyroid FNAs performed at the Walter Reed Army Medical Center during September 2001–August 2011 were reviewed.

A strict correlation between the biopsy site, location, and size of nodule on ultrasound (US) and pathology report was ensured. FNA results were classified as benign, atypical, follicular neoplasm/suspicious for follicular neoplasm (FN/SFN), suspicious for malignancy (SM), or malignant, and the pathology result was categorized as either benign or malignant. Nodules were analyzed by size: 0.5–0.9 cm (group A), 1.0–3.9 cm (group B), and ≥ 4 cm (group C). Incidental thyroid cancer was not included.

Results.—Of 3013 patients undergoing FNA, 667 (22.1%) had surgery. Patients were excluded for nodules < 0.5 cm, nondiagnostic FNA, or no preoperative US, leaving 540 patients with 695 nodules. Among patients referred for surgery, FNA results were benign in 417 nodules (60%), atypical in 22 (3.2%), FN/SFN in 122 (17.6%), SM in 77 (11.1%), and malignant in 57 (8.2%). Postoperative malignancy rates by FNA result were 7% if benign, 4.5% if atypical, 23% if FN/SFN, 33.8% if SM, and 78.9% if malignant. FNA accuracy was 60% in group A, 68.5% in group B, and 80.3% in group C ($p = 0.01$). False-negative rates for FNA were 7.0% overall, 15.8% in group A, 6.3% in group B, and 7.1% in group C ($p = 0.25$). Sensitivity and negative predictive value were highest in group B at 81.6% and 93.7%, respectively. The prevalence of malignancy was not different between groups.

Conclusion.—Our results show that the thyroid nodule size ≥ 4 cm increases neither the risk of false-negative FNA results, nor the overall risk of malignancy. We also show a tendency toward a higher false-negative rate in subcentimeter nodules. We conclude that a large nodule size should not prompt automatic referral for thyroidectomy. An increased awareness of potential sampling error in subcentimeter nodules is warranted.

▶ Fine-needle aspiration (FNA) is an excellent screening tool for thyroid nodules, with very high sensitivity and specificity. It has dramatically reduced the rate of explorative surgery for thyroid nodules and increased the incidence of finding cancer in operated patients, thus improving the yield of surgery. It has been reported that the accuracy of FNA declines with an increase in the size of the nodule, and when the nodule reaches the size of 4 cm (some studies have suggested greater than 3 cm), the rate of false-negative aspirates is "unacceptably high." When considered together with the clinical observation that tumors greater than 4 cm in diameter are more likely to be cancerous than smaller nodules, it has been recommended by more than one authority in the field to always perform an explorative operation to determine the nature of those nodules, regardless of the result of the FNA.

The authors of this selected study from a very reputable institution have taken this clinical approach head on, adding more controversy to an already controversial issue: In their very large series of fine-needle aspirates, confirmed surgically, they have found that 4 cm size of the thyroid nodule is neither associated with increased incidence of false-negative results nor with the increased overall risk of malignancy. To the contrary, they have shown that the rate of false-negative results is actually higher in subcentimeter-sized nodules.

M. Gapany, MD

Dual-Phase ^{99m}Tc Sestamibi Scintigraphy With Neck and Thorax SPECT/CT in Primary Hyperparathyroidism: A Single-Institution Experience

Ciappuccini R, Morera J, Pascal P, et al (Centre François Baclesse, Caen, France; Centre Hospitalo-Universitaire, Caen, France; et al)

Clin Nucl Med 37:223-228, 2012

Purpose.—To assess the diagnostic value of dual-phase ^{99m}Tc sestamibi scintigraphy with neck and thorax single-photon emission computed tomography/computed tomography (SPECT/CT) in patients with primary hyperparathyroidism, and to analyze the relationships between SPECT/CT data and serum calcium or parathyroid hormone (PTH) concentrations.

Materials and Methods.—^{99m}Tc sestamibi scintigraphy was performed in 94 consecutive patients. Images included early and delayed planar neck images and delayed neck and thorax SPECT/CT. Scintigraphy was scored positive or negative.

Results.—Fifty-nine sestamibi studies (63%) were positive. SPECT/CT demonstrated a single focus in 56 patients, in usual parathyroid sites in 80% of cases and in unusual sites in the remaining 20% (retrotracheal area, 7%; intrathyroidal, 9%; mediastinum, 4%), and double foci in 3. Serum calcium values were higher in patients with a positive scintigraphy than in those with a negative scintigraphy (2.80 vs. 2.66 mmol/L, $P = 0.001$) with similar figures for serum PTH values (129 vs. 107 pg/mL, $P = 0.0649$). In patients with a measurable parathyroid adenoma on integrated CT scan ($n = 43$), the greatest axial diameter of the adenoma was correlated to serum calcium ($r = 0.405$, $P < 0.0071$) or PTH concentrations ($r = 0.589$, $P < 0.0001$). Fifty-four patients underwent surgery, 45 with a positive, and 9 with a negative preoperative scintigraphy, resulting in a sensitivity of 92% (95% CI: 80–98) and a specificity of 83% (95% CI: 36–100).

Conclusions.—Dual-phase ^{99m}Tc sestamibi scintigraphy with SPECT/CT enables to identify a parathyroid adenoma in about two-thirds of patients with primary hyperparathyroidism and allows the surgeon to plan appropriate surgery. The likelihood of scintigraphy to be positive is affected by calcium or PTH concentrations.

▶ Success of minimally invasive parathyroidectomy relies on accurate preoperative localization of the parathyroid adenoma as well as intraoperative measurement parathyroid hormone levels. Technetium Tc 99m sestamibi single-photon emission computed tomography (SPECT) and sonography are used very successfully for preoperative localization. Both have comparable accuracy rates in identifying solitary adenomas but are less accurate in identifying multiple adenomas. Both studies can be complementary, and it is therefore common practice to obtain both a sonogram and a nuclear study for preoperative localization. However, several recent studies have suggested that it is perfectly adequate to use sonogram as the initial (and in most cases the only) study. But when it is inconclusive, what should be the next diagnostic step? Studies using first-generation hybrid equipment suggest that SPECT/computed tomography (CT) coregistration may be more accurate then SPECT alone in localizing parathyroid adenomas. This selected article reports the efficacy of new-generation hybrid SPECT/CT equipment for preoperative primary hyperparathyroidism workup. In my practice, sonogram remains the first-line study, with SPECT/CT reserved for initial localization failures.

M. Gapany, MD

A Combined Molecular-Pathologic Score Improves Risk Stratification of Thyroid Papillary Microcarcinoma

Niemeier LA, Kuffner Akatsu H, Song C, et al (Univ of Pittsburgh School of Medicine, PA; Univ of Pittsburgh, PA)

Cancer 118:2069-2077, 2012

Background.—Thyroid papillary microcarcinoma (TPMC) is an incidentally discovered papillary carcinoma that measures ≤1.0 cm in size. Most TPMCs are indolent, whereas some behave aggressively. The objective of the study was to evaluate whether the combination of v-raf murine sarcoma viral oncogene homolog B1 (*BRAF*) mutation and specific histopathologic features allows risk stratification of TPMC.

Methods.—A group aggressive TPMCs was selected based on the presence of lymph node metastasis or tumor recurrence. Another group of nonaggressive tumors included TPMCs matched with the first group for age, sex, and tumor size, but with no extrathyroid spread. A molecular analysis was performed, and histologic slides were scored for multiple histopathologic criteria. A separate validation cohort of 40 TPMCs was evaluated.

Results.—*BRAF* mutations were detected in 77% of aggressive TPMCs and in 32% of nonaggressive tumors ($P = .001$). Several histopathologic features differed significantly between the groups. By using multivariate regression analysis, a molecular-pathologic (MP) score was developed that included *BRAF* status and 3 histopathologic features: superficial tumor location, intraglandular tumor spread/multifocality, and tumor fibrosis. By adding the histologic criteria to *BRAF* status, sensitivity was increased from 77% to 96%, and specificity was increased from 68% to 80%. In the independent validation cohort, the MP score stratified tumors into low-risk, moderate-risk, and high-risk groups with the probability of lymph node metastases or tumor recurrence in 0%, 20%, and 60% of patients, respectively.

Conclusions.—*BRAF* status together with several histopathologic features allowed clinical risk stratification of TPMCs. The combined MP risk stratification model was a better predictor of extrathyroid tumor spread than either mutation or histopathologic findings alone.

▶ The incidence of thyroid papillary microcarcinoma (PTMC) is on the rise worldwide and is currently the most commonly diagnosed variant of thyroid cancer in the United States. It is considered to be a relatively well-behaved form of thyroid cancer, carrying a remarkably low incidence (0.3%) of disease-related death. Nevertheless, some of the PTMC show aggressive features, including local spread and regional metastases. Such tumors might benefit from more aggressive therapy.

This excellent study has explored the potential for risk stratification of PTMC using v-raf murine sarcoma viral oncogene homolog B1 (BRAF) mutation status together with several aggressiveness-predicting histopathologic features. The authors offer a relatively simple scoring algorithm, which includes the BRAF mutation status, superficial tumor location in respect to thyroid capsule, intra-glandular spread/tumor multifocality, and degree of fibrosis as parameters. It is interesting to note that using the proposed scoring system the authors were able to assign 65% of the tumors to the low-risk category, 25% to the intermediate category, and 10% to the high-risk category, which is consistent with the expected clinical behavior of PTMC and can serve as an indication for clinical relevance of this algorithm.

M. Gapany, MD

Outcomes

Aggressive Variants of Papillary Thyroid Cancer: Incidence, Characteristics and Predictors of Survival Among 43,738 Patients

Kazaure HS, Roman SA, Sosa JA (Yale Univ School of Medicine, New Haven, CT)

Ann Surg Oncol 19:1874-1880, 2012

Background.—The diffuse sclerosing (DSV) and tall cell (TCV) variants are considered aggressive subtypes of papillary thyroid cancer (PTC) for which data are limited.

Methods.—The Surveillance, Epidemiology, and End Results (SEER) database (1988–2008) was used to compare the incidence and clinical/pathologic characteristics of DSV and TCV with classic PTC. Prognostic factors associated with survival were analyzed by chi-square test, analysis of variance, log rank test, and Cox multivariate regression.

Results.—There were 261 DSV, 573 TCV, and 42,904 PTC patients. Compared to a 60.8% increase in classic PTC incidence, DSV and TCV incidence increased by 126% ($P_{trend} = 0.052$) and 158% ($P_{trend} = 0.002$), respectively. Aggressive variants were associated with higher rates of extrathyroidal extension, multifocality, and nodal and distant metastasis (all $P < 0.001$) compared to classic PTC. Nodal metastasis was more likely with DSV (72.2% vs. 66.8% TCV vs. 56.3% PTC, $P < 0.001$); distant metastasis was most common with TCV (11.1% vs. 7.3% DSV vs. 4.3% PTC, $P < 0.001$). After adjustment, DSV [hazard ratio (HR) 1.8, $P = 0.007$] and TCV (HR 1.9, $P < 0.001$) histologies were associated with significantly reduced survival (5-year overall: 87.5% DSV, 80.6% TCV vs. 93.5% PTC, $P < 0.001$). Tumor size independently predicted worse prognosis for TCV (HR 1.29, $P < 0.001$) but not DSV patients. Thyroid surgery and radioiodine improved survival of DSV and TCV patients (all $P < 0.05$). Patients with aggressive variants who received external-beam radiotherapy did not experience improved survival.

Conclusions.—DSV and TCV are rare, increasing in incidence, and have a worse prognosis than classic PTC. Patients with these variants should be treated aggressively with thyroidectomy and radioiodine, regardless of tumor size.

▶ This is the third Surveillance, Epidemiology, and End Results (SEER)-based epidemiologic study included in this year's selection. The goal of this selected study was to investigate the incidence, demographics, and clinical and pathologic characteristics of diffuse sclerosing and tall cell variants of papillary thyroid cancer based on a large data repository. It is generally accepted that diffuse sclerosing and tall cell variants of papillary thyroid carcinoma are associated with aggressive tumor behavior. It is, however, debatable whether the histologic pattern per se, or rather, other clinical-pathologic prognostic criteria are associated with worse outcome of these thyroid cancer variants. This study found that both papillary thyroid carcinoma variants were associated with high incidence of extrathyroidal extension, multifocality, and distant metastasis, which all appeared to be independent prognostic factors negatively affecting survival. Regional nodal metastasis, on the other hand, was not found to be of prognostic significance. Most importantly, total thyroidectomy and adjuvant radioiodine therapy appeared to be associated with improved survival in both papillary carcinoma variants.

M. Gapany, MD

Bilateral Subtotal Thyroidectomy Versus Hemithyroidectomy Plus Subtotal Resection (Dunhill Procedure) for Benign Goiter: Long-Term Results of a Prospective, Randomized Study

Rayes N, Steinmüller T, Schröder S, et al (Charité Campus Virchow, Berlin, Germany; DRK Westend, Berlin, Germany)
World J Surg 37:84-90, 2013

Background.—Two recent meta-analyses of mostly retrospective studies have shown high recurrence rates following subtotal resection of bilateral multinodular goiter. Therefore, many endocrine centers have changed their operative procedures in favor of thyroidectomy. Consequently, the rate of complications, especially hypoparathyroidism, has increased. Hemithyroidectomy plus subtotal resection (Dunhill operation) overcomes some disadvantages of bilateral subtotal resection (BST). We performed a prospective, randomized trial to compare the Dunhill operation (DO) and BST for benign goiters.

Methods.—Between October 1994 and March 1997, a total of 200 consecutive patients were randomized into two study groups. Primary outcome measure was the incidence of recurrent goiter. Secondary outcome measures were incidence of recurrent nerve palsy and hypoparathyroidism. In all patients, ultrasonography of the thyroid and measurement of serum calcium and parathyroid hormone were performed. Recurrent nerve function was analyzed by indirect laryngoscopy. Long term data (>10 years after surgery) were available in 70 DO patients and 65 BST patients. Mean follow-up was 11.3 ± 4.2 years (10–12 years).

Results.—No differences were seen in the operating times, transient and permanent hypoparathyroidism, or recurrent nerve palsy. In the long-term, mean thyroid volumes were significantly lower in the DO group (3.5 ± 3.5 vs. 6.4 ± 6.5 ml, $p = 0.01$). One reoperation was required in the BST group because of recurrence versus none in the DO group. 68 of 70 (97%) patients in group DO and 59 of 65 (91%) in group BST had ongoing thyroid hormone therapy with no significant differences in mean dosages of l-thyroxine.

Conclusions.—The Dunhill operation and BST are safe procedures. In case of small remnants, clinically significant recurrence is a rare event especially after the Dunhill operation.

▶ Recent studies have found that bilateral subtotal thyroidectomy for multinodular goiter is associated with unacceptably high rates of recurrence. The inevitable conclusion drawn from those studies was that total thyroidectomy was the operation of choice for multinodular goiter to prevent recurrence of the disease. On the other hand, total thyroidectomy is associated with a high complication rate when compared with bilateral subtotal thyroidectomy, especially when the operation is performed in low-volume centers. Hemithyroidectomy with contralateral subtotal thyroidectomy has been proposed as an alternative to total thyroidectomy.

This select, randomized, prospective study compared bilateral subtotal thyroidectomy with hemithyroidectomy plus contralateral subtotal thyroidectomy in terms of their safety and efficacy in prevention of recurrent goiter. The results of the study have shown that both are safe, with comparable complication rates and very low incidence of recurrence. The important point made by the authors is the significance of the size of the thyroid remnant: When small, the rate of recurrence is probably negligible. Just enough thyroid tissue has to be left to protect the parathyroid glands and recurrent laryngeal nerves.

M. Gapany, MD

Management of Grave's Disease Is Improved by Total Thyroidectomy

Annerbo M, Stålberg P, Hellman P (Uppsala Univ, Sweden)

World J Surg 36:1943-1946, 2012

Background.—A retrospective analysis was performed on 267 consecutive patients with Graves' disease (GD). The principal aim of this study was to evaluate the risk for recurrence and complications when changing the surgical method from subtotal (ST) to total thyroidectomy (TT).

Methods.—Information from 267 consecutive patients operated on for GD between 2000 and 2006 was collected at Uppsala University Hospital (143) and Falun County Hospital (128). There were 229 women and 38 men. Four patients were operated on twice. A total of 40 STs and 229 TTs were performed. Results were compared to those of a previous cohort from the same hospital, with a majority of STs (157/176) performed from 1980 to 1992.

Results.—The risk for relapse of GD was reduced from 20 to 3.3 % after the shift from ST to TT. In terms of surgical complications, 2.2 % demonstrated permanent vocal cord paralysis and 4.5 % had persistent hypocalcemia, not significant when compared to the previous cohort. In spite of TT, there were four recurrences, all due to remnant thyroid tissue high up at the hyoid bone. Changing the surgical method did not affect postoperative progression of dysthyroid ophthalmopathy (DO, 7.0 vs. 7.5 %). There were no differences in outcome with respect to which hospital the patients had their operation.

Conclusion.—Change from ST to TT dramatically reduced the risk for recurrence of GD without increasing the rate of complications. TT is not more effective than ST in hampering progression of DO as has been advocated by some. Careful surgical dissection up to the hyoid bone is necessary to avoid recurrence.

▶ This selected article comes from Sweden, where thyroid surgery plays a prominent role in managing Graves disease. Similar to the debate surrounding the extent of surgery and associated complication rate in managing multinodular goiter (see previous article in this YEAR BOOK's selection), in Graves disease, subtotal or near-total thyroidectomy is associated not only with increased rates of disease recurrence (as high as 20%) but possibly enhanced safety as well. In this retrospective study, the authors found that total thyroidectomy for Graves disease was not associated with statistically significant increase in complication rate compared with subtotal thyroidectomy. A word of caution to the American reader when interpreting Swedish data: In Sweden, thyroid surgery is performed in high-volume centers by specialized surgeons. Quality assurance (QA) is standard, and the outcomes are compared with the Scandinavian Quality Registry for Thyroid and Parathyroid Surgery. In the United States, on the other hand, thyroid operations are performed both by high- and low-volume surgeons in major centers and in private practice. Furthermore, QA through the American College of Surgeons National Quality Improvement Program is not universally used by QA programs in hospitals and medical centers across the country (except for the Veterans Affairs health care system). These factors have to be taken into consideration by low-volume thyroid surgeons when choosing an operation for Graves disease.

M. Gapany, MD

Is thyroidectomy in patients with Hashimoto thyroiditis more risky?

McManus C, Luo J, Sippel R, et al (Univ of Wisconsin, Madison)

J Surg Res 178:529-532, 2012

Background.—Hashimoto thyroiditis (HT) is an organ-specific autoimmune disease characterized by the production of antibodies such as antithyroperoxidase, which leads to the destruction of the thyroid gland and a decrease in normal thyroid function. Thyroidectomy is performed when the patient presents with symptoms or potential neoplastic degeneration occurs; however, surgery can be difficult because of the dense inflammatory process around the thyroid gland. We hypothesized that patients with HT may have a higher rate of complications after thyroid surgery.

Methods.—We identified 1791 consecutive patients who underwent thyroidectomy from May 1994 to December 2009. Patients with HT were compared with those without HT with regard to outcomes with analysis of variance and chi-square test (SPSS, Inc).

Results.—Patients with HT were significantly younger and more likely to be female. There was no significant difference between the two groups in the rate of malignancy. However, patients undergoing thyroidectomy with HT had a significantly higher postoperative complication rate. Specifically, the rates of overall, transient, and permanent complications were all increased in HT patients.

Conclusion.—Patients with HT had a higher rate of complications after thyroidectomy compared with those without HT. Therefore, careful consideration must be taken before pursuing operative treatment in patients with HT including providing adequate informed consent regarding the increased risks of surgery.

▶ Surgeons who operate on thyroid gland are well aware of the fact that presence of lymphocytic thyroiditis in the gland makes the operation more difficult, especially when thyroiditis was long-standing and advanced. The gland tends to be surrounded by inflammatory process that spills over into the surrounding tissues, making the dissection more difficult. It is also associated with increased bleeding, which makes the identification of critical structures such as recurrent laryngeal nerve and parathyroid gland more challenging.

This selected study has assessed in retrospective fashion the incidence of complications associated with thyroid surgery in the presence of lymphocytic thyroiditis as compared with thyroid glands without this disease process. The authors have found that the incidence of postoperative complications (both transient and permanent) was significantly higher in the presence of thyroiditis. Based on their findings, the authors recommend taking those higher complication rates into consideration when pursuing thyroid surgery in lymphocytic thyroiditis patients and counseling them appropriately as to the risks of the operation. I could not agree with them more!

M. Gapany, MD

A Novel Definition of Extrathyroidal Invasion for Patients With Papillary Thyroid Carcinoma for Predicting Prognosis

Hotomi M, Sugitani I, Toda K, et al (Cancer Inst Hosp, Tokyo, Japan)

World J Surg 36:1231-1240, 2012

Objectives.—Extrathyroidal invasion is one of the most significant risk factors for patients with papillary thyroid carcinoma (PTC). The purpose of this study was to evaluate a novel definition of extrathyroidal invasion for patients with PTC as a method for predicting a patient's prognosis.

Methods.—The prospective study was conducted for consecutive 930 patients with primary PTC who received surgery during 1993–2009. We defined only patients who had preoperative recurrent laryngeal nerve palsy or patients in whom the tumor had invaded to the mucosa of the trachea and/or esophagus as Ex3. Patients with minimal invasion were classified as Ex1, and patients with massive invasion, when we could shave off the tumors, were classified as Ex2. Patients without extrathyroidal invasion were classified as Ex0.

Results.—Patients classified Ex3 showed significantly shorter disease-free survival ($p = 0.03$) and disease-specific survival ($p = 0.007$) than patients classified Ex2. The time to recurrence at resection sites was shorter in patients classified Ex3 than in patients classified Ex2 ($p = 0.02$). The time to death due to distant metastasis of patients classified Ex3 was significantly shorter than that of patients classified Ex2 ($p = 0.02$). Within the patients classified Ex3, disease-specific survival of patients with invasion to other nearby structures was shorter than that of patients with invasion to only recurrent laryngeal nerve ($p = 0.008$).

Conclusions.—The degree and site of invasion is an important prognostic factor for PTC. Our novel classification of extrathyroidal invasion is valuable in predicting the prognosis of PTC.

▶ In this selected article, the authors propose a novel classification of extrathyroidal extension of well-differentiated thyroid carcinoma. Their data support classification of extrathyroidal extension into 3 categories: extrathyroidal extension with minimal tissue invasion (Ex1), massive but resectable invasion (Ex2), and massive invasion with involvement of tracheal and/or esophageal mucosa, hence unresectable without major organ sacrifice (Ex3). This classification has apparently been adopted by the Japanese Society of Thyroid Surgery and is used for additional risk stratification. In this article, such stratification by the degree of extrathyroidal extension allowed the authors to predict recurrence rates and distant metastases in addition to overall and disease-free survival rates. It is interesting to note that in their series, none of the tumors with resectable invasion (classified as Ex2) developed recurrences at the resection site, despite the fact that resections were macroscopic (defined as shave-resections).

For those of us who regularly review of the literature on thyroid cancer, it has long been evident that our Japanese colleagues have taken a radically different approach on treatment of well-differentiated thyroid cancer. Although use of radioiodine for well-differentiated thyroid cancer is standard in the United States, in Japan it is restricted by law, reflecting the national attitude toward use of radioactive materials for medical purposes. Furthermore, Japanese surgeons are more conservative when it comes to resecting the thyroid gland in tumors that are 2 cm or less in diameter, but they routinely perform cervical lymph node sampling as part of the operation for well-differentiated thyroid cancer.

This selected article is yet another example of such differences.

M. Gapany, MD

Characteristics of Inpatient Thyroid Surgery at US Academic and Affiliated Medical Centers

Stack BC Jr, Spencer HJ, Lee CE, et al (Univ of Arkansas for Med Sciences Thyroid Ctr, Little Rock; Univ of Mississippi Med Ctr, Jackson; et al)
Otolaryngol Head Neck Surg 146:210-219, 2012

Objective.—Describe data from patients undergoing thyroid surgeries for benign and malignant disease at US academic medical centers.

Study Design.—Retrospective, database search.

Setting.—The University Health System (UHC) Consortium (Oak Brook, Illinois) data compiled from discharge summaries.

Subjects and Methods.—Discharge data were collected from the first quarter of 2002 through the fourth quarter of 2009. Searching strategy was based on diagnosis of thyroid disease and patients undergoing thyroid surgery across all UHC facilities. Demographic information was collected as well as length of stay (LOS) and costs. Complications were evaluated in this analysis.

Results.—During the study period, 68,014 thyroidectomies were performed, with 27,200 for thyroid cancer. During the same period 6365 neck dissections were performed, with 1539 as stand-alone procedures. Total thyroidectomy was the procedure of choice for malignant disease. More total thyroidectomies and fewer hemithyroidectomies were being performed for benign thyroid disease in the inpatient setting. Almost all postoperative complications were more frequent after surgery for cancer except myocardial infarction and aspiration pneumonia. On average, LOS was longer for benign disease, but costs were higher for malignant disease.

Conclusion.—This is the largest series reporting inpatient LOS and mortality for thyroid surgery. The limitation of this study is that it reports patients whose stays were more than 23 hours, leaving out a significant number of thyroid surgeries that are performed as outpatients. Although the results contribute greatly to characterizing inpatient surgery, the results may not reflect current US trends for thyroid surgery.

▶ This large retrospective database review included only inpatient thyroid surgery performed in academic medical centers and thus was likely to include a higher percentage of advanced cases in a sicker patient population. Furthermore, the complication rate might have been affected because surgery was performed in a teaching environment, with the participation of trainees. But also, because of the teaching environment, it is fair to assume that the adherence to best medical practice guidelines were relatively more stringent. Nevertheless, the article is interesting to review because it provides some very important insights into the outcomes of thyroid surgery.

First, it is interesting to note that 49% of total thyroidectomies were performed for benign disease. Furthermore, the cost of total thyroidectomy was 33% more than for partial thyroidectomy. Second, neck dissection in conjunction with total thyroidectomy for thyroid malignancy has been steadily increasing in frequency, adding significantly to the hospital utilization and cost as well as to the incidence of complications such as hypocalcemia and hematomas, increasing the morbidity of the operation. Since the positive impact of neck dissection on the survival from well-differentiated thyroid cancer has not been proven, the data call for serious reevaluation of our current management of thyroid malignancy.

M. Gapany, MD

Prophylactic central lymph node dissection for clinically node-negative papillary thyroid microcarcinoma: Influence on serum thyroglobulin level, recurrence rate, and postoperative complications

So YK, Seo MY, Son Y-I (Inje Univ College of Medicine, Busan, South Korea; Sungkyunkwan Univ School of Medicine, Seoul, South Korea)

Surgery 151:192-198, 2012

Background.—In papillary thyroid microcarcinoma (PTMC), regional lymph node metastasis (LNM) is associated with a increased locoregional recurrence rate. Yet, prophylactic central lymph node dissection (CLND) targeting subclinical central LNM continues to be a matter of debate in the treatment of PTMC, which generally carries an excellent prognosis. The aim of our study was to investigate the benefits and risks of prophylactic CLND in patients with clinically node-negative PTMC.

Methods.—This study included 232 patients who underwent surgery for clinically node-negative PTMC from 1999 to 2006. Of these 232 patients, 113 underwent only total thyroidectomy (TT) and 119 underwent TT in conjunction with prophylactic bilateral CLND (TT with CLND). We then compared serum thyroglobulin (Tg) levels, recurrence rates, and postoperative complications between the 2 groups (TT only and TT with CLND).

Results.—The postoperative stimulated serum Tg level was significantly less in the TT with CLND group than in the TT only group (1.07 vs 2.24 ng/mL, respectively; $P = .022$). The stimulated Tg levels in the 2 groups became similar, however, after low-dose radioactive iodine treatment (0.44 ng/mL vs 0.69 ng/mL, respectively; $P = 0.341$). There was no significant difference in 3-year locoregional control rates after TT with CLND and TT only (98.3% vs 96.5%, respectively; $P = .368$). Although the frequency of permanent hypocalcemia was approximately 3 times greater in the TT with CLND group (5.6%) than in the TT only group (1.8%), this finding did not reach statistical significance.

Conclusion.—With prophylactic CLND, the postoperative Tg level can significantly decrease. However, prophylactic CLND is not helpful in decreasing short-term locoregional recurrence in patients with clinically node-negative PTMC. Finally, the risk of permanent hypocalcemia may increase after CLND.

► It is generally accepted that in papillary thyroid carcinoma, cervical lymph node metastases do not affect overall survival. However, presence of cervical lymph node metastases is associated with increased incidence of locoregional recurrence, justifying intraoperative removal of clinically or radiographically positive cervical lymph nodes in both lateral and central compartments. On the other hand, the issue of prophylactic cervical lymphadenectomy in clinically and radiographically negative cases remains subject to significant controversy. This holds particularly true for the prophylactic central compartment lymphadenectomy, which is associated with increased risk for recurrent laryngeal nerve injury and permanent hypoparathyroidism. The high incidence of central compartment micrometastases in clinically negative cases (50% to 60%) is often used by proponents of prophylactic neck dissection to justify their approach, while the detractors cite increased incidence of complications without proven benefit of survival or even change in the course of the disease to justify their objection. To make things even more confusing, the American Thyroid Association recently came out with a "recommendation" to consider lymph node dissection (basically leaving the decision to individual surgeon) in all patients undergoing thyroidectomy for papillary thyroid carcinoma, regardless of whether the nodes are enlarged. The results of this selected study showed that prophylactic central compartment neck dissection was not helpful in decreasing short-term local-regional recurrence in patients with papillary microcarcinomas and clinically negative necks. Furthermore, it was associated with increased risk for permanent hypoparathyroidism.

At this point, I would like to emphasize that many highly respected thyroid surgeons, based on their experience, their data, and their overall philosophy, recommend observation for clinically and radiographically a negative central compartment, and surgery only for clinically or radiographically positive nodes. In my practice, in addition to the above outlined philosophy, I use risk stratification to guide my surgical approach: prophylactic central compartment lymphadenectomy in high-risk patients and no lymphadenectomy in patients with low-risk scores.

M. Gapany, MD

A Population-Based Prospective Cohort Study of Complications after Thyroidectomy in the Elderly

Grogan RH, Mitmaker EJ, Hwang J, et al (Univ of Chicago Med Ctr, IL; Univ of California, San Francisco)

J Clin Endocrinol Metab 97:1645-1653, 2012

Context.—Data on the risk of postthyroidectomy complications in elderly patients are sparse, unclear, and conflicting.

Objective.—We sought to use a population-based cohort to determine whether thyroid operations in the elderly are as safe as those done in younger patients.

Design.—This was a prospective cohort study using the American College of Surgeons National Surgical Quality Improvement Program database from 2005 to 2008, with 30-d postoperative follow-up.

Setting.—The American College of Surgeons National Surgical Quality Improvement Program data set contains operative cases from a nationwide sampling of academic and community-based as well as high-volume and low-volume hospitals.

Patients.—All thyroidectomy and parathyroidectomy patients reported to the database during the study period were included in the analysis resulting in an experimental cohort of 7915 thyroidectomy cases and a control cohort of 3575 parathyroidectomy cases.

Main Outcome Measures.—We aggregated 83 complications into the following outcome measures: urinary tract infection, wound infection, systemic infection, cardiac complications, pulmonary complications, 30-d mortality, and total hospital length of stay.

Results.—Increased age is a risk factor for significant pulmonary, cardiac, and infectious complications after thyroidectomy. Elderly patients are twice as likely (odds ratio 2.1, 95% confidence interval 1.4–3.3), and the super-elderly are 5 times as likely (odds ratio 4.9, 95% confidence interval 2.5–9.6) to have a complication compared with their young counterparts. Preexisting comorbidities are effect modifiers and increase the risk of complications even further.

Conclusions.—Elderly thyroidectomy patients are at increased risk for major systemic complications. A systematic approach to the care of elderly thyroidectomy patients is necessary to minimize their risk of serious postoperative complications.

► This is a very important study for head and neck surgeons. The significance of this study is that it is based on the American College of Surgeons' National Surgical Quality Improvement Program (NISQUIP) database. The authors found the age of patients to be an independent (of comorbidities) risk factor for complications (primarily pulmonary) after thyroid surgery. It is very significant, because risk adjustment for systemic postoperative complications, as defined by NISQUIP criteria, addresses only comorbidities (as classified by American Society of Anesthesiologists). Although the focus of this study was thyroid surgery, its conclusions could be easily extrapolated to any major head and neck operation. Since introduction of NASQUIP criteria to monitor my Veterans Administration–based surgical head and neck oncology program, pulmonary complications were one of my high outliers. Prevalence of smoking among head and neck cancer patients was certainly a major contributing factor, usually addressed by American Society of Anesthesiologists classification, for which risk adjustment was provided. However, advanced patient age must have been another contributing factor, for which no risk adjustment was given. It is my hope that the data presented in this article will impact not only surgeons performing thyroid surgery but also policies of NISQIP when it comes to risk adjustment in elderly patients undergoing thyroid and other major head and neck surgery.

M. Gapany, MD

A Comparison of Outcomes for Younger and Older Adult Patients Undergoing Surgery for Primary Hyperparathyroidism

Kandil E, Majid DS, Carson KA, et al (Tulane Univ School of Medicine, New Orleans, LA; Johns Hopkins Bloomberg School of Public Health, Baltimore, MD; et al)

Ann Surg Oncol 19:1897-1901, 2012

Background.—In adolescents and young adults, primary hyperparathyroidism (PHPT) is an uncommon diagnosis. We compared the clinical characteristics of these patients to those of older adult patients with PHPT. We hypothesized that PHPT in adolescents and young adults is more often caused by single-gland disease and is amenable to minimally invasive parathyroidectomy (MIP).

Methods.—We retrospectively reviewed the medical records of 452 consecutive patients who had surgery for PHPT. Patients ranged in age from 13 to 94 years and were dichotomized into younger (age < 30 years, $n = 17, 3.8\%$) and older (age ≥ 30 years, $n = 435, 96.2\%$) patients. Continuous baseline and intraoperative and postoperative measures were not normally distributed and were summarized with medians and interquartile ranges (IQRs). Groups were compared using Wilcoxon rank sum test or Fisher exact test, and significance was set at $P < .05$.

Results.—Median [IQR] age was 24 [23–27] years for the younger group and 58 [51–66] years for the older group. Though not statistically significant, a smaller proportion of the younger patients compared with the older patients had a positive ^{99m}Tc-sestamibi scan (71%; 95% confidence interval [95% CI] = 44–90% vs. 83%; 95% CI = 79–86%) and showed a suspected parathyroid adenoma on ultrasound (65%; 95% CI = 38–86% vs. 80%; 95% CI = 76–83%). The younger and older age groups did not significantly differ on preoperative serum PTH levels (median [IQR]: 111 [76–145] pg/ml vs 110 [84–152] pg/ml; $P = .73$ respectively). The younger group had higher serum calcium levels (11.6 [11.1–12.2] mg/dl) compared with the older group (11.1 [10.7–11.5] mg/dl; $P = .01$). MIP was performed less frequently on the younger patients (70.6%) compared with older patients (88.7%; $P = 0.04$). Though the incidence of a single adenoma was somewhat more frequent in older patients (90%; 95% CI = 87–93%) than in younger patients (82%; 95% CI = 57–96%) it was the most frequent cause of PHPT in the younger patients. The younger and older groups did not significantly differ on percent drop from baseline for intraoperative PTH monitoring (81.7 vs 79.3%; $P = .46$), respectively.

Conclusions.—Younger patients with PHPT present with significantly higher serum calcium levels than older patients. However, younger patients are less likely to localize abnormal parathyroid glands on sestamibi or ultrasound. Though younger patients appear to have a higher incidence of hyperplasia compared with older patients, single gland disease is still the overall most frequent cause. Our data suggest that MIP should be more frequently considered in younger patients because of the high incidence of single gland disease.

▶ This selected study was undertaken to compare the outcomes for young adults and old adults undergoing surgery for primary hyperparathyroidism. Although the data of this study suggest that minimally invasive parathyroidectomy can be more frequently considered in young adults because of the high incidence of single gland disease, the most important finding was that young adult patients had similar overall cure rates as compared with old adults who underwent the same operative procedure.

The real debate concerning primary hyperparathyroidism, however, surrounds the issue of management of the so-called "asymptomatic" patient. The current recommendations for surgery, as defined by the Third International Workshop on Management of Primary Hyperparathyroidism (2008), calls for operation in asymptomatic patients younger than 50 and in patients with elevated serum calcium (> 1.0 mg/dL), reduced creatinine clearance (< 60 mL/min), and a bone density T-score of < −2.5 at any site or previous history of fracture. Hypercalciuria, in the absence of kidney stones, is no longer considered as an indication for parathyroid surgery.

The success of minimally invasive parathyroidectomy is highly dependent on preoperative localization studies. The standard preoperative localization studies (also used in this study) are ultrasound and Tc- sestamibi scan. When unsuccessful, however, localization studies could be supplemented with magnetic resonance imaging, computed tomography—positron emission tomography, and selective venous sampling for parathyroid hormone.

M. Gapany, MD

Surgical Technique

Postoperative Functional Voice Changes after Conventional Open or Robotic Thyroidectomy: A Prospective Trial

Lee J, Na KY, Kim RM, et al (Ajou Univ School of Medicine, Suwon, Korea; et al)

Ann Surg Oncol 19:2963-2970, 2012

Purpose.—To use objective and subjective voice function analysis to compare outcomes in patients who had undergone conventional open thyroidectomy or robotic thyroidectomy.

Methods.—The study involved 88 consecutive patients who underwent thyroid surgery between May 2009 and December 2009; 46 patients underwent a conventional open thyroidectomy, and 42 underwent a robotic thyroidectomy. Auditory perceptual evaluation was used to make subjective assessments of voice function, and videolaryngostroboscopy, acoustic voice analysis with aerodynamic study, electroglottography, and voice range profile were used to make objective assessments. Each assessment was made before surgery, and at 1 week and 3 months after surgery.

Results.—The conventional open and robotic thyroidectomy groups were similar in terms of age, gender ratio, and disease profile. We found that 18 (20.5%) of the 88 patients showed some level of voice dysfunction at 1 week after surgery; that the dysfunction resolved by 3 months after surgery in all cases; and that it was not permanent according to postoperative videolaryngostroboscopy. The conventional open and robotic thyroidectomy groups were found to have similar levels of dysfunction at 1 week after surgery, except for jitter, which was greater in the robotic group. For both groups, any such dysfunction spontaneously resolved by 3 months after surgery, and there were no significant differences between the groups in terms of any voice function parameter.

Conclusions.—Voice dysfunction was present after both open and robotic thyroidectomy (without any evident laryngeal nerve injury). However, function subsequently normalized to preoperative levels at 3 months after surgery in both groups. Voice function outcomes after robotic thyroidectomy are similar to those after conventional open thyroidectomy.

▶ Robotic thyroid surgery is gaining popularity. It offers several advantages over conventional open surgery, which include improved cosmetic outcomes, improved hemostasis, and reduced injury to surrounding tissues of the neck with resultant reduction in scarring. Similarly, other studies comparing minimally invasive video-assisted thyroidectomy with conventional open operation have shown reduced postoperative morbidity, primarily by lessening postthyroidectomy voice and swallowing impairment and possibly reducing postoperative pain.

This selected study prospectively evaluated voice dysfunction after conventional open thyroid surgery and robotic thyroidectomy. A range of subjective and objective measurements in this study have shown similar postoperative voice changes after both operations. Most importantly, those changes were transient.

This study has shown that robotic thyroidectomy is a safe operation when it comes to voice quality preservation and compares favorably with conventional open thyroidectomy. Given other advantages of robotic thyroidectomy over open thyroidectomy, the authors suggest that in the future, robotic operation might replace conventional surgery. I personally have my doubts about the final place of robotic thyroidectomy because of the cost of the equipment, its limited availability in medical centers that do not specialize in robotic surgery, and special training that is needed to perform this operation. Most importantly, minimally invasive video-assisted thyroidectomy offers all the advantages of robotic operation without the prohibitive cost.

M. Gapany, MD

Intraoperative Neuromonitoring does not Reduce the Incidence of Recurrent Laryngeal Nerve Palsy in Thyroid Reoperations: Results of a Retrospective Comparative Analysis

Alesina PF, Rolfs T, Hommeltenberg S, et al (Akademisches Lehrkrankenhaus der Universität Duisburg-Essen, Germany)

World J Surg 36:1348-1353, 2012

Purpose.—Recurrent laryngeal nerve (RLN) palsy is the major concern of reoperative thyroid surgery, and the introduction of neuromonitoring could reduce the rate of this complication. The present study is a retrospective analysis of the experience with completion thyroidectomy with and without neuromonitoring in a referral center.

Methods.—Between October 1999 and April 2011, 246 patients [37 men, 209 women; mean age, 55 ± 12.5 (range, 25–80) years] underwent 250 reoperations for recurrent goiter ($n = 203$), hyperthyroidism ($n = 26$), or recurrent thyroid cancer ($n = 17$). The mean interval between the initial and the reoperative procedure was 17.5 years. According to the availability of the neuromonitoring system and to the surgeon preference, 91 operations were performed with neuromonitoring (NM-group), whereas 159 were performed with direct nerve visualization (NV-group) alone. Patients' characteristics, perioperative data, and postoperative complications were collected in a prospectively maintained database.

Results.—In the NM-group, 51 unilateral and 40 bilateral resections were performed. The NV-group included 122 unilateral and 37 bilateral procedures. The number of nerves at risk after previous surgery was 128 (NM-group) and 161 (NV-group), respectively. We registered eight RLN palsy in the NM-group (6.2%) and four in the NV-group (2.5%; $p = 0.1$).

Conclusions.—The routine use of intraoperative neuromonitoring seems not to reduce the incidence of RLN during redo thyroid surgery, at least in the setting of a tertiary referral center.

▶ Intraoperative recurrent laryngeal nerve monitoring during thyroid surgery has become a fairly routine practice with both otolaryngologists and general surgeons who operate on the thyroid gland. In this retrospective analysis, the authors have shown that recurrent laryngeal nerve monitoring does not reduce the incidence of recurrent laryngeal nerve palsy in thyroid reoperations. I am not at all surprised by the results of this study. The real value of intraoperative recurrent laryngeal nerve monitoring is in assisting with its detection. Preservation of the nerve function is determined by meticulous surgical technique or the difficulty of the operation, such as the degree of scarring and the size and location of the tumor. On the other hand, the use of intraoperative recurrent laryngeal nerve monitoring can be of great value in an academic setting, with residents performing the operations under staff surgeons' supervision. The use of this monitoring technique may also have medico-legal ramifications similar to that of facial nerve monitoring for parotid gland surgery.

M. Gapany, MD

Early surgical outcomes comparison between robotic and conventional open thyroid surgery for papillary thyroid microcarcinoma

Lee S, Ryu HR, Park JH, et al (Yonsei Univ Health System, Seoul, South Korea)

Surgery 151:724-730, 2012

Background.—Robotic operations have enabled a safer and more meticulous approach to thyroidectomy with the notable benefit of improved cosmesis and decreases in postoperative pain and swallowing discomfort. The aim of this study was to document the early surgical outcomes of robotic thyroidectomy in patients with papillary thyroid carcinoma (PTC) by comparing it with conventional open thyroidectomy.

Methods.—From October 2007 to September 2008, 458 patients with PTC underwent thyroidectomy at the Yonsei University Health System. Of these patients, 266 patients were in the conventional open group and 192 patients were in the robotic group. These 2 groups were compared retrospectively with respect to clinicopathologic characteristics and surgical outcomes.

Results.—The mean follow-up period was 29.1 months. Mean tumor size, incidence of capsular invasion, multiplicity, and central nodal metastasis showed no significant difference between the 2 groups. Total thyroidectomy was performed more frequently in the open group. In terms of operation times, the robotic group had a significantly greater length of time for total thyroidectomy and subtotal thyroidectomy. The total number of retrieved central lymph nodes was greater in the open group (5.7 vs 4.6, $P = .004$). The 2 groups showed no differences in intraoperative and postoperative complications. The postoperative serum thyroglobulin levels were similar in both groups (0.25 vs 0.22 ng/mL, $P = .648$) and 2-year follow-up sonography of 433 patients revealed no recurrences. No abnormal I^{131} uptake was observed in whole-body scans in either group.

Conclusion.—Robotic thyroidectomy was similar to conventional open thyroidectomy in terms of early surgical outcomes but offers advantages. We conclude that robotic thyroidectomy offers a safe, feasible alternative to conventional open thyroidectomy in patients with PTC.

▶ There is no question that robotic surgery has become fashionable recently. In many fields, it has proven to be advantageous, especially when it comes to abdominal, pelvic, and thoracic surgery. Along with this advantage, however, comes the added cost in equipment, staff, and in-operating room time. It appears to me that when it comes to thyroid surgery, there is very little left to improve besides the cosmetic result. And even this aspect of thyroid surgery, when desired, can be addressed very successfully using an endoscopic technique. Even open total thyroidectomy for cancer, when performed by skillful surgeons, has been relegated to same-day surgery status, with an excellent record of safety and a very low complication rate. So what is the fuss about robotic thyroidectomy? Why do we need this safe, feasible alternative to conventional or, for that matter, endoscopic thyroidectomy? Do we really need to look for such alternatives, especially when they come with a very significant price tag attached?

M. Gapany, MD

Case-Controlled Comparison of Video-Assisted and Conventional Minimally Invasive Parathyroidectomy

Melck AL, Armstrong MJ, Yip L, et al (Univ of British Columbia Faculty of Medicine, Vancouver, Canada; Univ of Pittsburgh School of Medicine, PA)
Am Surg 78:125-132, 2012

Video-assisted parathyroidectomy (VAP) is a new approach to parathyroid exploration for primary hyperparathyroidism (PH). We examined the VAP learning curve and hypothesized that compared with conventional minimally invasive parathyroidectomy (MIS), VAP has similar complication rates and the added benefit of a shorter hospital length of stay. Using a case-control study design, patients with PH with single-focus imaging results undergoing VAP or MIS were compared during a 5-year VAP implementation period. VAP was possible in 18 per cent of patients undergoing initial parathyroid exploration. In comparing 125 VAP cases with 95 MIS control subjects, patients undergoing MIS had higher mean preoperative levels of calcium ($P = 0.007$) and parathyroid hormone ($P = 0.008$), greater mean adenoma weight ($P < 0.001$), and increased long-term mortality (4% MIS *vs* 0% VAP, $P = 0.03$). Mean operative time, in-house analgesia use, and operative complications did not differ. The rate of conversion from VAP to MIS was 14 per cent. Patients undergoing VAP were less likely to require an overnight hospital stay ($P = 0.01$). VAP is a safe surgical option for selected patients with PH, offering improved cosmesis with operative times comparable to conventional MIS. VAP can be done with a low conversion rate even during implementation and allows the added benefit of shorter hospital stay.

▶ With the introduction of video-assisted parathyroidectomy (VAP), the surgeons using this technique observed not only improved cosmetic outcomes, but more importantly reduced morbidity of the operation. Several recent studies have reported shortened hospital stays, decreased postoperative pain, and decreased postoperative voice and swallowing impairment, presumably from less extensive surgical dissection and injury to surrounding tissue. Very importantly, complication rate in VAP has been reported to be comparable to conventional surgery.

This selected study is a case-controlled comparison of VAP and conventional minimally invasive parathyroidectomy, based on preoperative localization of the adenoma and intraoperative parathyroid hormone level assessment. This study confirms previously reported feasibility of VAP, its safety in terms of complication rate, which was comparable to conventional operation. It also showed comparable operative time. The authors also found that VAP was easy to learn and incorporate into practice. Furthermore, it appeared to be even more conducive to same-day surgery. VAP, however, has not been used for bilateral 4-gland exploration for suspected multiple adenomas or in cases where localization studies have failed to identify the site.

M. Gapany, MD

General

A Review of Risk Factors and Timing for Postoperative Hematoma After Thyroidectomy: Is Outpatient Thyroidectomy Really Safe?

Lang BH-H, Yih PC-L, Lo C-Y (The Univ of Hong Kong, Hong Kong SAR, China)

World J Surg 36:2497-2502, 2012

Background.—Although postoperative hematoma after thyroidectomy is uncommon, patients traditionally have been advised to stay overnight in the hospital for monitoring. With the growing demand for outpatient thyroidectomy, we assessed its safety and feasibility by evaluating the potential risk factors and timing of postoperative hematoma after thyroidectomy.

Methods.—From 1995–2011, 3,086 consecutive patients underwent thyroidectomy at our institution; of these, 22 (0.7 %) developed a postoperative hematoma that required surgical reexploration (group I). Potential risk factors were compared between group I and those without hematoma (n = 3,045) or with hematoma but not requiring reexploration (n = 19; group II). Variables that were significant in the univariate analysis were entered into multivariate analysis by binary logistic regression analysis.

Results.—Group I was significantly more likely to have undergone previous thyroid operation than group II (27.3 vs. 8.2 %, $p = 0.007$). The median weight of excised thyroid gland (71.8 vs. 40 g, $p = 0.018$) and the median size of the dominant nodule (4.1 vs. 3 cm, $p = 0.004$) were significantly greater in group I than group II. Previous thyroid operation (odds ratio (OR) = 4.084; 95% confidence interval (CI), 1.105–15.098; $p = 0.035$) and size of dominant nodule (OR = 1.315; 95% CI, 1.024–1.687; $p = 0.032$) were independent factors for hematoma. Sixteen (72.7%) had hematoma within 6 h, whereas the other 6 (27.3%) had hematoma at 6–24 h.

Conclusions.—Previous thyroid operation and large dominant nodule were independent risk factors for hematoma requiring surgical reexploration. Given that a quarter of hematoma occurred between 6 to 24 h after surgery, routine outpatient thyroidectomy could not be recommended.

▶ Thyroid surgeons in the "modern era" are under a certain degree of pressure to perform thyroid operations as ambulatory procedures. Predicting and monitoring hypocalcemia in the ambulatory setting appears to be the main challenge. Although the focus is on serum calcium, I hope that the potential problem of postoperative hematoma is not overlooked. Admittedly, with the use of contemporary surgical hemostatic techniques, postoperative hematomas are quite rare. Notwithstanding, it is worthwhile to remember that postoperative hematomas that develop while the patient is in house usually pose a relatively minor problem. On the other hand, it can rapidly become a catastrophe if a hematoma develops while the patient is at home.

This selected article is worth reviewing. It should serve as a reminder that even after a technically well-performed thyroidectomy, the rate of postoperative hematoma is reported at 0.7%. Furthermore, 100% of all postoperative hematomas developed in the first 24 hours after the operation. Thus, 23-hour observation appears to be a much safer strategy than ambulatory operation when it comes to thyroid surgery.

M. Gapany, MD

The Role of Clinicians in Determining Radioactive Iodine Use for Low-Risk Thyroid Cancer

Haymart MR, Banerjee M, Yang D, et al (Univ of Michigan, Ann Arbor; et al)
Cancer 119:259-265, 2013

Background.—There is controversy regarding the optimal management of thyroid cancer. The proportion of patients with low-risk thyroid cancer who received radioactive iodine (RAI) treatment increased over the last 20 years, and little is known about the role played by clinicians in hospital-level RAI use for low-risk disease.

Methods.—Thyroid surgeons affiliated with 368 hospitals that had Commission on Cancer-accredited cancer programs were surveyed. Survey data were linked to data reported to the National Cancer Database. A multivariable analysis was used to assess the relation between clinician decision makers and hospital-level RAI use after total thyroidectomy in patients with stage I, well differentiated thyroid cancer.

Results.—The survey response rate was 70% (560 of 804 surgeons). The surgeon was identified as the primary decision maker by 16% of the surgeons; the endocrinologist was identified as the primary decision maker by 69%, and a nuclear medicine, radiologist, or other physician was identified as the primary decision maker by 15%. In a multivariable analysis controlling for hospital case volume and hospital type, when the primary decision maker was in a specialty other than endocrinology or surgery, there was greater use of RAI at the hospital ($P < .001$). A greater number of providers at the hospital where RAI was administered and having access to a tumor board also were associated with increased use of RAI ($P < .001$ and $P = .006$, respectively).

Conclusions.—The specialty of the primary decision maker, the number of providers administering RAI, and having access to a tumor board were associated significantly with the use of RAI for stage I thyroid cancer. The findings have implications for addressing nonclinical variation between hospitals, with a marked heterogeneity in decision making suggesting that standardization of care will be challenging.

► In my opinion, this selected article is important to review because it underscores the erratic and irrational way well-differentiated thyroid carcinoma is managed in the United States. Despite the fact that our Japanese colleagues over many years have consistently shown that, in patients with low-risk well-differentiated thyroid cancer, radioiodine therapy offers no disease-specific survival advantage over surgery alone, and despite the mounting evidence in the English-language literature that supports this observation, radioiodine is being routinely administered to low-risk thyroid cancer patients in this country. The findings in this study, which are particularly disheartening, are that in a multidisciplinary setting, where multiple subspecialists are involved in the decision-making process as well as in the tumor-board setting, the incidence of utilization of radioiodine is actually higher. Clearly, the specialty of the clinician influences radioiodine use, with nuclear medicine specialists and endocrinologists being the most likely experts to recommend its use; paradoxically, these are the specialists supposedly with the most expertise in the field!

M. Gapany, MD

Calcium Management after Thyroidectomy: A Simple and Cost-Effective Method

Singer MC, Bhakta D, Seybt MW, et al (Georgia Health Sciences Univ, Augusta)

Otolaryngol Head Neck Surg 146:362-365, 2012

Objective.—Hypocalcemia is one of the principal complications of total or completion thyroidectomy. A number of different protocols for managing this potential complication have been published. Our simple postoperative regimen is described and the safety and cost-effectiveness assessed.

Study Design.—Case series with planned data collection.

Setting.—Academic medical center.

Subjects and Methods.—All patients undergoing total or completion thyroidectomy from January 2008 through June 2010 were evaluated. Data collected included age; gender; procedure performed; levels of ionized calcium, parathyroid hormone, and vitamin D; complications; and need for readmission. Standard descriptive statistics were used to summarize these data.

Results.—In total, 526 patients had thyroid surgery during the 30-month study period. Of these, 307 underwent completion or total thyroidectomy and were prescribed a 3-week tapering course of calcium carbonate postoperatively. Twenty-three patients (7.5%) experienced symptoms of hypocalcemia that were managed on an outpatient basis with additional doses of oral calcium. Two patients (0.7%) required readmission. The cost of a 3-week regimen of calcium carbonate is approximately $15. This is considerably less expensive than either the cost of overnight admission or published laboratory protocols that are designed to predict the risk of hypocalcemia.

Conclusions.—Prophylactic calcium supplementation without routine laboratory assessment proved to be a safe and costeffective method of preventing and managing postoperative hypocalcemia following total or completion thyroidectomy.

► The current trend in thyroid surgery is reducing it to ambulatory surgery or 23-hour observation level. To this end, algorithms have been developed to monitor and predict postoperative hypocalcaemia through serial measurement of postoperative ionized calcium or parathyroid hormone (PTH) levels using rapid PTH assay. In this selected article, the authors describe their simple and cost-effective method of routine calcium and vitamin D supplementation in all thyroidectomy patients without the need for any postoperative hospital observation. They routinely prescribe a 3-week taper course of calcium carbonate and 200 IU of cholecalciferol along with very thorough written instructions to patients on how to monitor clinical symptoms of emerging hypocalcaemia and the proper course of action in case such symptoms occur. This information is reinforced through a repeated perioperative educational effort. The cost of such a prophylactic therapy appears to be negligible compared with 23-hour hospital observation and the cost of repeated laboratory studies. Furthermore, this method has been shown by the authors as effective and safe.

M. Gapany, MD

Abandoning Unilateral Parathyroidectomy: Why We Reversed Our Position After 15,000 Parathyroid Operations

Norman J, Lopez J, Politz D (Norman Parathyroid Ctr, Tampa, FL)

J Am Coll Surg 214:260-269, 2012

Background.—Our group championed the techniques and benefits of unilateral parathyroidectomy. As our experience has matured, it seems this limited operation might be appropriate only occasionally.

Methods.—A single surgical group's experience with 15,000 parathyroidectomies examined the ongoing differences between unilateral and bilateral techniques for 10-year failure/recurrence, multigland removal, operative times, and length of stay.

Results.—With limited experience, 100% of operations were bilateral, decreasing to 32% by the 500th operation ($p < 0.001$), and long-term failure rates increased to 6%. Failures were 11 times more likely for unilateral explorations ($p < 0.001$ vs bilateral), causing gradual increases in bilateral explorations to 97% at the 14,000th operation ($p < 0.001$). Ten-year cure rates are unchanged for bilateral operations, and unilateral operations show continued slow recurrence rates of 5% ($p < 0.001$). Removal of more than one gland occurred 16 times more frequently when 4 glands were analyzed ($p < 0.001$), increasing cure rates to the current 99.4% ($p < 0.001$). Of 1,060 reoperations performed for failure at another institution, intraoperative parathyroid hormone levels fell >50% in 22% of patients, yet a second adenoma was subsequently found. Operative times decreased with experience; bilateral operations taking only 5.9 minutes longer on average (22.3 vs 16.4 minutes; $p < 0.001$), which is 25 minutes less than unilateral at the 500th operation ($p < 0.001$). By the 1,000th operation, incision size (2.5 ± 0.2 cm), anesthesia, and hospital stay (1.6 hours) were identical for unilateral and bilateral procedures.

Conclusions.—Regardless of surgical adjuncts (scanning, intraoperative parathyroid hormone), unilateral parathyroidectomy will carry a 1-year failure rate of 3% to 5% and a 10-year recurrence rate of 4% to 6%.

Allowing rapid analysis of all 4 glands through the same 1-inch incision has caused us to all but abandon unilateral parathyroidectomy.

▶ This article is a must-read for otolaryngologists who operate on parathyroid glands. The authors of this study, who once were instrumental in coining the current paradigm for parathyroid adenoma surgery, are challenging the concept of unilateral surgery based on localization studies and intraoperative parathyroid hormone level measurement. Their argument for exploration in all cases of suspected primary hyperparathyroidism is based on their unmatched experience and skill in performing this operation: 1-inch midline incision, 16-minute unilateral exploration, 22-minute bilateral exploration, and long-term cure rates of 96%—such level of mastery can be achieved only in centers that specialize in performing only 1 operation. But for the rest of us "mortals" who have to make a living by practicing the whole spectrum of head and neck surgery, localization using a combination of ultrasound and Tc 99M Sestamibi scanning and unilateral 20-minute operation with intraoperative parathyroid hormone level measurement (additional 20 minutes of operating room time) that results in a success rate of about 90% does seem like an acceptable alternative to traveling 3000 miles across the country to improve the success rate by 6%.

M. Gapany, MD

Article Index

Chapter 1: Allergy and Immunology

Chapter 2: Head and Neck Surgery and Tumors

Chapter 3: Laryngology

Chapter 4: Otology

Chapter 5: Pediatric Otolaryngology

Chapter 6: Rhinology and Skull Base Surgery

Chapter 7: Thyroid and Parathyroid

Author Index

M

N

O

P

Q

R

S

FSC
www.fsc.org
MIX
Papier | Fördert
gute Waldnutzung
FSC® C083411

Kolibri 360 GmbH
Ferdinand-Jühlke-Straße 7
99095 Erfurt, Deutschland
produktsicherheit@kolibri360.de